INFLAMMATORY BOWEL DISEASE

CLINICAL GASTROENTEROLOGY

George Y. Wu, SERIES EDITOR

INFLAMMATORY BOWEL DISEASE

DIAGNOSIS AND THERAPEUTICS

Edited by

RUSSELL D. COHEN, MD

*The University of Chicago Medical Center,
Chicago, IL*

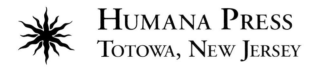

HUMANA PRESS
TOTOWA, NEW JERSEY

© 2003 Humana Press Inc.
999 Riverview Drive, Suite 208
Totowa, New Jersey 07512

humanapress.com

For additional copies, pricing for bulk purchases, and/or information about other Humana titles,
contact Humana at the above address or at any of the following numbers: Tel: 973-256-1699;
Fax: 973-256-8341; E-mail: humana@humanapr.com or visit our Website at humanapress.com

Due diligence has been taken by the publishers, editors, and authors of this book to ensure the accuracy of the
information published and to describe generally accepted practices. The contributors herein have carefully
checked to ensure that the drug selections and dosages set forth in this text are accurate in accord with the
standards accepted at the time of publication. Notwithstanding, as new research, changes in government regu-
lations, and knowledge from clinical experience relating to drug therapy and drug reactions constantly occurs,
the reader is advised to check the product information provided by the manufacturer of each drug for any change
in dosages or for additional warnings and contraindications. This is of utmost importance when the recommended drug herein is a new or infrequently used drug. It is the responsibility of the health care provider to
ascertain the Food and Drug Administration status of each drug or device used in their clinical practice. The
publisher, editors, and authors are not responsible for errors or omissions or for any consequences from the
application of the information presented in this book and make no warranty, express or implied, with respect
to the contents in this publication.

This publication is printed on acid-free paper. ∞
ANSI Z39.48-1984 (American National Standards Institute)
Permanence of Paper for Printed Library Materials.

Production Editor: Mark J. Breaugh.

Cover Illustration: (Background): Single-contrast lower GI study demonstrating a shortened featureless
"lead pipe" colon typical of chronic UC. *See* Fig. 4 on p. 96; (Left): Large, irregular Crohn's disease ulcer
of the colon. Courtesy of Dr. Russell D. Cohen; (Center): Crohn's ileitis. *See* Fig. 6 on p. 336; (Right): Large
Pyoderma gangrenosum affecting the anterior tibial surface on the lower extremity in a patient with Crohn's
disease. Courtesy of Dr. Russell D. Cohen.

Cover design by Patricia F. Cleary.

Printed in the United States of America.   10 9 8 7 6 5 4 3 2 1

Library of Congress Cataloging-in-Publication Data

Inflammatory Bowel Disease : diagnosis and therapeutics / edited by Russell D. Cohen.
      p. cm. -- (Clinical gastroenterology)
   Includes bibliographical references and index.
   ISBN 0-89603-909-9 (alk. paper): 1-59259-311-9 (ebook)
    1. Inflammatory bowel diseases. I. Cohen, Russell D. II. Series.

   RC862.I53 I527 2003
   616.3'44--dc21

                                                                       2002032874

PREFACE

One of the most vivid memories from my medical school training was seeing my first surgical operation on a patient with Crohn's disease. The senior surgeon at Mount Sinai Hospital in New York City, the same institution at which Burrill Crohn, Leon Ginzburg, and Gordon Oppenheimer had first described the disease "terminal ileitis," had undoubtedly done countless operations on patients with inflammatory bowel disease in the past. Yet as we both gazed down into the patient's open abdomen, at the "creeping fat" that seemed to be wrapping its sticky fingers around the young man's intestines, he stated, "this is the mystery of Crohn's disease—no two patients are ever the same."

What is it about the inflammatory bowel diseases, Crohn's disease, and ulcerative colitis, that we find so intriguing? Is it the young age of the patients, many who are younger than even the medical students attending to them? Or is it the elusive etiology, the theory of a "mystery organism" that has yet to be identified? Perhaps it is the familial pattern of disease, where many patients have relatives with similar diseases, yet in some instances only one of a pair of identical twins is affected.

Regardless of the cause, these chronic diseases with a typically early age of onset, result in a long-term commitment of the patient, their families, friends, health care providers, researchers, employers, and even health care insurers and other health-related industries. Each of these groups have their own areas of interest and understanding of these diseases, with a need to know particular details, as well as how to find out additional information.

It is precisely with this in mind that we set out to write *Inflammatory Bowel Disease: Diagnosis and Therapeutics*. Our goal is to provide a comprehensive but concise overview of the myriad of issues surrounding the inflammatory bowel diseases, written in a language targeted to those both within and outside of the medical community. The intent of many of the chapters is also to provide resources on how to get more information on a particular topic, with web page addresses, phone numbers, and addresses of various sources

Who should read this book? Patients, their friends, and families, will find answers to many of the questions that they have about the disease.

Physicians, surgeons, nurses, ostomy specialists, social workers, pharmacists, and other medical professionals will find the information helpful in treating their patients and providing answers to many of the questions that are often thrown to them. Laboratory and clinical scientists will be provided with state-of-the-art information on the diseases and future directions of research. Members of the health care, insurance, and pharmaceutical industries will find a comprehensive review of the economics of these diseases, which should be valuable in the development of sensible health care policies toward these patients. And finally, students of the medical, biological, and social sciences should read this book, as they hold the promise for future advances in our understanding and treatment of inflammatory bowel disease.

I would like to thank Centocor Inc., Procter & Gamble Pharmaceuticals, Shire US Inc., Prometheus Laboratories Inc., and Salix Pharmaceuticals, who have made it possible to include color photographs in this book.

Russell D. Cohen, MD

CONTENTS

vii

CONTRIBUTORS

WILLIAM M. BAUER, MD • *Department of Gastroenterology, The Cleveland Clinic Foundation, Cleveland, OH*

CHARLES N. BERNSTEIN, MD • *Department of Medicine, University of Manitoba, Winnipeg, Canada*

JAMES F. BLANCHARD, MD, PhD • *Department of Community Health Sciences, University of Manitoba, Winnipeg, Canada*

JUDY CHO, MD • *Department of Medicine, The University of Chicago Medical Center, Chicago, IL*

RUSSELL D. COHEN, MD • *Section of Gastroenterology, Department of Medicine, The University of Chicago Medical Center, Chicago, IL*

JANICE C. COLWELL, RN, MS, CWOCN • *The University of Chicago Hospitals, Chicago, IL*

THEMISTOCLES DASSOPOULOS, MD • *Section of Gastroenterology, Department of Medicine, Johns Hopkins University, Baltimore, MD*

MARLA C. DUBINSKY, MD • *Inflammatory Bowel Disease Center, Cedars Sinai Medical*

JAMES J. FARRELL, MB • *Division of Digestive Diseases, UCLA School of Medicine, Los Angeles, CA*

ARUNAS E. GASPARAITIS, MD • *Department of Radiology, The University of Chicago Medical Center, Chicago, IL*

RANJANA GOKHALE, MD • *Section of Pediatric Gastroenterology, Hepatology, and Nutrition, The University of Chicago Children's Hospital, Chicago, IL*

STEPHEN HANAUER, MD • *Section of Gastroenterology, Department of Medicine, The University of Chicago Medical Center, Chicago, IL*

JOHN HART, MD • *Department of Pathology, The University of Chicago Medical Center, Chicago, IL*

TODD E. H. HECHT, MD • *Department of Medicine, University of Pennsylvania School of Medicine, Philadelphia, PA*

ROGER D. HURST, MD • *Department of Clinical Surgery, University of Chicago Pritzker School of Medicine, Chicago, IL*

SUNANDA V. KANE, MD • *Section of Gastroenterology, Department of Medicine, The University of Chicago Medical Center, Chicago, IL*

JEANETTE NEWTON KEITH, MD • *Section of GI/Nutrition, Department of Internal Medicine, The University of Chicago Medical Center, Chicago, IL*

BARBARA S. KIRSCHNER, MD • *Section of Pediatric Gastroenterology, Hepatology, and Nutrition, The University of Chicago Children's Hospital, Chicago, IL*

JOSEPH B. KIRSNER, MD, PhD, DSCI (HON) • *Department of Medicine, The University of Chicago Medical Center, Chicago, IL*

BRET A. LASHNER, MD • *Department of Gastroenterology, The Cleveland Clinic Foundation, Cleveland, OH*

GARY R. LICHTENSTEIN, MD • *Division of Gastroenterology, Department of Medicine, University of Pennsylvania School of Medicine, Philadelphia, PA*

PETER M. MACENEANEY, FRCR • *Department of Radiology, The University of Chicago Medical Center, Chicago, IL*

ELENA RICART, MD • *Division of Gastroenterology, Hospital de Sant Pau, Barcelona, Spain*

WILLIAM J. SANDBORN, MD • *Division of Gastroenterology and Hepatology, Mayo Clinic, Rochester, MN*

BRUCE E. SANDS, MD • *Gastrointestinal Unit, Massachusetts General Hospital, Harvard Medical School, Boston, MA*

MICHAEL SITRIN, MD • *Section of GI/Nutrition, Department of Internal Medicine, The University of Chicago Medical Center, Chicago, IL*

CHINYU G. SU, MD • *Division of Gastroenterology, Department of Medicine, Presbyterian Medical Center, University of Pennsylvania School of Medicine, Philadelphia, PA*

STEPHAN R. TARGAN, MD • *Inflammatory Bowel Disease Center, Cedars Sinai Medical Center, Los Angeles, CA*

1

Inflammatory Bowel Disease (Ulcerative Colitis, Crohn's Disease)

Early History, Current Concepts, and 21st Century Directions

Joseph B. Kirsner, MD, PhD, DSCI

CONTENTS

ULCERATIVE COLITIS

The early history of ulcerative colitis is lost in the obscurities of past centuries and in the mix of the infectious colitides *(1)*. During the latter years of the 19th century, individual descriptions of a noncontagious illness labeled "simple ulcerative colitis," manifested by diarrhea, rectal bleeding, abdominal pain, fever, and multiple complications, appeared in Great Britain and northern Europe. Clinical information on 317 patients collected between 1888 and 1907 from seven London hospitals formed the basis of a major symposium in 1909. At a time of active microbiological discovery, bacterial infection, including bacillary dysentery, seemed a likely cause *(2)*. Specific enterocolonic infections (e.g.,

From: *Clinical Gastroenterology:*
Inflammatory Bowel Disease: Diagnosis and Therapeutics
Edited by: R. D. Cohen © Humana Press Inc., Totowa, NJ

shigella, salmonella, *E. histolytica*) gradually were excluded from the ulcerative colitis category. Ulcerative colitis steadily increased in clinical recognition and in geographic distribution. An early view emphasized the "nonspecificity" of the inflammation *(3)*.

CROHN'S DISEASE

In 1612, pathologist W. H. Fabry of Germany found at autopsy in a teenage boy, who had died after a brief illness with fever and abdominal pain, a thickened and obstructed terminal ileum *(4)*. In 1769, G. B. Morgagni of Italy described ulceration and perforation of an inflamed, thickened distal ileum and enlarged mesenteric lymph nodes in a man of 20 who had experienced diarrhea and fever *(5)*. The anatomic findings in both instances were consistent with later descriptions of Crohn's disease. Other possible early instances of Crohn's disease have been recorded by H. I. Goldstein *(6)*. Early in the 20th century, at a time of limited abdominal surgery, similar instances, presenting with an abdominal (inflammatory) mass, were dismissed as "inoperable neoplasms" *(7)*. In 1913, T. K. Dalziel *(8)* of Glasgow described 13 patients with recurrent ileal inflammation, in one instance clinically dating back to 1903. The illness was compared to the then recently described Johne's mycobacterial (*M. paratuberculosis*) infection of cattle, a relationship unsupported by recent evidence *(9)*. In 1932, at a meeting of the American Medical Association, Crohn, Ginzburg and Oppenheimer of New York, excluding specific infections, particularly intestinal tuberculosis, described similar findings in 14 patients *(10)*. Popular usage established the designation of Crohn's disease for this second form of "nonspecific" inflammatory bowel disease. Beginning in the 1960s, the term idiopathic inflammatory bowel diseases (IBD) was applied to both conditions.

Epidemiology and Demography

Acknowledging earlier diagnostic limitations, the prominence of ulcerative colitis during the first half and of Crohn's disease during the second half of the 20th century, encompassing varying geographic, ethnic and cultural patterns and differing health care systems over lengthy time periods, indicated environmentally-influenced disorders *(11)*. Incidence and prevalence figures for IBD varied throughout the century, reflecting not only differences in clinical awareness but also a rising prevalence of Crohn's disease *(12)*. Current estimates for the United States approximate an incidence of 20 per 100,000 population per year for both and a prevalence of 300, equally divided between the two diseases. In some countries, IBD (CD) is more common among

Jewish inhabitants; in Israel more frequently among Ashkenazi (European) Jews than among Sephardic (North African) Jews *(13)*. Today, IBD affects ethnic groups worldwide. Yet often involving children and young adults, males and females equally, many IBD patients today are older (50–80 yr). The scarcity of life-long cigarette smokers and the many ex-smokers in the ulcerative colitis population, [also in Parkinson's disease and adult celiac disease *(14)*] contrast with the many active cigarette smokers among patients with Crohn's disease *(15)*.

Additional epidemiologic issues awaiting clarification include:

1. The "birth-cohort pattern," *(16)* implicating environmental risk factors;
2. Onset circumstances of IBD in children and teenagers (measles, mumps infections early *(17,18)*, antibiotic excess);
3. Risk factors among individuals acquiring IBD after moving from low-risk rural to higher-risk urban areas, and;
4. "Geographic epidemiology," (status of local agriculture, water supply, industrial pollutants) possibly associated with high- and low-risk IBD prevalence.

CLINICAL FEATURES

The clinical manifestations of ulcerative colitis have changed partially throughout the century. Massive hemorrhage, toxic dilatation of the colon, bowel perforation, and malnutrition are less common now because of earlier diagnosis and improved supportive therapy. Population surveys indicate a rising incidence of proctitis *(19,20)*. Among the complications, the association between ulcerative colitis and primary sclerosing cholangitis (PSC) is noteworthy because of the increased risk for colon cancer and for pouchitis in those patients undergoing colectomy and ileoanal J-pouch anastomosis. More frequent colonoscopies, expert biopsy recognition of dysplasia, and earlier colectomy for patients not responding to medical treatment or requiring excessive amounts of steroids have reduced the urgency of the colorectal cancer problem.

The clinical manifestations of Crohn's disease also have changed. The previous "tumor-like" and "acute appendicitis" presentations are less common now. Earlier phases of the disease (e.g., mucosal inflammation) are being recognized. The prevalence of Crohn's disease in cooler, industrialized, urban areas, its paradoxical infrequency in underdeveloped countries with a high incidence of enteric infections and parasitic infestations, and its frequency in "westernized" ("cleaner") countries are significant environmental features. The infrequency of experimental intestinal inflammation in animals previously exposed to helminthic parasites suggests an acquired "protection" of the intestinal mucosal immune system, *(21)* perhaps by suppression of the TH1 inflammatory response *(22)*. The aphthoid erosions overlying M cells located in the epithelium overlying Peyer's patches in the small intestine implicate these specialized cells as portals of entry of "pathogens" *(23)*. Risk factors for IBD recurrence include a positive family history of IBD, upper respiratory infections, possibly an early measles virus infection, the use of aspirin and related compounds, enteric infections, the discontinuation of cigarette smoking (ulcerative colitis), the oral ingestion of penicillin-type antibiotics, and emotional stress. Recurrent Crohn's disease postoperatively, at the neoterminal ileum immediately proximal to the ileal-colonic surgical anastomosis, healing after diverting ileostomy, implicates the intestinal contents in the pathogenesis of Crohn's disease *(24)*.

ETIOLOGIC CONSIDERATIONS

Lactose, fructose, and sorbitol sensitivities, idiosyncrasies to food additives and the occasional immunologic reactions to foods among infants and young children *(25)*. notwithstanding, foods (e.g., cornflakes, refined sugars, and margarine) do not cause Crohn's disease. The uncontrolled psychosomatic hypotheses of the 1930s and 1940s ("ulcerative colitis personality") have been replaced by integrating intestinal neuroimmunohumoral mechanisms mediating the intestinal response to emotional stress *(26)*. Earlier immunologic assumptions (defective immunity, "autoimmunity") have been supplanted by "dysregulation" of the gut mucosal immune system and increased vulnerability of the intestinal epithelium to inflammation *(27)*. Microbiological possibilities in Crohn's disease in addition to the intestinal microflora include new pathogenic organisms (e.g., adherent-invasive *Eschericia coli*). The role of childhood paramyxovirus (measles) and mumps coinfections as antecedents to Crohn's disease remains uncertain *(28)*. The intestinal inflammatory reaction now is recognized as a complex sequence of molecular events involving alterations in the intestinal epithelial barrier, an increasing assortment of biological molecules (granulysins, *[29]* integrins, *[30]* defensins, claudins *[31]*, aquaporins, microcins *[32]*), and immune and nonimmune cells (endothelial, mesenchymal, nerve cells). The lower incidence of appendectomy in patients with ulcerative colitis and the "protective" effect of neonatal appendectomy against experimental ulcerative colitis await immunologic clarification.

UC VS CD

Ulcerative colitis (UC) and Crohn's disease (CD) with overlapping clinical features and responsiveness to similar (nonspecific) therapeutic agents are emerging as independent entities *(33)*. The tendency of Crohn's disease to irregularly affect the entire gastrointestinal tract differs from the limitation of ulcerative colitis to the colon and rectum. Histologically, the diffuse mucosal–submucosal involvement of ulcerative colitis contrasts with the focal transmural inflammation of Crohn's disease, though focal inflammation is observed in healing ulcerative colitis. The M cell in the epithelium overlying Peyer's patches, the prominent lymphoid aggregates, dilated submucosal lymphatics, and the granulomas distributed throughout the bowel wall, not observed in ulcerative colitis *(34)*, are pathogenetically significant features of Crohn's disease. The recurrence of Crohn's disease after bowel resection and reanastomosis contrasts with the "cure" of ulcerative colitis following total colectomy and ileostomy or ileoanal anastomosis with J pouch, but pouchitis is an increasing problem *(35)*.

Perinuclear antineutrophil cytoplasmic autoantibodies (UC) and antibodies to saccharomyces cerevisiae (CD) contribute to the clinical differentiation of the two entities *(36)* though their biological significance is unclear. The increased titers of serum antineutrophil cytoplasmic antibodies *(37)* and antibodies against goblet cells are typical of patients with ulcerative colitis and their first degree relatives. On the other hand, antisaccharomyces cerevisiae mannon antibodies, antibodies to a trypsin-sensitive antigen in pancreatic juice, and antiendothelial cell antibodies characterize Crohn's disease *(38)*. As noted by MacDonald et al. *(39)*. "Crohn's disease tissue manifests an ongoing T-helper cell type I response with excess interleukin 12 (IL-12), interferon-γ and tumor necrosis factor α (TNFα), directed against the normal bacterial flora. In ulcerative colitis tissue, the lesion represents an antibody-mediated hypersensitivity." Interleukin 2 (IL-2) messenger RNA is increased in the intestinal lesions of Crohn's disease, but not in ulcerative colitis. Microvascular endothelial adhesiveness for leukocytes is increased in both ulcerative colitis and Crohn's disease *(40)*.

ANIMAL MODELS

Early models of IBD induced by carrageenan, mecholyl, Freund's adjuvant, and dextran, made possible limited histologic studies of intestinal injury and repair. Kirsner's 1955 immune complex colitis in rabbits provided an early indication of immune mechanisms. Transgenic techniques have created experimental models of intestinal inflamma-tion more closely resembling the human disease *(41–43)*.

The ability to genetically engineer mice (transgenic methodology) emerged in the early 1970s with the technical ability to microinject individual mouse oocytes (eggs) with solutions of purified DNA *(44–47)*. Improving molecular cloning techniques allowed scientists to link regulatory gene segments with different structural genes, and experiments could be designed in which structural genes encoding growth factors, inflammatory molecules, or other proteins directed to a particular tissue or cell type. The profound impact of gene targeting experiments on the understanding of intestinal inflammation began in 1993, with the observation that mutations or deletions in four different genes [IL-2, interleukin 10 (IL-10), TGF-B1 and T-cell receptor β] resulted in progressively severe bowel inflammation, evidence that T cells and the protein products (lymphocyte-specific proteins) of all three genes are essential for maintaining the limited inflammation in the intestine ("physiologic inflammation").

Fuss and Strober *(48)* describe a TH_1-T cell driven tissue reaction resembling Crohn's disease in immunodeficient (SCID) mice immuno-logically reconstituted by the transfer of naive CD45RB[high] T cells, with the overproduction of IL-12 and interferon γ. On the other hand, IL-2 and IL-10 knockout mice and T-cell antigen receptor (TCR)-a-chain knockout mice, with the overproduction of IL-4, develop a TH_2-T cell driven tissue reaction resembling ulcerative colitis. The two models are characterized by an immunologic imbalance (dysregulation), but not an immunologic deficiency *(49)*. An intestinal germ-free environment pre-vents or attenuates the experimental colitis, implicating the intestinal microflora in the inflammation *(50)*. The microbially-induced alter-ation of mucosal barrier function *(51)* and the large microbial load to the gut-associated lymphoid tissue disrupt normal intestinal mucosal im-mune balances, resulting in an unregulated TH_1 or TH_2 response ("a failure of oral tolerance"). The prevention of colitis and its response to antibiotics in the IL-10 gene-deficient mouse associated with an increased number of mucosal adherent colonic bacteria is of interest in this regard *(52)*. Boirivant et al. *(53)* describe a rapidly developing colitis confined to the distal half of the colon in SJL/J mice following the rectal instillation of the haptenating agent, oxazolone; characterized by mixed neutrophil/lymphocyte infiltration and ulceration limited to the superficial layer of the mucosa, resembling UC. Oxazolone colitis is a T-helper cell type 2 (TH_2)-mediated process associated with greatly increased amounts of interleukin 4 and 5 (IL-4) and (IL-5); anti-IL-4 administration ameliorates the disease. Mice lacking Stat-3 in T cells (a signal transducer and activator of transcription-3 gene of macrophage origin) do not develop enterocolitis, indicating the role of activated macrophages in the process *(54)*.

CURRENT ETIOLOGIC CONSIDERATIONS

Current etiologic concepts revolve around altered gut mucosal immunologic and intestinal epithelial cytoprotective mechanisms, immune and nonimmune cellular and cytokine patterns of inflammation, a possible measles virus-related vasculitis) in Crohn's disease, *(55)* the essentiality of the intestinal microflora in IBD, and genetic influences in both diseases *(56)*. As summarized by C. Elson, *(57)*. IBD is a "dysregulated mucosal immune response particularly a CD4+ T-cell response to antigens of the enteric bacterial flora in a genetically susceptible (decreased oral tolerance) host" *(58,59)*.

UC and CD each result from the conjunction of multiple etiologic factors (genetic vulnerability, altered intestinal defenses, increased epithelial permeability, abnormal gut mucosal immune system, and an etiologic agent within the intestinal microflora) (anaerobic bacterial antigen) *(60)*. Earlier negative microbiological studies notwithstanding, today's molecular techniques *(61,62)* may yet identify an infectious agent in IBD. The focal, crypt-sparing tissue reaction of Crohn's disease suggests cellular-site (M cell, dendritic cell) entry of a pathogen into the intestinal lymphatic network, inducing an endolymphangitis. The diffuse colonic inflammation of ulcerative colitis is consistent with a surface epithelial injury, perhaps microbially initiated and immune-driven. Precipitating factors for each IBD include environmental "triggers" (bacteria, viruses, industrial and water pollutants, and chemicals) and "pathophysiological stress downregulating the cellular immune response," *(63)* circumstances not limited to any geographic area or to any ethnic group. The complex inflammatory reaction involves an unbalanced profusion of proinflammatory biological molecules, with important contributions from immunological cells (T cells, B cells, and lymphocytes), activated macrophages and inflammatory cells (polymorphonuclear cells, eosinophils, mast cells, and Paneth cells), and non-immune cells (e.g., fibroblasts).

The genetic influence in IBD, stronger in Crohn's disease than in ulcerative colitis, is reflected in the frequency of IBD among first-degree family members, the increased concordance rates for monozygotic IBD twins (CD), and the increased frequency of intestinal epithelial antigens in healthy first-degree relatives of patients with IBD *(64)*.

Multiple "susceptibility loci," including loci common to both ulcerative colitis and Crohn's disease (1,3,7,12,16* loci) *(65,66)* have been identified in genetic linkage studies. An association between ulcerative colitis and rare VNTR alleles of the human intestinal mucin gene, MUC-3, also has been reported *(67)*.

The recognition of a vulnerability gene on chromosome 1 in the highly inbred Chaldean (Iraq) immigrant population (located near Detroit) *(68–70)* and the expanding genetic studies are promising developments. "Genetic anticipation in CD," *(71)* that is, the progressively earlier onset and increasing severity of disease in successive generations, supports a genetic influence in IBD but more studies are desirable *(72)*. Orchard et al. *(73)* suggest that between 10 and 20 genes may be involved in Crohn's disease. Currently, five genome-wide searches for disease susceptibility genes and two abstracts have been reported. Potential loci have been identified in at least six regions (chromosomes *1p*, *4q*, *6p*-MHC region, *12*, *14q*, and *16*).

Many issues relating to the pathogenesis of IBD await clarification: the precise role of the gut microflora in CD, *(74,75)* the possible involvement of viruses, *(76)* the possible role of emerging infectious disease, *(77)* the immunologic integrity of the gastrointestinal epithelium (oral tolerance), the role of macrophages in intestinal inflammation, *(78)* the epithelial cytoprotective effects of intestinal IgA, *(79)* heat-shock proteins, and other intracellular protective agents (trefoil peptides, and growth factors), the role of powerful biologic molecules, such as TNFα *(80)*, the brain-mast cell connection *(81)*, the pathogenetic implications of "indeterminate IBD," the IBD-tobacco enigma, and the nature of the genetic influence in IBD.

EARLY TREATMENT

The absence of an established etiology of IBD during the early 1900s encouraged unusual treatments of ulcerative colitis, including calomel, tincture of hamamelis, and rectal instillations of boracic acid, silver nitrate, iron pernitrate or kerosene *(82)*. Therapy later included the rectal insufflation of oxygen, narco-analysis, roentgen irradiation of the abdomen (Crohn's disease), thiouracil drugs, liver extracts, detergents, and "extracts" of hog stomach and intestine. Russian approaches included the oral administration of dried coliform bacteria *(83)*, strawberry juice *(84)*, cooling the rectal mucosa *(85)*, oxygenating it *(86)*, irradiating it *(87)*, and exposing it to the topical application of Borzhom mineral water *(88)*, all to no avail. "Pelvic autonomic neurectomy" *(89)* and distal vagotomy in the 1950s were futile surgical efforts to correct an alleged "parasympathetic overactivity." Thymectomy *(90)* was performed in the 1960s to "correct an unidentified immune abnormality" in ulcerative colitis. Psychotherapy, including psychoanalysis, prominent in IBD therapy between 1930 and 1960, now is limited to individuals with serious psychiatric problems. Electrocoagulation or procaine injection of the "prefrontal lobes" of the brain utilized in France during the 1950s to disrupt connections between the frontal lobe and the thalamo-hypothalamic region was an extreme, fortunately temporary, support for psychogenic hypotheses *(91)*

Treatment of the inflammatory bowel diseases today, though nonspecific and variably effective, *(92)* is much improved. Increased medical resources include improved nutrition, limited administration of steroids, selected antiinflammatory drugs, and immunosuppressant compounds (6MP, Imuran) *(93)*, methotrexate to maintain remission of Crohn's disease *(94)*, and more potent antiinflammatory agents (e.g., oral Tacrolimus [FK506] monoclonal chimeric antibodies to a pivotal proinflammatory cytokine:human TNFα) *(95,96)*. Indications for operation are clearer and surgical procedures are improved, including the operation of total colectomy and ileoanal anastomosis with J pouch for ulcerative colitis and the limited intestinal resections for Crohn's disease.

The recent administration of "probiotic organisms" [*lactobacilli sp.*, *bifidobacteria*] *(97,98)* presumably to "correct" an "abnormal" intestinal microflora, protect against recurrent Crohn's disease after surgery, and even against toxigenic *E. coli* infections *(99)* is an intriguing development. Investigation of the molecular basis of intestinal inflammation has identified targeted "biologic" therapeutic agents (e.g., antisense oligonucleotides) *(100)*. As Podolsky and Fiocchi *(101)* note, "In theory the use of biologic mediators with antiinflammatory activity should be ideal because they are already produced and used physiologically by the body to control excessive immune reactivity and protect against inflammation." The impressive antiinflammatory effect of antibodies to TNFα *(102)* in Crohn's disease is a major advance in this direction. An important role also can be expected of the inhibitor$_\kappa$B (I$_\kappa$B)/nuclear factor$_\kappa$B (NF$_\kappa$B) family of pleiotropic transcription factors (including PPAR [proxisone proliferator-activated receptor]), controlling the expression of proinflammatory molecules: IL-1, TNFα, adhesion molecules and acute-phase proteins and other promoters of proinflammatory cytokines *(103,104)*. An intriguing possibility involves novel vaccination strategies using DNA for the induction of mucosal immunity *(105)*.

Treatment during the 20th century was directed chiefly toward nonspecifically downregulating the inflammatory response and inhibiting the production of immune and inflammatory mediators *(106)*. Therapeutic strategy in the 21st century will seek also to restore the cytokine imbalance of IBD via the generation of antigen-specific suppressor T lymphocytes [oral tolerance *(107)*] and the antimicrobial granulysins of cytolytic T cells *(108,109)* to control the intestinal inflammatory reaction, the potential benefit of "adjusting" the "abnormal" intestinal microflora of Crohn's disease with probiotics (e.g., lactobacillus bifidobacteria), protection of the intestinal epithelium by the secretory immune system, (goblet cells, immunoglobulins), and by endogenous antiinflammatory molecules *(110)*, the role of B-defensins *(111,112)*, the restoration of normal intestinal epithelial permeability, the therapeutic potential of glucagon-like peptide 2 *(113)*, and butyrate *(114)*, trophic to the intestinal epithelial mucosa, heparin to promote both endothelial and mucosal healing *(115)*, new antiinflammatory agents such as recombinant human TNF receptor attached to immunoglobulin protein (etanercept) *(116)*, the development of immunologic strategies for the treatment of autoimmune disorders including IL-10 *(117)* and mechanisms inducing oral tolerance. The increasing identification of key biological molecules involved in intestinal inflammation will accelerate the advance from the nonspecific management of the past century to the biologically more specific therapy of the 21st century *(118)*.

ACKNOWLEDGMENT

This work was based in part on "Nonspecific" Inflammatory Bowel Disease (Ulcerative Colitis and Crohn's disease) after 100 Years—What Next? Italian Journal of Gastroenterology and Hepatology 31:651–658, 1999 (with permission).

REFERENCES

1. Kirsner JB. Historical basis of the idiopathic inflammatory bowel diseases. J Inflamm Bowel Dis 1995;1:2–26.
2. Cameron HC, Rippman CH. Statistics of ulcerative colitis from London hospitals. Proc Roy Soc Med 1909;2:100–106.
3. Sloan WP Jr., Bargen JA, Gage RP: Life histories of patients with chronic ulcerative colitis. Review of 2000 cases. Gastroenterology 1950;16:25–38.
4. Fabry W. Ex scirrho et ulcere cancioso in intestino cocco exorta iliaca passio. In Opera observatio LXI centuriae I. cited by Fielding JF: Crohn's disease and Dalziel's syndrome. J Clin Gastroenterology 1988;10:279–285.
5. Morgagni GB. The seats and causes of disease investigated by anatomy. In Johnson B., Payne W., eds. Five Books Containing a Great Variety of Dissections with Remarks. Translated from Latin by B. Alexander, A. Millar, T. Cadell, London, U.K., 1769.

6. Goldstein HI: The history of regional enteritis (Saunders - Abercrombie–Crohn) ileitis. In Victor Robinson Memorial Volume (Essays on History of Medicine). Froben, New York, 1948:99–104, ch. 8.

7. Shapiro R. Regional ileitis - Summary of the literature. Am J Med Sci 1939;198:269.

8. Dalziel TK: Chronic interstitial enteritis. Brit Med J 1913;2:1068–1070.

9. Van Kruiningen HJ. Lack of support for a common etiology in Johne's disease of animals and Crohn's disease in humans. J Inflamm Bowel Dis 1999;5:183–191.

10. Crohn BB, Ginzburg L, Oppenheimer GD. Regional ileitis - a pathologic and clinical entity. JAMA 1932;99:1323–1329.

11. Kirsner JB. Inflammatory bowel disease. Part I. Nature and pathogenesis. Part II. Clinical and therapeutic aspects. Disease-a-Month (Masters in Medicine) 1991;37:610–666, 673–746.

12. Bernstein CN, Rawsthorne P, Wajda P, et al.: The high prevalence of Crohn's disease in a central Canadian province: A population based epidemiologic study. Gastroenterology 1997;112:A932.

13. Gilat T, Grossman A, Fireman Z, Rozen P: Inflammatory bowel disease in Jews. Front Gastrointest Res 1986;11:135–140.

14. Snook JA, Dwyer L, Lee-Elliott C, et al. Adult coeliac disease and cigarette smoking. Gut 1996;39:60–72.

15. Logan R: Smoking and inflammatory bowel disease. In Inflammatory Bowel Disease - Current Status and Future Approaches. MacDermott RP, ed. Elsevier Science Publishers, New York, 1988, pp. 663–670.

16. Delco F, Sonnenberg A. Exposure to risk factors for ulcerative colitis occurs during an early period of life. Am J Gastroenterol 1999;94:679–684.

17. Montgomery SM, Morris DL, Pounder RE, Wakefield AJ. Paramyxovirus infections in childhood and subsequent inflammatory bowel disease. Gastroenterology 1999;116:796–803.

18. Pardi DS, Tremaine WJ, Sandborn WJ, et al. Measles infection is associated with the development of inflammatory bowel disease. Am J Gastroenterol 2000; 95:1480–1484.

19. Ekbom A, Helmick C, Zack M, Adami HO. The epidemiology of inflammatory bowel disease. A large population-based study in Sweden. Gastroenterology 1991;100:350–358.

20. Meucci G, Vecchi M, Astegiano M, et al. The natural history of ulcerative proctitis: A multicenter, retrospective study. Am J Gastroenterol 2000;95:469–478.

21. Elliott DE, Li J, and others incl. Weinstock JV. Exposure to helminthic parasites protects mice from intestinal inflammation (abstract). Gastroenterology 1999;116(part 2):A706.

22. Fox JG, Beck P, Dangler CA, et al. Concurrent enteric helminth infection moldulates inflammation and gastric immune responses and reduces helicobacter-induced gastric atrophy. Nature Medicine 2000;6:536–542.

23. Fujimura Y, Owen R. The intestinal epithelial M cell properties and functions. In: Kirsner JB, ed. Inflammatory Bowel Disease, Fifth Edition. W. B. Saunders, Philadelphia, PA, 1999.

24. D'Haens GR, Geboes K, Peeters M, Baert F, Penninckx F, Rutgeerts P. Early lesions of recurrent Crohn's disease caused by infusion of intestinal contents in excluded ileum in Crohn's disease. Gastroenterology 1998;114:262–267.

25. Sampson HA, Anderson JA. Summary and recommendations: Classification of gastrointestinal manifestations due to immunologic reactions to foods in infants and young children. J Pediatr Gastroenterol Nutr (Conclusion of Proc Workshop JPFN 2000;30(Suppl. 1):587–597.

26. Sternberg EM. Neural-immune interactions in health and disease. J Clin Invest 1997;100:2641–2647.
27. Campbell N, Yio, XY, So LP, Li J, Mayer L. The intestinal epithelial cell: Processing and presentation of antigen to the mucosal immune system. Immunol Rev 1999;172:315–324.
28. Pardi DS, Tremaine WJ, Sandborn WJ, et al. Perinatal exposure to measles virus is not associated with the development of inflammatory bowel disease. J Inflamm Bowel Dis 1999;5:104–106.
29. Stenger S, Hanson DA, Teitelbaum R, et al. An antimicrobial activity of cytolytic T cells mediated by granulysin. Science 1998;282:121–125.
30. Etziori A. Integrins: The molecular glue of life. Hospital Practice Mar 15, 2000; 102–111.
31. Kinugasa T, Sakaguchi T, Gu X, Reineiker HC Claudins regulate the intestinal barrier in response to immune mediators. Gastroenterology 2000;118:1001–1011.
32. Khnel IA Microcins, peptide antibiotics of enterobacteria: Genetic control of synthesis, structure and model of action. Russian J Genet 1999;35:1–10.
33. Rubin PH, Marion J, Present DH. Differential diagnosis of chronic ulcerative colitis and Crohn's disease of the colon - One, two or many diseases? In: Kirsner JB, ed. Inflammatory Bowel Disease, Fifth Edition. W. B. Saunders, Philadelphia, PA, 1999.
34. Taraka M, Riddell RH, Saito H, et al. Morphologic criteria applicable to biopsy specimens for effective distinction of inflammatory bowel disease from other forms of colitis and of Crohn's disease from ulcerative colitis. Scand J Gastroenterol 1999;34:55–67.
35. Sandborn W. Pouchitis in the Kock continent ileostomy and the ileoanal pouch. In: Kirsner JB, ed. Inflammatory Bowel Disease, Fifth Edition. PW. B. Saunders, Philadelphia, PA, 1999.
36. Quinton JF, Sendid B, Reumaux D, et al. Anti-saccharomyces cerevisiae mannan antibodies combined with anti-neutrophil cytoplasmic autoantibodies in inflammatory bowel disease: Prevalence and diagnostic role. Gut 1998;42:788–791.
37. Shanahan F, Duerr RH, Rotter JI, Yang H, Sutherland LR, McElree C, et al. Neutrophil autoantibodies in ulcerative colitis: Familial aggregation and genetic heterogeneity. Gastroenterology 1992;103:456–461.
38. Sawyer AM, Pottenger BE, Wakefield AJ: Serum anti-endothelial cell antibodies are present in Crohn's disease but not ulcerative colitis. Gut 1990;31:A1169.
39. MacDonald TT, Monteleone G, Pender SLF. Recent developments in the immunology of inflammatory bowel disease. Scand. J. Immunol. 2000;51:2–9.
40. Binion DG, West CA, Volk EE, Drazba JA, Ziats NP, Petras RE, et al. Acquired increase in leukocyte binding by intestinal microvascular endothelium in inflammatory bowel disease. Lancet 1998;352:1742–1746.
41. Elson CO, Sartor RB, Tennyson GS, Riddell RH. Experimental models of inflammatory bowel disease. Gastroenterology 1995;109:1344–1367.
42. Fedorak R, Madsen KL. Naturally occurring and experimental IBD. In: Kirsner JB, ed. Inflammatory Bowel Disease, Fifth Edition. W. B. Saunders, Philadelphia, PA, 1999.
43. Blumberg RS, Saubermann LJ, Strober W. Animal models of mucosal inflammation and their relation to human inflammatory bowel disease. Curr Opin Immunol 1999;11:648–656.
44. Adams JM, Harris AW, Pinkert CA, Corcoran LM, Alexander WS, Cory S, et al. The c-myc oncogene driven by immunoglobulin enhancers induces lymphoid malignancy in transgenic mice. Nature 1985;318:533–538.

45. Sadlack B, Merz H, Schorle H, Schimpl A, Feller AC, Horak I. Ulcerative colitis-like disease in mice with a disrupted interleukin-2 gene. Cell 1993;75:253–261.
46. Ma A, Datta M, Margosian E, Chen J, Horak I. T cells, but not B cells, are required for bowel inflammation in interleukin-2-deficient mice. J Exp Med 1995; 182:1567–72.
47. Kuhn R, Lohler J, Rennick D, Rajewsky K, Muller W. Interleukin 10-deficient mice develop chronic enterocolitis. Cell 1993;75:263–274.
48. Fuss IJ, Strober W. Animal models of inflammatory bowel disease: Insights into the immunopathogenesis of Crohn's disease and ulcerative colitis. Currt Opin Gastroenterol 1998;14:476–482.
49. Strober W, Ludviksson BR, Fuss IJ: The pathogenesis of mucosal inflammation in murine models of inflammatory bowel disease and Crohn's disease. Ann Int Med 1998;128:848–856.
50. Sartor RB. Microbial factors in the pathogenesis of ulcerative colitis and Crohn's disease. In: Kirsner JB, ed. Inflammatory Bowel Disease, Fifth Edition. W. B. Saunders, Philadelphia, PA, 1999.
51. Garcia-Lafuente A, Antolin M, Guarner F, et al. Derangement of mucosal barrier function by bacteria colonizing the rat colonic mucosa. European J Clin Investigat 1998;28:1019–1026.
52. Madsen KL, Doyle JS, Tavernini MM, et al. Antibiotic therapy attenuates colitis in interleukin 10 gene-deficient mice. Gastroenterology2000;118:1094–1105.
53. Boirivant M, Fuss IJ, Chu A, Strober W. Oxazalone colitis: A murine model of T helper cell type 2 colitis treatable with antibodies to interleukin 4. J Exp Med 1998;188:1929–1939.
54. Takeda K, Clausen BE, Kaisho T, et al. Enchanced TH1 activity and development of chronic enterocolitis in mice devoid of Stat3 in macrophages and neutrophils. Immunity 1999;10:39–49.
55. Wakefield AJ, Sankey EA, Dhillon AP, et al. Pathogenesis of Crohn's disease: Multifocal gastrointestinal infarction. Lancet 1989;2:1057–1062.
56. Fiocchi C. Inflammatory bowel disease: Etiology and pathogenesis. Gastroenterology 1998;115:182–205.
57. Elson C. The immunology of IBD. In Kirsner JB, ed. Inflamm Bowel Dis, Fifth Edition. W. B. Saunders, Philadelphia, PA, 1999.
58. Weiner H. The nature of oral gastrointestinal tolerance. In Kirsner JB, ed. Inflamm Bowel Dis, Fifth Edition. W. B. Saunders, Philadelphia, PA, 1999.
59. Strober W, Kelsall B, Marth T. Oral tolerance. J Clin Immunol 1998;18:1–30.
60. Mayer LF. Current concepts of IBD etiology and pathogenesis. In: Kirsner JB ed. Inflamm Bowel Dis, Fifth Edition. W. B. Saunders, Philadelphia, PA, 1999.
61. Relman DA. The search for unrecognized pathogens. Science 1999;284: 1308–1310.
62. Meng J, Doyle MP. Emerging and evolving microbial foodborne pathogens. Bull Inst Pasteur 1998;96:151–164.
63. Rabin BS. Stress, immune function and health - the connection. Wiley-Liss, New York, 1999.
64. Kirsner JB. Genetic aspects of inflammatory bowel disease. Clin Gastroenterol 1973;2:557–576.
65. Duerr RH, Barmada MM, Zhang L, et al. Linkage and association between inflammatory bowel disease and a locus on chromosome 12. Am J Human Genetics 1998;63:95–100.
66. Ma Y, Ohmen JD, Zhiming L, et al. A genome-wide search identifies potential new susceptibility loci for Crohn's disease. J Inflamm Bowel Dis 1999;5:271–278.

67. Kyo K, Parkes M, Takei Y, Nishimori H, Vyas P, Satsangi J, et al. Association of ulcerative colitis with rare VNTR alleles of the human intestinal mucin gene, MUC-3. Human Mol Genet 1999;8:307–311.

68. Cho JH, Brant SR. Genetics and genetic markers in IBD. Curr Opin Gastroenterol 1988;14:283–288.

69. Cho JH, Nicolae DL, Gold LH, et al. Identificatin of novel susceptibility loci for inflammatory bowel disease on chromosomes lp, 3q and 4q: Evidence for epistasis between 1p and IBD1. Proc Natl Acadm Sci USA 1998;95:7502–7507.

70. Hampe J, Schreiber S, Shaw SH, et al. A genome-wide analysis provides evidence for novel linkages in inflammatory bowel disease in a large European cohort. Am J Human Genet 1999;64:808–816.

71. Polito JM 2nd, Rees RC, Childs B, Mendeloff AI, Harris ML, Bayless TM. Preliminary evidence for genetic anticipation in Crohn's disease. Lancet 1996;347:798–800.

72. McInnes MG: Anticipation: An old idea in new genes. Am J Human Genet 1996;59:973–979.

73. Orchard TR, Satsangi J, Van Heel D, Jewell DP: Genetics of inflammatory bowel disease: A Reappraisal. Scand J Immunol 2000;51:10–17.

74. Onderdonk A: The intestinal microflora and inflammatory bowel diseases. In: Kirsner JB, ed. Inflammatory Bowel Disease, Fifth Edition. W. B. Saunders, Philadelphia, PA, 1999.

75. Schultsz C, Van Den Berg FM, TenKate FW, et al. The intestinal mucus layer from patients with inflammatory bowel disease harbors high numbers of bacteria compared with controls. Gastroenterology 1999;117:1089–1097.

76. Bernstein CN, Blanchard JF. Viruses and inflammatory bowel disease: Is there evidence for a causal association? J Inflamm Bowel Dis 2000;6:34–39.

77. Daszak P, Cunningham AA, Hyatt AD. Emerging infectious diseases of wildlife. Threats to biodiversity and human health. Science 2000;287:443–449.

78. Machida YR. The key role of macrophages in the immunopathogenesis of inflammatory bowel disease. J Inflammatory Bowel Disease 2000;6:21–38.

79. Mestecky J, Russell MW, Elson CO: Intestinal IgA. Novel views on its function in the defense of the largest mucosal surface. Gut 1999;44:2–5.

80. Kollias G, Douni E, Kassiotis G, et al. The function of tumour necrosis factor and receptors in models of multi-organ inflammation, rheumatoid arthritis, multiple sclerosis and inflammatory bowel disease. Ann Rheum Dis 1999;58(Suppl 1):132–139.

81. Peck OC, Wood JD. Brain-gut interactions in ulcerative colitis (Corresp). Gastroenterology 2000;118:807–8.

82. Kirsner JB. Historical antecedents of inflammatory bowel disease therapy. J Inflamm Bowel Dis 1996;2:73–81.

83. Ratner SI, Fain O, Mashilov VP, Mitrofanova VC, Khudiakova GK, Vil'Shanskala FL. Treatment of patients with nonspecific ulcerative colitis with dried coliform bacteria. Klin Med 1963;41:102–109. Cited by Goligher JC, deDombal FT, Watts JMcK, Watkinson G: Ulcerative Colitis. Williams and Wilkins, Baltimore, MD, 1968:215.

84. Tashev T, Nedkova N, Balabanov G. On the etiology, clinic and treatment of chronic ulcerative colitis. Gastroenterologia 1956;86:760–762. Cited by Goligher JC, de Dombal FT, Watts JMcK, Watkinson G: Ulcerative Colitis. Baltimore, MD: Williams and Wilkins, 1968:215.

85. Mandache F, Prodescu V, Mateescu D, Lutescu I, Kover G, Stanciulescu P, et al. Rectal hypothermia, indications, technic and results in ulcerative haemorrhagic

anorectitis and rectocolitis. J Int Coll Surg 1965;44:128–135. Cited by Goligher JC, deDombal FT, Watts JMcK, Watkinson G: Ulcerative Colitis. Williams and Wilkins, Baltimore, MD, 1968:215.

86. Felsen J. Intestinal oxygenation in idiopathic ulcerative colitis. Arch Int Med 1931;48:786–792.

87. Sitkowski W, Plocker L, Szymanowski J. Three cases of ulcerative colitis successfully treated by x-ray. Pol Tyg Lek 1962;17:2040–3. Cited by Goligher JC, deDombal FT, Watts JMcK, Watkinson G: Ulcerative Colitis. Williams and Wilkins, Baltimore, MD, 1968:215.

88. Trauri MP. Protein fractions of the blood serum in chronic colitis and their change under the influence of submerged lavage with Borzhom mineral water. Tec Arkh 1962;34:112–114.

89. Schlitt RJ, McNally JJ, Shafiroff BGP, Hinton JW. Pelvic autonomic neurectomy for ulcerative colitis. Gastroenterology 1951;19:812–816.

90. Cesnick H. Thymectomy in ulcerative colitis: Promising results in seven patients. Langenbecks Arch Klin Dir 1968;321:86–98.

91. Sanpanet R, Bucaille M. Procaine injection of the prefrontal lobe of the brain. Technic and present indications. Ann Surg 1955;141:388–397.

92. Kirsner JB. Limitations in the evaluation of therapy in inflammatory bowel disease: Suggestions for future research. J Clin Gastroenterology 1990;12:516–524.

93. Sandborn WJ. Preliminary report on the use of oral tacrolimus (FK506) in the treatment of complicated proximal small bowel and fistulizing Crohn's disease. Am J Gastroenterol 1997;92:876–879.

94. Feagan BG, Fedorak RN, Irvine J, et al. A comparison of methotrexate with placebo for the maintenance of remission in Crohn's disease. New Engl J Med 2000;342:1627–1632.

95. Targan SR, Hanauer SB, Van Deventer SJ, Mayer L, Present DH, Braakman T, et al. A short-term study of chimeric monoclonal antibody cA2 to tumor necrosis factor alpha for Crohn's disease. New Engl J Med 1997;337:1029–1035.

96. Hanauer SB, Kane S: The pharmacology and pathogenetic rationale of anti-inflammatory drugs in inflammatory bowel disease. In: Kirsner JB, ed. Inflammatory Bowel Disease, Fifth Edition. W. B. Saunders, Philadelphia, PA, 1999.

97. Campieri M, Gionchetti P. Probiotics in inflammatory bowel disease: New insight to pathogenesis or a possible therapeutic alternative. Gastroenterology 1999; 116:1246–1249.

98. Madsen KL, Doyle JS, Jewell LD, et al. Lactobacillus species prevents colitis in interleuken-10 gene-deficient mice. Gastroenterology 1999;116:1107–1114.

99. Paton AW, Morona R, Paton JC. A new biological agent for treatment of shiga toxigenic escherichia coli infections and dysentery in humans. Nature Med. 2000;6:265–270.

100. Agrawal S, Kandimalla ER. Anti-sense therapeutics: Is it as simple as complementary base recognition? Mol Med Today 2000;6:72–81.

101. Fiocchi C, Podolsky DK. Cytokines and growth factors in inflammatory bowel disease. In: Kirsner JB, ed. Inflamm Bowel Dis, Fifth Edition. W. B. Saunders, Philadelphia, PA, 1999.

102. Rutgeerts PJ, Targan SR, eds: New advances in inflammatory bowel disease: A focus on infliximab. Alimen Pharmacol Therapeut 1999;13(Suppl 4):1–38.

103. Neurath MF, Becker C, Barbulescu K. Role of NFKB in immune and inflammatory responses in the gut. Gut 1998;43:856–60.

104. Schmid RM, Adler G. NFKB/Rcl/IKB: Implications in gastrointestinal diseases. Gastroenterology 2000;118:1208–1228.

105. McCluskie MF, Davis HL: Novel strategies using DNA for the induction of mucosal immunity. Crit Rev Immunol1999;19:303–329.
106. Kirsner JB. The influence of 20th century biomedical thought upon the origins of IBD therapy. Kluwer Academic, Dordrecht, Holland, 2000.
107. Wardrop RM III, Whitacre CC: Oral tolerance in the treatment of inflammatory autoimmune diseases. Inflamm Res 1999;48:106–119.
108. Stenger S, Hanson DA, Teitelbaum R, et al. An anticmicrobial activity of cytolytic T cells mediated by granulysin. Science 1998;282:121–125.
109. Krensky AM. A novel antimicrobial peptide of cytolytic lymphocytes and natural killer cells. Biochem. Pharmacol 2000;59:317–320.
110. Si-Tahar M, Merlin D, Sitaraman S, Madara JL. Constitutive and regulated secretion of secretory leukocyte proteinase inhibitor by human intestinal epithelial cells. Gastroenterology 2000;118:1061–1071.
111. Ouellette AJ, Selsted ME. Paneth cell defensins: Endogenous peptide components of intestinal host defense. Faseb J 1996;10:1280–1289.
112. Diamond G, Bevins CL. B-defensins: Endogenous antibiotics of the innate host defense response. Clin Immunol Immunopathol 1998;88:221–225.
113. Munroe DG, Gupta AK, Kooshesh F, et al. Prototypic G-protein-coupled receptor for the intestinotrophic factor glucagon-like peptide 2. Proc Natl Acad Sci USA 1999;96:569–573.
114. Inan MS, Rasoulpour RJ, Yin L, et al. The luminal short-chain fatty acid butyrate modulates NFKB activity on a human colonic epithelial cell line. Gastroenterology 2000;118:724–734.
115. Korzenik JR. Heparin: An emerging, counterintuitive therapy for inflammatory bowel disease. Curr Treat Opt Gastroenterol 2000;3:95–98.
116. Lovell DJ, Gianniri EH, Reiff A, et al. Etanercept in children with polyarticular juvenile rheumatoid arthritis. New Eng J Med 2000;342:763–769.
117. Romagnani S. Th1/Th2 cells. J Inflamm Bowel Dis 1999;5:285–294.
118. Sands BE. Therapy of inflammatory bowel disease. Gastroenterology 2000;118:S68–S82.

Epidemiology of Inflammatory Bowel Disease

Charles N. Bernstein, MD
and James F. Blanchard, MD, PhD

CONTENTS

INTRODUCTION

Despite progress in understanding the immunoinflammatory response of the bowel and in therapeutic options in inflammatory bowel disease (IBD), there is still much to learn about disease etiology. Epidemiological studies examining differences in occurrence in different places and among different age groups, as well as at different times, can provide clues as to factors that influence the origin of these diseases. Also, new hypotheses regarding etiology can be generated. Defining disease epidemiology also leads to an appreciation of the magnitude of public health concern a disease poses. Epidemiological data about IBD have highlighted important public health concerns. For instance, the highest incidence of disease is seen in young adults. Thus, morbidity relating to disease and its therapy (i.e., surgery) will affect school and work productivity and possibly socialization and personal and family development. Furthermore, ulcerative colitis and Crohn's colitis are associated

From: *Clinical Gastroenterology:*
Inflammatory Bowel Disease: Diagnosis and Therapeutics
Edited by: R. D. Cohen © Humana Press Inc., Totowa, NJ

with an increased risk for intestinal cancer and the associated increased mortality risk. Finally, the morbidity of these conditions is associated with considerable expenditure of health care resources and large indirect costs.

METHODOLOGICAL ISSUES

The validity of early epidemiological studies (of periods prior to the early 1970s) is problematical as diagnostic techniques (in particular, colonoscopy) have improved substantially over the past three decades and categorization of different forms of IBD continues to evolve. This particularly applies to distinguishing Crohn's colitis from ulcerative colitis *(1,2)*. Modern era studies are required, particularly because it has been suggested that the incidence of Crohn's disease of the colon (as opposed to small bowel disease) was increasing in the 1970s *(3–6)* and in some areas markedly increasing in the 1980s *(7)*.

Regarding specific epidemiological approaches to studying IBD, a main problem has been the lack of population-based approaches. Often, hospital-based data have been used to represent the population as a whole. For a number of these studies, the investigators supplemented their hospital-based data with surveys of community physicians and with perusal of community radiology, pathology, and chart records. In the era of the 1950s through the early 1970s, hospital-based data likely gave much more reasonable estimates of true disease incidence than they would for the past 15 yr. The advent of corticosteroids and other effective therapies between 1950 and the ensuing two decades might have precipitated increased referral by general practitioners to more specialized centers and therefore, inclusion in their hospital-based studies. With the proliferation of high-quality endoscopic technology, IBD has become easier to diagnose and treatment options have also become more varied. Furthermore, community clinicians have become more educated regarding diagnosis and therapy, as the understanding of these diseases and their differences has expanded and as the medical community has become bombarded by marketing of various new therapies. These changes have all led to IBD becoming more of an outpatient problem and fewer new diagnoses require hospitalization. Therefore, modern epidemiological studies have not relied solely on hospital-based data and have had broad access to population-based data.

INCIDENCE AND PREVALENCE RATES

Owing to the early average age of onset and chronicity of IBD, the prevalence generally ranges from 10 to 20 times higher than the incidence. In areas of high incidence such as the United Kingdom and northern Europe, it has been estimated that as many as 1 in 100 people will develop IBD in their lifetime *(8)*. Epidemiological data in IBD generally reflect only detected cases. One interesting study from the United Kingdom using mass screening for fecal occult blood suggested that as many as 33% of IBD cases may be undetected at one time in the community *(9)*.

Ulcerative Colitis

Much of the available epidemiological information about IBD is from northern Europe. The incidence in that area of the world of ulcerative colitis ranges from approx 1.8/100,000 person-years in Finland (1956–1961) *(10)* to 15.1/100,000 person-years in North Tees, England (1971–1977) *(4)*. Generally, the incidence varies from 6.3 to 15.1/100,000 person-years *(4,11–19)*. The estimated prevalence rates in Northern Europe ranges from 58/100,000 person-years in Leiden, Holland (1983) *(16)* to 157/100,000 person-years in the Faroe Islands (1983) *(17)*. The most recent Scandinavian data are from Norway which reveal an incidence rate of 13.6/100,000 for the years 1990–1993 *(20)*. This was a study of four Norwegian counties and the incidence varied from 11.7/100,000 to 18.6/100,000. These more recent data reflect a higher incidence rate than that which had previously been reported from northern Europe. This is particularly noteworthy because it had been considered that the incidence of ulcerative colitis had somewhat plateaued through the 1970s and the 1980s. Incidence rates in more southern areas have been much lower, closer to 1.5–5.8/100,000 person-years *(21–26)*.

In North America there is a paucity of population-based data. In the United States incidence rates are less homogeneous, although few data are available. In 1973, the incidence of first hospitalizations in 15 different geographic centers was 0–14.3/100,000 person-years, with a mean incidence of 3.5/100,000 person-years *(27)*. This type of study is skewed to reporting only severe or complicated cases, since they represent the cases likely to have been hospitalized. In Olmsted County, MN (Mayo Clinic catchment area), the incidence reported for the years 1960–1979 was 15/100,000 person-years, with a prevalence of 225/100,000 person-years *(28)*. The incidence rates remained stable throughout the 1980s up until 1993. The reported prevalence rate in 1993 was 229/100,000 *(29)*. This contrasts to a lower incidence of 2.8/100,000 person-years reported from urban Baltimore in the early 1960s *(30)*. Recent studies based on hospitalization data from United States Medicare discharge data and from a group of United States Veterans' hospitals *(31,32)* have both suggested an increased prevalence of ulcerative colitis in the northern United States compared with the southern United States.

Just north of the United States border, two Canadian studies have yielded very disparate prevalence rates in ulcerative colitis. In the northern areas of the province of Alberta around 1980, the prevalence rate was 37.5/100,000 *(33)*. In southern Alberta prevalence rates were less than 25/100,000 *(34)*. Patients were identified for these studies through hospital discharge records and through private gastroenterologists' charts, and may have underestimated the true prevalence. Data from the early 1990s in the province of Manitoba, whose population ethnicity is similar to that of Alberta's reveals a prevalence rate in 1994 of 167/100,000 *(35)*. This study was population-based and may more accurately reflect the modern epidemiology of this disease. This study found that 20% of patients were being regularly followed by a family physician and nearly 20% (particularly in rural areas) were being followed by general surgeons. This points out the potential flaw in assessing disease burden by solely pursuing gastroenterologists' practices. The incidence of ulcerative colitis in 1990–1994 was 14.5/100,000 in Manitoba.

Crohn's Disease

The incidence of Crohn's disease in northern Europe ranges from 0.8/100,000 person-years in Oxford, England (1951–1960) *(11)* to 6.1/100,000 person-years in Uppsala, Sweden (1965–1983) *(19)*. Generally, the incidence rates have varied between 1.6–5.4/100,000 person-years with prevalence rates of 27–48/100,000 person-years *(12,16,36–45)*. A recent update of the data from Northern Scotland found an overall mean incidence of 5.4/100,000 person-years in Aberdeen in the years from 1955 through 1987. However, for the years of 1985 through 1987 the mean incidence for this area was 11.6/100,000 person-years *(7)*. There was a trend toward higher rates in the later years of most studies, but incidence rates in general have remained less than that seen with ulcerative colitis. Incidence rates in Stockholm County between 1955–1989 also appear to have plateaued at a rate of approx 4.6/100,000 through the 1970s and 1980s *(45)*. Incidence rates for southern areas including Spain, Italy, Cuba, and South America are <1.0/100,000 person-years *(46)* and from central Israel 1.3 /100,000 person-years *(47)*. The most recent Scandinavian data are from Norway that reveal an incidence rate of 5.8/100,000 for the years 1990–1993 *(48)*. This was a study of four Norwegian counties and the incidence varied among the counties from 4.7/100,000 to 8.7/100,000.

In the United States, incidence rates for Olmsted County were reported as 4.3/100,000 person-years in 1978–1982 *(49)*. A recent update of these data revealed an incidence rate that was 5.8/100,000 (and essentially unchanged over the 30 yr between 1964–1993) whereas

the prevalence rate in 1993 was 144/100,00 *(50,51)*. First, hospitalizations in the 15 different American geographic areas varied from 0–4.9/
100,000 person-years *(27)*. Data from the recent United States Medicare
and Veterans' studies show an increased prevalence in the northern United
States compared with southern United States for Crohn's disease, as well
(31,32). Interestingly, the lowest rate among the fifteen states was in
Minnesota, which somewhat corroborates the much lower rate in Olmsted
County than in Manitoba, a nearby Canadian province *(35)*.

The Alberta studies revealed a slightly higher prevalence of Crohn's
disease than ulcerative colitis, 44.4/100,000 in the north *(33)* and up to
63.7/100,000 for females in the south *(34)*. The highest incidence and
prevalence rates for Crohn's disease yet to be reported were data from
Manitoba *(35)*. The incidence rate was 15/100,000 in 1990–1994 and
the prevalence rate of Crohn's disease in 1994 was 198/100,000 *(35)*. In
support of these widely disparate data from Alberta and Manitoba a
decade apart are data generated by Statistics Canada from hospital discharge diagnoses across the country. Discharge rates for Crohn's disease and ulcerative colitis from hospitals across Canada between 1971
and 1989 for Crohn's disease approx tripled from 9 to 25/100,000 in
males and from 12 to 36/100,000 in females *(52)*. Furthermore, a population-based cohort in Britain initiated in 1970 was assessed in 1996 for
the prevalence of IBD among the 26 yr olds in the cohort *(53)*. The rate
for Crohn's disease was 214/100,000 and for ulcerative colitis was 122/
100,000 for all confirmed cases. These authors attributed these higher
rates than that reported previously from the United Kingdom to either
enhanced accrual secondary to a population basis of the cohort or to the
high likelihood that by examining young persons the prevalence rate
was high.

An important and unresolved epidemiological issue, globally, are the
trends in incidence of both Crohn's disease and ulcerative colitis *(46,54)*.
For ulcerative colitis in Northern Europe alone, the incidence into the
1970s was thought to be rising in Norway and Scotland, falling in
Stockholm and stable in Britain, Denmark, and Finland. In the 1970s,
the incidence of Crohn's disease was thought to be rising in Britain and
Denmark and falling or stabilized in Stockholm and Scotland. The incidence rates in Scotland and in Copenhagen County, Denmark, in the
1980s had been rising considerably *(7,44)*. Among other nations,
Crohn's disease is thought to be on the rise in Israel, South Africa, and
Japan, and in other countries where traditionally IBD was rarely seen.
For instance the hospital prevalence of Crohn's disease increased by
approx eight-fold between 1986 and 1993 in the Singapore Chinese
population *(55)* Overall, the incidence rates of Crohn's disease in the

1970s were rising greater than the rates for ulcerative colitis. Although these diseases share many common features, the epidemiological data help to define that they are very distinct entities.

POTENTIAL CLUES TO ETIOLOGY BASED ON THE EPIDEMIOLOGY
Geographic Variation

A potentially important issue that might provide clues to IBD etiology is that the highest incidence and prevalence rates are in the northern hemisphere and areas with generally colder climates. Studies from Australia *(23)*, South African whites *(56,57)*, central Israel *(22,47)*, and smaller studies from southern Europe and the South Pacific revealed low incidence and prevalence rates of either ulcerative colitis or Crohn's disease *(25,26,46,54,58)*. One aspect of the north–south issue is the imbalance in data collection methods *(59)*. Northern countries such as in Scandinavia and in the United Kingdom have well-established population-based registries, whereas these types of data collection are not available in southern Europe or other southern hemisphere countries. An important lesson on the ability to extrapolate epidemiological data in terms of geographic variation comes from Manitoba and Minnesota. The only population-based North American data of IBD epidemiology come from these two neighboring areas separated by the 49th parallel. In the early 1990s, the incidence of Crohn's disease was 15/100,000 in Manitoba but only 7/100,000 in Olmsted County. How can these rates be reconciled considering a distance of less than 500 miles between the Manitoba border and Olmsted County? The incidence of 15/100,000 is the average incidence in the province. Based on postal forward sortation areas we found a seven-fold variation in age-adjusted incidence for ulcerative colitis *(60)* and a six-fold variation in Crohn's disease incidence *(60)*. Although some of these differences likely reflect differences in demographic mix, they also suggest the presence of environmental influences as well. It is also interesting to note that there is a geographic correlation between Crohn's disease and ulcerative colitis incidence rates *(60)* in Manitoba that is consistent with the existence of some common environmental risk factors. These data also suggest that the clues to disease etiology might be derived from studying small area variations in incidence.

Age and Gender

Almost uniformly, epidemiological studies reveal a peak incident age in the second through third decades of life. Many studies report a bimodal incidence, particularly for ulcerative colitis, with a second incident peak in the sixth through seventh decades. The second and third decades are the ages of social expansion, family development and significant economic contribution to society. Thus, chronic debilitating disease in this age range may have broader societal implications. Age differences may reflect specific alterations in the immune systems that evolve with aging. Crohn's disease is rarely seen under age 5. However, the peak incidence in the second and third decades suggests that exposure to important environmental causes are likely to be experienced in early life *(61)*. Crohn's disease that presents after age 60 often has a different phenotypic pattern of expression, with a predilection for the left colon as opposed to more typical terminal ileal disease of younger patients. Thus, immunological alterations identified in IBD might best be analyzed in the context of the age of the subjects in whom they are discerned.

Regarding gender, there is an approximate excess of females by 30% in Crohn's disease, but on average no gender preference in ulcerative colitis. Data from Manitoba similarly revealed a 30% excess of females with Crohn's disease and no gender predilection in ulcerative colitis *(35)*. However, on analysis of birth cohorts an interesting finding was that of a reversal in the gender predilection for males born between 1968 and 1981 who presented with Crohn's disease by the age of 20. This led us to consider what environmental factors might have accounted for such a male predominance. One hypothesis is that in Manitoba females were vaccinated against rubella prior to 1981, but males were not. On exploring the incidence rates of Crohn's disease in comparison to incidence rates of rubella revealed an interesting parallel (Fig. 1). This has led to a pursuit of infection rates of rubella and other paramyxoviruses in the Manitoba IBD population compared to a matched population based control group. Gender differences may point to the potential importance of the sex hormone milieu in either the initiation or perpetuation of the disease.

Elsewhere, recently an emerging male predominance has been shown. A review of Crohn's disease patients presenting to clinics in Athens found a male: female ratio of 1.58 *(62)*. It is noteworthy that most recent reports of incident pediatric Crohn's disease reveal a male predominance. The male:female ratio was reported as 4:1 in children in Wales for the years 1995–1997 *(63)*. In a study of all newly diagnosed children presenting to a New York hospital the ratio was 1.51 *(64)*. Perhaps the changing gender pattern from female to male predominance may provide some etiologic clues.

Race and Ethnicity

Although the clinical features do not exhibit significant racial differences *(65)*, populations of European ancestry are thought to be at great-

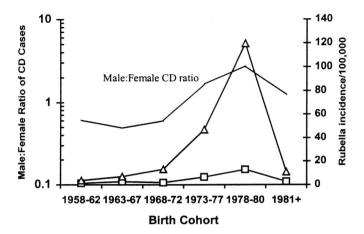

Fig. 1. Male:female ratio (—) of incident cases of CD between ages 10–19 and the gender-specific incidence of rubella (1990–97) (△ males, □ females), by birth cohort.

est risk for developing IBD. This is supported by data showing lower rates among the Maoris in New Zealand *(66)*, the Japanese *(67)* and possibly in the black and Native American Indian populations of the United States *(68,69)*. The study from urban Baltimore, however, suggested an incidence among urban blacks that approaches (but is still somewhat less than) that for whites *(30)*, however, these data are nearly 40 yr old. A recent study from a large Health Maintenance Organization in California revealed that the hospitalization rate for IBD in the black population was comparable to the rate seen in whites *(70)*. In this study, there was a much lower rate of hospitalization for IBD in the Hispanic and Asian populations. One paper from South Africa, where there is thought to be a low incidence in the black population, reported a rising incidence among black urbanites in Johannesburg *(57)*. Racial differences highlight the potential importance of genetics on disease etiology. The population-based data from Manitoba and Olmsted County mostly reflect populations of mostly northern European origins.

There is an increased incidence of IBD among Jews. This was found to be true in studies from United States Veterans in the 1950s *(71)*, from a United States college in the 1970s *(72)*, and from Baltimore *(30)*, South Africa *(56)*, and Sweden *(39,40)*. Because studies from central Israel suggested a lower incidence among the population there (all Jews) than incidence rates reported for the rest of the Western world, this challenged the notion of a Jewish predilection. However, the rates among Ashkenazie Jews (versus Sephardic or Oriental Jews) and among those born in the United States and western Europe who immigrated to Israel approached those of the United States and northern European studies *(22,47)*. Furthermore, a more recent study from southern Israel revealed higher incidence rates approaching those previously reported from the United States and Europe *(24)*. Nonetheless, the early Israeli data raised potential etiologic questions, including considerations of climate, culture, or diet that may have accounted for the different rates among Jews in Israel compared with western and northern European and American Jews. Some authors have advocated that future epidemiological studies in IBD must address environmental issues *(7,61)*.

An interesting aspect of studying ethnicity is to examine the epidemiological trends among ethnic groups of typically low incidence in their homeland in comparison to the incidence rates for these groups when they migrate to areas of typically high incidence. In Leicestershire, the incidence of ulcerative colitis among second-generation South Asian migrants was significantly higher than that among native Europeans by a factor of nearly 2.5-fold *(73)*. It had previously been shown that South Asians immigrants in Leicestershire had a higher prevalence of ulcerative colitis than native Europeans, whereas the prevalence of Crohn's disease among the South Asian group was lower *(74)*.

Birth Cohort

Changes in incidence rates based on birth cohort may point to some environmental factors. The existence of a birth cohort phenomenon implies an exposure to an environmental risk factor early in life which plays a crucial role in the development of a disease. Alternatively, it may relate to an exposure that affects individuals at a specific age and occurred at only specific intervals. For instance, investigators in northern Europe have assessed eras of measles and mumps epidemics and correlated this with changes in IBD incidence rates *(75–77)*. The birth cohort of people born in 1945–1954 was thought to be at increased risk in Uppsala, Sweden *(19)* and in Stockholm, Sweden *(40)*, but no birth cohort effect was found in studies from Cardiff, Wales *(6)* or from Copenhagen, Denmark *(12)*. An interesting report from six different western countries revealed a similar peak mortality rate from ulcerative colitis for the birth cohort born between 1880–1890. These authors speculated that perhaps enhanced infant hygiene in that period led to increased rates of ulcerative colitis (and ultimately deaths attributed to ulcerative colitis). Nonetheless, the long periods of follow up and consistency of the data across countries pointed to the importance of an environmental factor(s) *(78)*.

Socioeconomic Factors

There is a suggestion of predilection among single versus married people but these data are complicated by a potential effect that the disease may have on a patient's likelihood of marrying. Urbanites have a greater incidence in Baltimore *(30)*, Olmsted County *(29)*, Uppsala, Sweden *(19)*, Northern Scotland *(7)*, and Manitoba *(35)*. In Alberta studies where the prevalence rates were as low as 44/100,000 the rates were 234.1/100,000 in 30–39-yr-old urban dwelling females *(33)* and 373/100,000 in urban-dwelling Jewish males *(34)*. Obviously issues regarding gender, ethnicity, and possibly other confounding factors affect these high rates.

There are conflicting data as to whether patients with IBD are more likely to have a higher socioeconomic standard of living and there are data that suggest a greater likelihood of attaining postsecondary education among patients with IBD *(79–81)*. Much of these data have come from tertiary referral centers which undoubtedly see a selected population. Epidemiological data gathering regarding ethnicity, marital status, urban versus rural living, and socioeconomic standard of living may be confounded by the specific health care utilization patterns of the different groups. This is particularly true in the American health care system of the past four decades where access has been unequal, but less of a problem in studies from Scandinavia where health care access is more universal. This would also be less of a problem in Canada. The Manitoba data suggest that in fact there are few socioeconomic differences between patients with IBD and matched controls *(82)*.

SUMMARY

There are a variety of reasons as to why it is essential to pursue population-based epidemiological studies in IBD. First, it is important to quantify the magnitude of the problem. This helps health planners understand the resources that are necessary to manage these patients. Trends in the epidemiology more importantly can lead to disease etiology clues. Currently in Manitoba we are utilizing our population-based database to pursue studies of possible microbial factors. Ultimately, when one is searching for etiological clues whether they are environmental such as microbial, or related to ingestion of toxins such as cigarette smoke or the oral contraceptive *(83–87)*, or whether one is simply pursuing genetic studies it is critical to define the appropriate population of both patients and controls.

Based on data from Manitoba derived from nearly 5000 subjects with IBD in 1995 in a population of 1.1 million, we believe there are over

120,000 Canadians and well over 1 million Americans with IBD. Furthermore, our data suggest that incidence rates are among the highest in the world in our area (Manitoba), and that prevalence rates are continuing to rise in Crohn's disease. These diseases will continue to be among the more challenging faced by gastroenterologists and our estimates point to an increasing burden of these challenges in gastroenterology practices over the next several years.

REFERENCES

1. Bernstein CN, Shanahan F, Anton PA, Weinstein WM. Patchy involvement, including rectal sparing, occurs in ulcerative colitis (UC):A prospective study. Gastrointest Endosc 1995;42:232–237.
2. Lewin KJ, Riddell RH, Weinstein WM, eds. Idiopathic inflammatory bowel disease. In:*Gastrointestinal Pathology and Its Clinical Implications.* Igaku-Shoin, New York, 1992, 834–989.
3. Kyle J, Stark G. Fall in the incidence of Crohn's disease. Gut 1980;21:340–343.
4. Devlin HB, Datta D, Dellipiani AW. The incidence and prevalence of inflammatory bowel disease in North Tees Health District. World J Surg 1980;4:183–193.
5. Shivananda S, Pena AS, Nap M, Weterman IT, Mayberry JF, Ruitenberg EJ, Hoedemaeker Ph J. Epidemiology of Crohn's disease in Regio Leiden, The Netherlands. Gastroenterol 1987;93:966–974.
6. Rose JDR, Roberts GM, Williams G, Mayberry JF, Rhodes J. Cardiff Crohn's disease jubilee:The incidence over 50 years. Gut 1988;29:346–351.
7. Kyle J. Crohn's disease in the Northeastern and Northern Isles of Scotland:An epidemiological review. Gastroenterol 1992;103:392–399.
8. Logan RFA. Inflammatory bowel disease incidence:up, down or unchanged? Gut 1998;42:309–311.
9. Howarth GF, Robinson MHE, Jenkins D, Hardcastle JD, Logan RFA. High prevalence of undetected inflammatory bowel disease (IBD);Data from the Nottingham faecal occult blood (FOB) screening trial.
10. Moller C, Linden G. Ulcerative colitis in Finland:I. Cases treated at Central hospitals, 1956–1967. Dis Col Rect 1971;14:259–263.
11. Evans JG, Acheson ED. An epidemiological study of ulcerative colitis and regional enteritis in the Oxford area. Gut 1965;6:311–324.
12. Binder V, Both H, Hansen PK, Hendriksen C, Kreiner S, Torp-Pedersen K. Incidence and prevalence of ulcerative colitis and Crohn's disease in the county of Copenhagen, 1962 to 1978. Gastroenterol 1982;83:563–568.
13. Sinclair TS, Brunt PW, Mowat NAG. Nonspecific proctocolitis in Northeastern Scotland:A community study. Gastroenterol 1983;85:1–11.
14. Morris T, Rhodes J. Incidence of ulcerative colitis in the Cardiff region 1968–1977. Gut 1992;33:256–258.
15. Srivastava ED, Mayberry JF, Morris TJ, et al. Incidence of ulcerative colitis in Cardiff over 20 years:1968–87. Gut 1992;33:256–258.
16. Berner J, Kiaer T. Ulcerative colitis and Crohn's disease on the Faroe Islands 1964–83. A retrospective epidemiological survey. Scand J Gastroenterol 1986;21:188–192.
17. Shivananda S, Pena AS, Mayberry JF, Ruitenberg EJ, Hoedemaeker Ph J. Epidemiology of proctocolitis in the region of Leiden, The Netherlands. Scand J Gastroenterol 1987;22:993–1002.

18. Haug K, Schrumf E, Barstad S, et al. Epidemiology of ulcerative colitis in Western Norway. Scand J Gastroenterol 1988;23:517–522.
19. Ekbom A, Helmick C, Zack M, Adami H-O. The epidemiology of inflammatory bowel disease: a large population-based study in Sweden. Gastroenterol 1991;100:350–358.
20. Moum B, Vatn MH, Ekbom A, et al. Incidence of ulcerative colitis and indeterminate colitis in four counties of southeastern Norway, 1990–1993. Scand J Gastroenterol 1996;31:362–366.
21. Gower-Rousseau C, Salomex JL, Dupas JL, et al. Incidence of inflammatory bowel disease in northern France (1988–1990). Gut 1994;35:1433–1438.
22. Gilat T, Ribak J, Benaroya Y, Zemishlany Z, Weissman I. Ulcerative colitis in the Jewish population of Tel-Aviv Jafo. I. Epidemiology. Gastroenterol 1974;66:335–342.
23. McDermott FT, Whelan G, St John JB, et al. Relative incidence of Crohn's disease and ulcerative colitis in six Melbourne hospitals. Med J Aust 1987;146:525–529.
24. Odes HS, Fraser D, Krawiec J. Ulcerative colitis in the Jewish population of Southern Israel 1961–1985:epidemiological and clinical study. Gut 1987;28:1630–1636.
25. Vucelic B, Korac B, Sentic M, et al. Ulcerative colitis in Zagreb Yugoslavia:incidence and prevalence 1980–1989. Int J Epidemiol 1991;20:1043–1047.
26. Probert CSJ, Jayanthi V, Mayberry JF. Inflammatory bowel disease in Indian migrants in Fiji. Digestion 1991;50:82–84.
27. Garland CF, Lilienfield AM, Mendeloff AI, Markowitz JA, Terrell KB, Garland FC. Incidence rates of ulcerative colitis and Crohn's disease in fifteen areas of the United States. Gastroenterol 1981;81:1115–1124.
28. Stonnington CM, Phillips SF, Melton LJ III, Zinsmeister AR. Chronic ulcerative colitis:incidence and prevalence in a community. Gut 1987;28:402–409.
29. Loftus EV, Silverstein MD, Sandborn WJ, Tremaine WJ, Harmsen WS, Zinsmeister AR. Ulcerative colitis in Olmsted County, Minnesota 1940–1993; incidence, prevalence and survival. Gut 2000;46:336–343.
30. Monk M, Mendeloff AI, Siegel CI, Lilienfeld A. An epidemiological study of ulcerative colitis and regional enteritis among adults in Baltimore. Gastroenterol 1967;53:198–210.
31. Sonnenberg A, McCarty DJ, Jacobsen SJ. Geographic variation of inflammatory bowel disease within the United States. Gastroenterol 1991;100:143–149.
32. Sonnenberg A, Wasserman IH. Epidemiology of inflammatory bowel disease among U.S. military veterans. Gastroenteroly 1991;101:122–130.
33. Pinchbeck BR, Kirdeikis J, Thomson ABR. Inflammatory bowel disease in Northern Alberta. An epidemiologic study. J Clin Gastroenterol 1988;10:505–515.
34. Pinchbeck BR, Kirdeikis J, Thomson ABR. Effect of religious affiliation and education status on the prevalence of inflammatory bowel disease in northern Alberta. Can J Gastroenterol 1988;2(Suppl A):95A–100A.
35. Bernstein CN, Blanchard JF, Rawsthorne P, Wajda A. The epidemiology of Crohn's disease and ulcerative colitis in a central Canadian province:a population-based study. Am J Epidemiol 1999;149:916–924.
36. Fahrländer H, Baerlocher CH. Clinical features and epidemiological data on Crohn's disease in the Basle area. Scand J Gastroenterol 1971;6:657–662.
37. Norlen BJ, Krause U, Bergman L. An epidemiological study of Crohn's disease. Scand J Gastroenterol 1970;5:385–390.
38. Miller DS, Keighley AC, Langman MJS. Changing patterns in epidemiology of Crohn's disease. Lancet 1974;II:691–693.
39. Brahme F, lindstrom C, Wenckert A. Crohn's disease in a defined population. An epidemiological study of incidence, prevalence, mortality, and secular trends in the city of Malmö, Sweden. Gastroenterol 1975;69:342–351.

40. Hellers G. Crohn's disease in Stockholm County 1955–1974. Acta Chir Scand 1979;490:1–84 (Suppl 1).
41. Mayberry J, Rhodes J, Hughes LE. Incidence of Crohn's disease in Cardiff between 1934 and 1977. Gut 1979;20:602–608.
42. Lee FI, Costello FT. Crohn's disease in Blackpool - incidence and prevalence 1968–1980. Gut 1985;26:274–278.
43. Jayanthi V, Probert CSJ, Pinder D, Wicks ACB, Mayberry JF. Epidemiology of Crohn's disease in Indian migrants and the indigenous population in Leicestershire. Q J Med 1992;82:125–138.
44. Munkholm P, Langholz E, Haagen Nielsen O, Kreiner S, Binder V. Incidence and prevalence of Crohn's disease in the county of Copenhagen, 1962–87:A sixfold increase in incidence. Scand J Gastroenterol 1992;27:609–614.
45. Lapidus A, Bernell O, Hellers G, Persson P-G, Lofberg R. Incidence of Crohn's disease in Stockholm County 1955–1989. Gut 97;41:480–486.
46. Calkins BM, Mendeloff AI. Epidemiology of inflammatory bowel disease. Epidem Rev 1986;8:60–91.
47. Rozen P, Zonis J, Yekutiel P, Gilat T. Crohn's disease in the Jewish population of Tel-Aviv-Yafo. Epidemiologic and clinical aspects. Gastroenterol1979;76:25–30.
48. Moum B, Vatn MH, Ekbom A, et al. Incidence of Crohn's disease in four counties of southeastern Norway, 1990–1993. A prospective population-based study. Scand J Gastroenterol 1996;31:355–361.
49. Gollop JH, Phillips SF, Melton LJ III, Zinsmeister AR. Epidemiologic aspects of Crohn's disease:a population based study in Olmstead County, Minnesota, 1943–1982. Gut 1988;29:49–56.
50. Loftus EV, Silverstein MD, Sandborn WJ, Tremaine WJ, Harmsen WS, Zinsmeister AR. Crohn's disease in Olmsted County, Minnesota, 1940–1993; incidence, prevalence, and survival. Gastroenterol 1998;114:1161–1168.
51. Loftus EV. The epidemiology of Crohn's disease. Gastroenterology 1999;116: 1502–1506 (reply).
52. Riley R. Crohn's disease and ulcerative colitis-Morbidity and mortality:The Canadian experience. Can J Gastroenterol 1994;8:145–150.
53. Montgomery SM, Morris DL, Thompson NP, Subhani J, Pounder RE, Wakefield AJ. Prevalence of inflammatory bowel disease in British 26 year olds:national longitudinal birth cohort. Brit Med J 1998;316:1058–1060.
54. Whelan G. Epidemiology of inflammatory bowel disease. Med Clin N 1990;74:1–12.
55. Law NM, Lim CC, Chong R, Ng HS. Crohn's disease in the Singapore Chinese population. J Clin Gastroenterol 1998;26:27–29.
56. Novis BH, Marks IN, Bank S, Louw JH. Incidence of Crohn's disease at Groote Schuur Hospital during 1970–1974. S Afr Med J 1975;49:693–697.
57. Segal I. Intestinal tuberculosis, Crohn's disease and ulcerative colitis in an urban Black population. S Afr Med J 1984;65:37–44.
58. Ruiz V. Crohn's disease in Galacia, Spain. Scand J Gastroenterol 1989;24 (suppl 170):29–31.
59. Shivinada S, Lennard-Jones J, Logan R, et al. Incidence of inflammatory bowel disease across Europe:is there a difference between north and south? Results of the European collaborative study on inflammatory bowel disease (EC-IBD). Gut 1996;39:690–697.
60. Blanchard JF, Bernstein CN, Wajda A, Rawsthorne P. Small area variations socio-demographic correlates for the incidence of Crohn's disease and ulcerative colitis. Amer J Epidemiol 2001;154:328–335.
61. Lashner BA. Epidemiology of inflammatory bowel disease. Gastroenterol Clin N Am 1995;24:467–74.

62. Triantafillidis JK, Emmanouilidis A, Manousos O, Nicolakis D, Kogevinas M. Clinical patterns of Crohn's disease in Greece: a follow up study of 155 cases. Digestion 2000;61:121–128.

63. Hassan K, Cowan FJ, Jenkins HR. The incidence of childhood inflammatory bowel disease in Wales. Eur J Pediatr 2000;159:261–263.

64. Weinstein TA, Levine M, Pettei M, Gold DM, Kessler BH. The influence of age and family history in the presentation of pediatric inflammatory bowel disease. Gastroenterol 2000;118:A531.

65. Straus WL, Eisen GM, Sandler RS, Murray SC, Sessions JT, for the Mid-Atlantic Crohn's Disease Study Group. Crohn's disease: does race matter? Am J Gastroenterol 2000;95:479–483.

66. Wigley RD, MacLaurin BP. A study of ulcerative colitis in New Zealand, showing a low incidence in Maoris. Br Med J 1962;2:228–231.

67. Matsunaga F. Clinical studies of ulcerative colitis and its related diseases in Japan, in Proceedings of the World Congress on Gastroenterol Baltimore, Md, Williams and Wilkins, 1958.

68. Mendeloff AI, Dunn JP. Digestive diseases. American Public Health Association Vital and Health Statistics Monograph. Cambridge, MA: Harvard University Press, 1971.

69. Congilosi SM, Rosendale DE, Herman DL. Crohn's disease-A rare disorder in American Indians. West J Med 1992;157:682 (letter).

70. Kurata JH, Kantor-Fish S, Frankl H, Godby P, Vadheim CM. Crohn's disease among ethnic groups in a large Health Maintenance Organization. Gastroenterology 1992;102:1940–1948.

71. Acheson ED. The distribution of ulcerative colitis and regional enteritis in United States Veterans with a particular reference to the Jewish religion. Gut 1960;1:291–293.

72. Gelpi AP. Inflammatory bowel disease among college students. West J Med 1978;129:369–373.

73. Carr I, Mayberry JF. The effects of migration on ulcerative colitis:a three year prospective study among Europeans and first- and second-generation South Asians in Leicester (1991–1994) Am J Gastroenterol 1999;94:2918–2922.

74. Probert CSJ, Jayanthi V, Hughes AO, Thompson JR, Wicks ACB, Mayberry JF. Prevalence and family risk of ulcerative colitis and Crohn's disease: an epidemiological study among Europeans and South Asians in Leicestershire. Gut 1993; 34:1547–1551.

75. Ekbom A, Wakefield AJ, Zack M, Adami HO. The role of perinatal measles infection in the aetiology of Crohn's disease: a population-based epidemiological study. Lancet 1994;344:508–510.

76. Montgomery SM, Björnsson S, Jóhannsson JH, Thjodleifsson B, Pounder RE, Wakefield AJ. Concurrent viral epidemics in Iceland are a risk for inflammatory bowel disease. Gut 1998;42:A41.

77. Montgomery SM, Morris DL, Pounder RE, Wakefield AJ. Paramyxovirus infections in childhood and subsequent inflammatory bowel disease Gastroenterology 1999;116:796–803.

78. Delco F, Sonnenberg A. Birth-cohort phenomenon in the time trends of mortality from ulcerative colitis. Am J Epidemiol 1999;150:359–366.

79. Rogers BHJ, Clark LM, Kirsner JB. The epidemiologic and demographic characteristics of inflammatory bowel disease-An analysis of a computerized file of 1400 patients. J Chronic Dis 1971;24:743–773.

80. Grace M, Priest G. The epidemiology of inflammatory bowel disease, in Inflammatory Bowel Disease:Crohn's Disease and Chronic Ulcerative Colitis. ABR Thomson, ed. Canadian Public Health Association, Ottawa, Canada, 1982, pp. 52–66.

81. Monk M, Mendeloff AI, Siegel CE, et al. An epidemiological study of ulcerative colitis and regional enteritis among adults in Baltimore. II. Social and demographic factors. Gastroenterology 1969;56:947–957.
82. Bernstein CN, Kraut A, Blanchard JF, Rawsthorne P, Yu N, Walld R. The relationship between inflammatory bowel disease and socioeconomic variables. Amer J Gastroenterol 2001;96:2117–2125.
83. Harries AD, Baird A, Rhodes J. Non-smoking: a feature of ulcerative colitis. Brit Med J 1982;284:706.
84. Somerville KW, Logan RFA, Edmond M, Langman MJS. Smoking and Crohn's disease. BMJ 1984;289:954–956.
85. Tragnone A, Hanau C, Bazzocchi G, et al. Epidemiological characteristics of inflammatory bowel disease in Bologna, Italy - incidence and risk factors. Digestion 1993;54:183–188.
86. Boyko EJ, Koepsell TD, Perera DR, et al. Risk of ulcerative colitis among former and current cigarette smokers. N Engl J Med 1987;316:707–710.
87. Lesko SM, Kaufman DW, Rosenberg L, et al. Evidence for an increased risk of Crohn's disease in oral contraceptive users. Gastroenterology 1985;89:1046–1049.

3 Etiology and Pathogenesis of Inflammatory Bowel Disease

James J. Farrell, MB and Bruce E. Sands, MD

Contents

INTRODUCTION

Despite improved understanding of the mechanisms of intestinal inflammation, the etiology and pathogenesis of inflammatory bowel disease (IBD) remain obscure. Hence, the approaches to the diagnosis and management of both Crohn's disease (CD) and ulcerative colitis (UC) have been largely empiric. However, progress in IBD research has fostered development of new agents that target pivotal processes in disease pathogenesis *(1)*. This chapter addresses the etiology and pathogenesis of IBD, including the latest developments in animal models. It will serve as a basis for understanding current and future therapeutic development.

There is increasing evidence that CD and UC represent a heterogeneous group of diseases that have a common final pathway (Table 1). No

From: *Clinical Gastroenterology:*
Inflammatory Bowel Disease: Diagnosis and Therapeutics
Edited by: R. D. Cohen © Humana Press Inc., Totowa, NJ

Table 1
Distinguishing Features of UC and CD Pathogenesis

Component	Ulcerative Colitis	Crohn's Disease
Environmental factors	Beneficial effect of smoking	Detrimental effect of smoking
	No beneficial effect of diet	Symptoms improved by selected diets
Familial factors	High concordance among monzygotic twins	Very high concordance among monzygotic twins
	Normal intestinal permeability in healthy relatives	Increased intestinal permeability in healthy relatives
Genetic factors	Large contribution of the HLA class II region	Small contribution of the HLA class II region
	Linkage with chromosomes 3,7, and 12	Linkage with chromosomes 3,7, and 12
	Linkage with chromosome 6	No linkage with chromosome 6
	No linkage with chromosome 16	Linkage with chromosome 16
	No association with TNFa2b1c2d4e1	Increased association with TNFa2b1c2d4e1
	Decreased TNFα-308 allele 2	No linkage TNFα-308 allele 2
	Increased IL-1Ra allele 2 in extensive disease	
Microbial factors	Limited role of bacterial flora	Important role of bacterial flora
	No association with *M. paratuberculosis*	Association with *M. paratuberculosis*
	No association with measles virus	Some association with measles virus
Humoral immunity	Prominent antibody secretion	Moderate antibody secretion
	Increased IgG1 secretion	Increased IgG2 secretion
	Evidence for autoimmunity	Limited evidence for autoimmunity
	Strong association with pANCA	Weak association with pANCA
	Weak association with ASCA	Strong association with ASCA
Cell-mediated immunity	Prominent mucosal neutrophil infiltration	Prominent mucosal T-cell infiltration
	Normal/hyporeactive T cells	Hyperreactive T cells
	Normal T-cell apoptosis (?)	Resistance of T cells to apoptosis (?)
	*Fas-Fas*L-mediated T cell apoptosis important	*Fas-Fas*L-mediated T-cell apoptosis less important
	Th2-like profile	Th1-like profile
Cytokines and mediators	Cytokine increase limited to involved mucosa	Cytokine increase in involved and uninvolved mucosa
	Prominent production of eicosanoids	Moderate production of eicosanoids
	High substance P/receptor expression limited to involved mucose but not to enteric neurons.	?High substance P/receptor expression in involved and uninvolved mucosa as well as enteric neurons.

HLA, human leukocyte antigen; ANCA, antineutrophil cytoplasmic antibodies; ASCA, anti-*Saccharomyces cerevisiae* antibodies.
Adapted from: Fiocchi C. Inflammatory Bowel Disease: Etiology and Pathogenesis. Gastroenterology 1988;115:182–205.

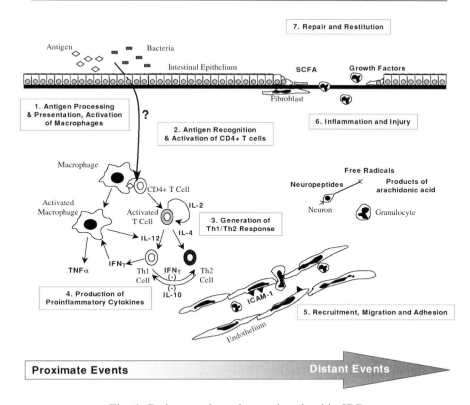

Fig. 1. Pathogenetic pathways involved in IBD.

one agent or single mechanism can account for all aspects of IBD, and several distinct factors are likely to result in either CD or UC. The pathogenesis of CD and UC involves an interplay of environmental, genetic, microbial, immune, and nonimmune factors, which, in combination, result in chronic intestinal inflammation (Fig. 1). These factors are discussed later.

Environmental Risk Factors

The incidence and prevalence of IBD continues to rise, suggesting an important role played by the environment in its pathogenesis. However, the relative importance of environmental compared to genetic factors in the initiation or progression of UC and CD remains unclear and controversial. Smoking, childhood infections, oral contraceptives, diet, prenatal events, breastfeeding, hygiene, microbial agents, occupation, pollution, and stress have all been suggested as possible environmental factors.

Cigarette smoking appears beneficial in UC, whereas it is detrimental in CD *(2)*. Harries initial study found that smoking protected against UC, with the risk of developing UC among current smokers only 40% that of nonsmokers *(3)*. No gender difference with this protective effect was seen in UC. In contrast, several studies have demonstrated a twofold increase in the risk of CD in smokers *(4,5)*. However, unlike UC, women smokers were four times more likely to develop CD recurrence than non-smokers, whereas male smokers were at less of an increased risk *(6)*. Smoking also appears to be an independent risk factor for recurrence in CD, especially following medically-induced remission *(7)*.

Several explanations exist to explain this relationship, including differences in colonic mucus and proinflammatory cytokine levels. Initial studies revealed that colonic mucus in UC was both quantitatively and qualitatively abnormal, and that mucus production in UC patients who smoked was similar to that of healthy controls *(8,9)*. This suggests that smoking restores a normal pattern of mucus production in UC. However, more recent studies have found similarities in the composition of colonic mucus in nonsmoking UC patients and controls *(10)*. Likewise, reductions in the colonic mucosal concentrations of proinflammatory cytokines interleukin 1β (IL-1β) and interleukin 8 (IL-8) have been observed in smokers with UC compared to nonsmokers with UC. The opposite effect is seen in healthy controls. It is of interest that IL-8 levels alone are reduced in smokers with CD compared with nonsmokers with CD, with no significant reduction in IL-1β levels *(11)*. In addition, nicotine has been shown to have an inhibitory effect in vivo on T-helper 2 cell (Th2) function (the predominant cytokine pattern of UC) cell function as measured by inhibition of IL-10 production. Nicotine does not appear to have any effect on T-helper 1 cell function (the predominant cytokine pattern of CD) as indicated by IL-2 and tumor necrosis factor-alpha (TNFα) production *(12)*. Finally, the thrombogenic properties of cigarette smoking may contribute to vascular changes reported to be present in CD.

To date, no specific dietary factors has been clearly linked to IBD. The association between the consumption of cola drinks, chewing gum, and chocolate with CD, and cola drinks and chocolate with UC, may simply be the expression of a "modern lifestyle" representing unknown risk factors, as opposed to playing a causal role. Zinc and selenium deficiencies are common in CD; and it is possible that these deficiencies contribute to immunological dysfunction seen in IBD *(13)*. Although there have been a number of uncontrolled studies assessing the efficacy of elemental diets in CD, which suggest some degree of clinical improvement, most controlled studies have found that enteral nutrition is less effective than steroids and aminosalicylates *(14,15)*. Meta-analyses reveals that the overall remission rates for diet- and steroid-treated patients were 58% and 80%, respectively *(16,17)*. Some data suggest that elemental diet may improve CD by reducing intestinal permeability. It has also been suggested that elemental diet may result in beneficial alterations in bowel flora *(18)*. In contrast to Crohn's disease, elemental diet does not appear to be beneficial in ulcerative colitis. The reason for this discrepancy in response is not known.

Certain medications, including oral contraceptives and NSAIDs, have also been implicated in the pathogenesis of IBD. There are several reports linking the use of oral contraceptives and the development of IBD. In a case control study, the relative risk for CD among oral contraceptive users was 1.9 (95% confidence intervals (CI), 1.0 to 3.5) when compared to persons who had never used these drugs *(19)*. Moreover, the magnitude of the risk was proportional to the duration of use of oral contraceptives. The data for UC is less clear. Vessey et al. found the relative risk for UC to be 2.5 (95% CI, 1.1 to 5.6) in women using oral contraceptives, but Lashner et al. found no increased risk *(20,21)*. In addition to causing exacerbations of preexisting IBD, NSAID use can occasionally induce a colitis *de novo (22)*. Recent studies indicate that fecal pH is more acidic in patients with IBD than in healthy controls. Fecal pH is reduced in the indomethacin model of chronic ileitis in rats, which is similar in some respects to human IBD *(23)*. In this model, indomethacin significantly changed microcirculation parameters causing a twofold increase in leucocyte adherence and a threefold increase in leucocyte migration, thus providing a possible pathophysiological mechanism for the observations mentioned above. Finally, the increasing use of antibiotics in human and veterinary medicine over the last 50 yr has paralleled the increase in CD. Hence, it has been exposure of intestinal flora to sublethal antibiotics that may induce a capacity for toxin production in bacteria, or can make them invasive. It is conceivable that CD is caused in genetically susceptible persons by intestinal bacteria whose biological (but not morphological) properties have been altered by antibiotics *(24)*.

There is epidemiological evidence showing an increased frequency of childhood infections and tonsillectomies in patients with IBD. Patients with CD are more likely to report an increased frequency of childhood infections in general (odds ratio 4.67) and pharyngitis specifically (odds ratio 2.14), whereas patients with UC reported an excess of infections generally (odds ratio 2.37) *(25)*. Curiously, the ileum is the most prevalent location of disease in CD patients with previous tonsillectomy. Furthermore, it has been found that appendectomy is protective for the development of UC. Patients with UC are less likely to have undergone an appendectomy (0.6%) than age- and sex-matched control (25.4%) *(26)*. This difference was highly significant with an odds ratio of 59.1 compared with an odds ratio of getting the disease in nonsmokers of 2.95. No similar protective effect of appendectomy has been noted in CD, although appendectomies may be occasionally performed in cases of yet undiagnosed CD. It has been speculated that the appendix serves as an important site of antigen presentation within the gut, being a blind-ended organ with dense bacterial growth and replete with antigen presenting cells and lymphoid tissue. This may also account for the frequent finding of appendiceal and peri-appendiceal inflammation, even remotely, from distal ulcerative colitis.

There is evidence to suggest a relationship between stress and increased illness behavior and possibly between stress and infectious pathology. Stress has been associated with decreases in functional immune measures (proliferative response to mitogens and natural killer activity), percent of circulating white blood cells, immunoglobulin levels, and antibody titers to herpesviruses *(27)*. This may offer some explanation for a recent study showing a significant proportion of 247 women with IBD who thought that they may have acquired their disease from stress and emotional issues (UC 40% and CD 29%) and internalizing issues (2.3%) *(28)*. Animal models support this suggesting that stress reactivates experimental colitis by facilitating entry of luminal contents that activate previously sensitized CD4 cells in the colon *(29)*. However, future controlled studies are required to elucidate the role that stress-related factors may play in both the pathogenesis and expression of IBD.

Vascular injury with focal arteritis, fibrin deposition, arterial occlusion, leading to tissue infarction or neovascularization has been documented in intestinal resection specimens form patients with IBD, especially Crohn's disease *(30)*. Furthermore, 85% of identified granulomas in CD have a vascular localization, suggesting that changes in the intestinal microvasculature may be an early element in the pathogenesis of CD *(31)*. Wakefield and colleagues have proposed a unifying "vascular theory" by which smoking, the oral contraceptive pill, and measles virus may potentiate a tendency for focal thrombosis, and, hence, contribute to the pathogenesis of CD *(32)*.

GENETIC FACTORS

Multiple epidemiologic studies have documented significant ethnic and familial predisposition to IBD. There is a high incidence of CD and UC among family members of the index case (up to 40% in first degree family members) *(33)*. Concordance rates in twins provide the strongest evidence that both genetic and environmental factors are important in IBD pathogenesis. There is a higher rate of concordance found for monozygotic twins with CD or UC compared with dizygotic twins, with the genetic contribution for CD considerably greater than that for UC *(34)*. Similarly, the relatively high concordance of clinical characteristics between the index case and family members with regard to age, site of inflammation, and type of clinical manifestations, coupled with the concept of "genetic anticipation", defined by a progressively earlier disease onset in successive generations further supports the relevance of genetics and genetic predisposition in IBD pathogenesis *(35,36)*. Ultimately, however, it has been difficult to distinguish between the genetic and environmental contributions to IBD pathogenesis. Other potential familial factors explored include an abnormal immune response, exemplified by abnormal activation of complement via the alternate pathway in both patients with IBD and their relatives, a high prevalence of antibodies to intestinal epithelial antigens in healthy first-degree relatives of IBD patients, and increased intestinal permeability in healthy first-degree relatives of CD patients. Increased intestinal permeabilty, resulting in increased uptake of antigenic material by the mucosal immune system, can initiate and perpetuate inflammation and has been postulated to play a pathogenic role in the development of CD. However, increased intestinal permeability appears to predate clinical relapse and can normalize after surgery, implying that it may simply be a phenomenon secondary to inflammation *(37–39)*.

Current thinking, based on the epidemiological data, the clinical variability of presentation of IBD and results of genetic marker studies suggest that IBD is a number of complex polygenic diseases, each sharing some, but not all susceptibility genes. This complex model incorporates both polygenic inheritance and genetic heterogeneity, and could explain not only the variability of clinical presentation, but also ethnic differences in disease prevalence *(40)*. Two complementary strategies have been used to identify genes involved in determining susceptibility to disease and disease behavior. The candidate gene directed strategy presumes an understanding of disease pathophysiology and uses either population-based association studies, family-based studies such as linkage analysis, or the transmission disequilibrium test. By contrast, the relatively new technique of genome wide scanning involves a systematic analysis of the entire human genome, and is directed at identifying the chromosomal location of susceptibility loci. Genome-wide scanning currently uses family-based linkage analysis for "coarse" mapping and both population-based studies and larger family studies for "finer" mapping.

Candidate gene studies have investigated the contribution of genes involved in the regulation of the immune response, particularly the major histocompatibility complex (MHC), which is situated in the human leucocyte antigen (HLA) region in humans. There appears to be considerable heterogeneity, not only between CD and UC, but also within both CD and UC, with heterogeneity between different populations a further confounding factor. The evidence for a contribution of the HLA region to genetic susceptibility in IBD is strongest in UC. Significant linkage between the HLA Class II region and UC has been demonstrated in European Caucasian families *(41)*. Allelic associations have been reported in Japanese, North American, and European studies. Allelic association studies are most consistent in the Japanese population, where the HLA-DRB1*1502 allele (DR2) is associated with susceptibility to UC, and alleles representing DR4 are associated with decreased susceptibility to UC. Although the negative association with DR4 has been widely reported in both Jewish and non-Jewish Caucasian populations, the positive association with DR2 has been demonstrated in Californian patients (a mixed Jewish/non-Jewish population), but not in the majority of European studies (mostly non-Jewish). Population-based association studies suggest that the relatively rare HLA class II gene DRB1*0103 may be predictive of severe UC disease behavior, particularly with the need for colectomy. Further data from Caucasian populations also suggest that the HLA class II genotype may influence disease extent and the presence of extra-intestinal manifestations, particularly arthropathy *(42–46)*. The recent discovery of the first Crohn's disease susceptibility gene, the Nod 2 gene, has opened the door to further investigations into the role of this exciting finding, as well as other candidate genes.

The contribution of genes encoding cytokines or cytokine antagonists have also been studied by both association studies and linkage analysis. Although strong associations have been reported in Jewish populations between polymorphisms of the gene encoding the interleukin 1 receptor antagonist (IL-1RA) and susceptibility to UC, data from non-Jewish Caucasian populations are contradictory. Similarly, although association between susceptibility to CD and tumor necrosis factor α polymorphisms are reported in Californian populations, northern European studies found little evidence for this association. Genes encoding IL-2, IL-6, IL-10 are also currently being studied. There is particular interest in the contribution of genes encoding intestinal mucins. In total, nine mucin genes have been characterized, designated MUC1 to MUC9. Recent molecular genotyping data have provided preliminary evidence that inherited polymorphisms of MUC2 and MUC3 may be involved in disease pathogenesis. Other candidates genes are those encoding adhesion molecules, trefoil peptides, and proteins involved in intra-cellular signalling *(47–50)*.

The application of genome-wide scanning to IBD has been more successful to date than in many other complex disorders. Hugot et al. reported the first genome screening in CD patients. The genome was systematically screened using polymorphic microsatellite markers distributed on all autosomes. Using nonparametric linkage analysis, they identified a susceptibility locus in the pericentromeric region of chromosome 16, designated IBD1 by the authors. Putative candidate genes within this region include the gene encoding the IL-4 receptor, and CD11 integrin, but recently the Nod 2 gene has emerged as the Crohn's disease susceptibility gene. This locus, which appears to be important in CD, but not in UC, has been corroborated by many investigators. Subsequently, Satsangi et al, reported the results of a genome-wide scan involving 186 affected sibling pairs with IBD. The data provides the strongest evidence to date that CD and UC are related polygenic disorders. They demonstrated linkage between IBD overall and regions on chromosome 12, 7, and 3. Linkage with CD was noted with the pericentromeric region on chromosome 16, although linkage with UC was noted with individual markers on chromosome 2 and 6 (HLA region). Although the linkage between susceptibility to IBD and the region on chromosome 12 has been replicated in North America and Europe, recently Rioux et al., found no evidence for linkage between IBD and selected susceptibility loci on chromosome 3, 7,12, or 16 *(51–55)*.

MICROBIAL FACTORS

Because both CD and UC closely mimic defined intestinal infections and occur in areas of highest luminal bacterial concentrations, investigators have long searched for a transmissable agent responsible for IBD. Although several pathogens, including the measles virus, *Mycobacterium paratuberculosis*, and *Listeria monocytogenes* have been suggested as etiologic agents in CD, the possibility that normal enteric flora play a role in initiating or maintaining IBD is also possible. For example, common anerobes are capable of inducing inflammatory cytokines, including transforming growth factor beta (TGF β, which leads to intestinal fibrosis in colitic rats. In humans, *Escherichia coli* isolated from CD ileal mucosa adhere to intestinal cells and synthesize cytotoxins, which may cause disruption of the intestinal barrier. Recently, fecal hydrogen sulfide (H_2S), a volatile, highly toxic but relatively uncommon sulfide product of sulfate-reducing bacteria, has been proposed to play an etiologic role in UC. H_2S release by UC feces has been shown to be three to four times higher compared with normal feces. This increased H_2S may reflect abnormalities of the fecal bacteria and/or substrate availability *(56)*.

Of direct clinical relevance to the relation between bacteria and IBD, antibiotics continue to be evaluated in the treatment of UC and CD, but results remain equivocal. A recent 6-mo study of ciprofloxacin in addition to 5-aminoslicylates and corticosteroids suggested clinical benefit in patients with UC, particularly those failing under corticosteroid treatment *(57)*.

Further clinical evidence of the importance of normal enteric flora has been the role of the fecal stream in the pathogenesis of IBD. Patients with CD with a diverting ileostomy fail to develop recurrent disease until reanastomosed, and infusion of a CD patients's ileostomy effluent into the excluded normal ileal loop of the same patient rapidly induces local immune activation and *de novo* inflammation. Therefore, some components of the fecal stream, possibly normal flora, may promote inflammation *(58,59)*.

The most compelling support for a crucial role of normal enteric bacteria in IBD comes from studies in experimental animals. Intestinal inflammation is absent in animals raised in germ-free conditions, but appears when the gut is repopulated with normal defined flora, particularly anaerobes. In one of these animal models, the C3H/HeJBir mouse, mucosal T cells proliferate in vitro when exposed to cecal bacteria, but not to food or intestinal epithelial cell antigens. Interestingly, these T cells when transferred to other mice are capable of inducing colitis, establishing a strong link among flora, immune reactivity, and gut inflammation *(60)*.

Other pathogens, such as measles virus and *M. paratuberculosis* have been suggested to play significant roles in the pathogenesis of IBD. However, recent studies found neither molecular nor epidemiologic evidence supporting an etiologic or pathogenic link between either organism and CD. Results of trials with anti-tuberculous therapy have been disappointing *(61,62)*. *L. monocytogenes* has also gained prominence as another candidate pathogen in CD. Antigen for this organism was found in macrophages and giant cells beneath mucosal ulcers, adjacent to fistulae, near abscesses, and within the lamina propria, granulomas, and mesenteric lymph nodes of 75% of CD patients, compared with 13% of UC patients and 0% of control subjects *(63)*. The significance of these observations remains to be determined, because *Listeria* is a relatively frequent environmental contaminant, and 83% of the patients with positive results had immunohistochemical evidence of coexistent *E. coli* or streptococcal antigen, suggesting nonspecific secondary invasion of ulcerated tissues by luminal organisms.

Although much emphasis has been placed on the harmful effects of bacteria, there is growing interest in the beneficial effects of other components of the intestinal flora. Although only very limited data exist to suggest differences between the microbial ecology of UC and CD patients and normal individuals, there is evidence to suggest that some components of the normal enteric flora downregulate inflammation. This regulatory function may be lost or abnormal in IBD, and probiotic therapy may help restore microbial homeostasis in the gut. A probiotic formula has been shown to increase fecal IgA levels in infants and perhaps enhance mucosal resistance *(64)*. In patients with chronic pouchitis, Venturi et al., have recently reported that a probiotic mixture of lactobacilli, bifidobacteria, and streptococci is quite effective in maintaining clinical remission *(65)*.

IMMUNOLOGY OF IBD

Three hypotheses exist to explain the interaction between possible antigenic triggers and the host immune response, at both the mucosal and systemic level, in IBD. One hypothesis suggests that the antigenic triggers are microbial pathogens that have not yet been identified because of fastidious culture requirements. According to this hypothesis, the immune response in IBD is an appropriate but ineffective response to these pathogens. Such a "hypoactive" immune response could lead to proliferation and persistence of microbial agents. The second hypothesis proposes that the antigenic trigger in IBD is some common dietary antigen or nonpathogenic microbial agent against which the patient mounts an abnormal immune response, mediated by CD4+ T cells, which results in inappropriate tissue damage. The third hypothesis is that the antigenic trigger is expressed on the patient's own cells, particularly the intestinal epithelial cells. In this "autoimmune" theory, the patient mounts an appropriate immune response against some luminal antigen, either dietary or microbial; however, because of similarities between proteins on the epithelial cells and the lumenal antigen, the patient's immune system also attacks the epithelial cells, destroying it by either antibody-dependent cellular cytotoxicity or direct cell-mediated cytoxicity.

At present, two autoantibodies appear to be more specific for UC, and may play a role in the pathogenesis of the disease. These are perinuclear antineutrophil cytoplasmic antibodies, pANCA, and the antibodies directed to tropomyosin. A series of reports has confirmed the high prevalence (approx 80%) of pANCA antibodies in UC and an even higher prevalence in patients with associated primary sclerosing cholangitis *(66)*. A related finding is the increased incidence of pANCAs in healthy relatives of patients with UC *(67)*. In addition to being a potential marker of susceptibility and genetic heterogeneity in UC, pANCAs may define subsets of patients with IBD with studies suggesting a higher prevalence of pANCAs among patients with aggressive UC, and in those who develop chronic pouchitis after ileal pouch-anal anastomosis *(68,69)*.

A 40-kiloDalton size colonic protein exclusively recognized by IgG eluted from colons affected by UC has been proposed as an autoantigen in UC. This putative autoantigen appears to be the fraction 5 of the tropomyosin family of cytoskeletal proteins, and is codeposited with IgG1 and complement on UC colonocytes. Monoclonal autoantibodies against this antigen identified a shared epitope in human colon, skin, biliary epithelium, eyes, and joints, locations compatible with the extraintestinal manifestations of UC. More recently, mucosal mononuclear cells from UC, but not CD, have been shown to produce autoantibodies against epithelial cell-derived isoforms (hTM1 and hTM5) of tropomyosin. The true relevance of these autoantibodies in UC is unclear, and whether they initiate or perpetuate damage to intestinal tissue remains unknown *(70)*.

IMMUNE CELLS AND PATHOGENESIS

Human intestinal mucosal T-lymphocytes are found predominantly in the lamina propria and to a lesser extent in the epithelium (intraepithelial lymphocytes). Although exposure of peripheral blood T-lymphocytes to luminal antigens leads to their activation, normal mucosal T-lymphocytes do not become similarly activated. However, in active IBD, mucosal T-cells show an activated phenotype (increased expression of IL-2 receptors, the 4F2 antigen, the T9 transferrin receptor (CD71), and an increased $CD4^+/CD8^+$ cell ratio). This activation appears to be in response to luminal microorganisms. It is likely that these activated T-lymphocytes are derived from the circulation and they can be seen as an example of the response of the systemic immune system occurring in the intestinal mucosa *(71)*.

Subsets of $CD4^+$ T cells have been defined on the basis of cytokine profiles as they relate to immune function. Th1 $CD4^+$ T cells produce IFNγ and IL-2 and mediate cell-mediated immunity, while Th2 $CD4^+$ T cells produce IL-4, IL-5, IL-10, IL-13, and mediate humoral immunity. More recently, Th3 and Tr1 cells, distinguished by TGF-b and IL-10 production, respectively, have been shown to provide critical regulation of immune homeostasis in the mucosa. In the normal intestine, the regulatory subsets (Th3) are dominant over the effector (Th1, Th2) subsets. In IBD, the effector cells dominate. In most animal models of colitis, Th1 CD4⁺ subsets are predominant and mediate the disease. In other models, predominant Th2 CD4⁺ T-cell activity in the mucosa may also result in colitis. Experimental data from animal models (see later) support therapeutic strategies whereby the effector CD4⁺ T-cell subsets, which cause inflammation (Th1 or Th2) are inhibited, or the regulatory CD4⁺ T cell subsets, which in turn inhibit the effectors, are stimulated. Depletion of global perturbation of CD4⁺ T cells may also prove effective, but raise concern about substituting an immunodeficiency state for the original disease in man.

Mucosal T cells in children with CD display an exceedingly strong proliferative response to IL-2 regardless of disease location, duration, clinical activity, or treatment of the disease. This aberration is detected even in areas free of inflammation. Compared with circulating T cells, mucosal T cells are more susceptible to *Fas*-mediated apoptosis, a physiologic process of cell death that, if altered, could contribute to IBD. In support of this possibility is the strong expression of the *Fas* ligand (*Fas*L) by T cells in active UC, but not CD lesions, suggesting that *Fas*-*Fas*L-mediated apoptosis may be important in UC pathogenesis. Although the intricacies of mucosal immunity in IBD remain to be fully elucidated, additional proof for the dominant role of the immune system over intrinsic gut factors in CD is provided by long-lasting clinical remissions among patients who have had replacement of their immune system by virtue of allogeneic bone marrow transplantation *(72,73)*.

B-lymphocytes in the lamina propria are derived from lymphoid aggregates (such as Peyer's patches) where they are primed with antigen. They produce secretory IgA that is transported via epithelial cells to the mucus layer and the lumen. Secretory IgA provides protection by inhibiting interaction of microbes and their products with epithelial cells. In active IBD, there is an increase in the mucosal B-cell and plasma cell population, which are largely derived from the systemic circulation and secrete predominantly IgG. Previous studies have demonstrated IgG subclass differences between UC and CD with higher levels of IgG1 in UC and higher levels of IgG2 in CD. The reason for this difference is unclear, but distinct immune regulatory mechanisms or genetically conditioned differences may be responsible. In addition, there has also been interest in the capacity of the immunoglobulins to induce or exacerbate the disease via autoantibodies *(74–76)*.

Polymorphonuclear (PMN) cells represent a rapid-response component of the host-systemic response to infection and injury. PMN cells are usually confined to the systemic circulation in healthy individuals. In active IBD, PMNs migrate between the vascular endothelial cells into the lamina propria. The majority of these cells subsequently migrate into the lumen via the intestinal epithelium, manifesting as cryptitis and crypt abscesses. It is likely that in IBD, their presence is predominantly a consequence of increased epithelial permeability and penetration of luminal microorganisms and/or their products. They are, therefore, often characteristically seen in diseases affecting the colon and terminal ileum, but not so prominent in the proximal small bowel, which is usually relatively sterile. Polymorphonuclear cells are capable of mediating potent antimicrobial activity via a variety of mechanisms including release of reactive oxygen metabolites and proteolytic enzymes. The release of such enzymes is likely to be responsible for damaging the basement membrane and lamina propria matrix. Measures to avoid such damage, while retaining the host protective function of these cells, could be therapeutically beneficial. An increase of eosinophils, IgE-positive cells, activated mast cells, mucosal, and intestinal secretions level of histamine, has been reported in both CD and UC. However, this probably represents a secondary nonspecific event associated with inflammation.

Platelets have proinflammatory as well as prothombotic properties. Increased platelet numbers, aggregation, and activation are well-recognized indicators of disease activity in IBD. This leads to an increased release of inflammatory mediators from platelets such as platelet activating factor, thromboxanes, serotonin, and oxygen-free radicals, as well as the recruitment, chemotaxis, and modulation of the activity of neutrophils, monocytes, and other inflammatory cells. Platelet activation in the gut vasculature could conceivably contribute to the pathogenesis of CD by promoting local microinfarction. Whereas aminosalicylates may act to inhibit platelet aggregation and activation, clinical trials with specific thromboxane synthesis inhibitors and platelet activating factor antagonists have produced disappointing results in IBD *(77)*.

Macrophages are present in large numbers in the lamina propria of normal intestinal mucosa and they are especially prominent below the surface epithelium. In active IBD, the macrophages are phenotypically and functionally different from normal macrophages. Activated macrophages have an enhanced capacity to present antigen to T lymphocytes, secrete proinflammatory cytokines, and release oxygen radicals, resulting in perpetuation of chronic intestinal inflammation and tissue damage. Accumulating evidence suggests that these activated macrophages are derived from circulating monocytes, which, after migration into the lamina propria, are exposed to T-cell derived cytokines such as

IL-2 and IFN-γ and luminally derived bacterial products such as lipopolysaccharide via a disrupted epithelial barrier. Therapeutic agents that inhibit macrophage activation directly or indirectly (e.g., by enhancing epithelial barrier function and reducing penetration of microbial products into the lamina propria) are likely to be of benefit in patients with IBD *(78,79)*.

NONIMMUNE CELLS IN THE PATHOGENESIS OF IBD

The importance of nonimmune cells in the pathogenesis of gut inflammation is increasingly appreciated. Epithelial cells, for example, can modulate local immune responses in IBD. Their role may be seen in increased epithelial expression of IL-1 receptor antagonist, a natural antiinflammatory cytokine, and upregulation of other mediators, including transforming growth factor (TGF)-β1 and IL-15, before the onset of mucosal inflammation, suggesting an early involvement of the epithelium in gut inflammation. The proposal that epithelial cells undergo apoptotic death at a high rate in IBD remains unproven. Recent studies in *Helicobacter pylori*-induced gastritis demonstrate that bacteria-induced, *Fas*-mediated apoptosis does occur in vivo. Colonic epithelial cells undergo apoptosis in vitro after bacterial invasion, however, evidence for a similar event in IBD remains to be confirmed *(80,81)*.

Mesenchymal cells and their products also actively participate in intestinal inflammation. When exposed to proinflammatory stimuli, both mucosal fibroblasts and muscles cells proliferate and produce IL-1β, IL-6, and tumor necrosis factor (TNF). Activated mesenchymal cells produce a variety of extracellular matrix proteins responsible for collagen deposition and metalloproteinases responsible for tissue remodeling. This production is altered in IBD where there is increased production of collagen type III in strictured areas of CD, and increased production of collagen by muscularis propria cells. Mesenchymal cells are also susceptible to regulation. The immunosuppressive cytokine IL-10 inhibits metalloproteinase production in bacterial superantigen-stimulated fetal intestinal cultures, and antibiotics prevent collagen deposition in experimental colitis. These reports demonstrate a dynamic interaction between immune activation, bacteria, and fibrosis in IBD *(82,83)*.

Leucocyte-endothelial interactions regulate the number and type of immune cells that move from the intravascular into the interstitial space. Enhanced leucocyte binding by human intestinal microvascular endothelial cells (HIMEC) in IBD has been reported; but is unclear whether this is a primary or a secondary phenomenon. In a follow-up study, the same investigators studied HIMEC from both the uninvolved and the involved mucosa of one UC and two CD patients. After activation with

IL-1β or lipopolysaccharide, HIMEC from inflamed mucosa bound twice as many leucocytes as HIMEC from histologically normal IBD mucosa. Thus, HIMEC-enhanced capacity to bind inflammatory cells in IBD is an acquired defect, probably conditioned by continuous exposure to inflammation. Once established, this high binding capacity may contribute to the chronicity of IBD (84,85).

Disruption of the enteric nervous system is also a consistent histopathological feature in CD and UC. Neuronal cell bodies in the myenteric and submucosal enteric nervous system plexuses are damaged and the networks of nerve fibers extending from the submucosal plexuses have been shown to be altered in both CD and UC. Qualitative abnormalities of nerve fibers in IBD tissue have long been recognized, and quantitative changes in the expression of several neuropeptides have also been demonstrated in the inflamed mucosa. Although these changes may be secondary to inflammation, there is also evidence of different concentrations and receptor density expression for substance P in UC compared to CD-involved mucosa. Furthermore, because neuropeptides interact with and influence the function of lymphocytes and macrophages, alterations in their expression could also underlie proposed links between psychological stress and relapse. It is conceivable that modulation of neuropeptide expression may explain the reported beneficial effect of local anesthetic in refractory distal UC (86–88).

CYTOKINES

Cytokines are a large and growing family of low-molecular-weight glycosylated proteins that can be secreted by many different cell types. They mediate cellular function by interacting with specific cell-surface receptors on both the cells that secrete them (autocrine effect) and also on adjacent cells (paracrine effect). Cytokines are important in the regulation of inflammatory and immunological responses and can be divided on the basis of their major biological functions into proinflammatory and antiinflammatory cytokines, Th1 and Th2 cytokines and chemokines. Proinflammatory cytokines include IL-1, IL-6, IL-8, and TNF and contribute to many of the characteristic attributes of IBD: neutrophil infiltration (IL-8), T-cell activation (IL-1), expression of adhesion molecules (IL-1 and TNF), enhanced epithelial permeability (IFN-γ), and epithelial injury (TNF and IFN-γ). IL-1 is produced early in the inflammatory cascade and has numerous actions. The balance of production of IL-1 vs IL-1 receptor antagonist (IL-1ra), a naturally occurring molecule that blocks binding of IL-1 to both of the identified IL-1 receptors, can determine the overall contribution of IL-1 to an inflammatory process. Casini-Raggi et al., demonstrated an imbalance in the production of these two molecules (increased IL-1: IL-1ra ratio) in Crohn's colitis and UC compared to healthy controls, perhaps contributing to the chronicity of IBD. This defect may be mediated at a transcriptional level because IL-1ra mRNA levels are decreased in CD patients relative to infectious controls. IL-1ra is effective in reducing inflammation in a rabbit model of colitis *(89,90)*.

Cytokines that have a predominant antiinflammatory effect include IL-4, IL-10 and TGF-β. Mouse models suggest that IL-10 and TGF-β, the products of CD4$^+$ Tr1 and Th3 cells, respectively, play a major role as immunoregulatory cytokines in the downregulation of responses to luminal antigens, failure of which may lead to chronic inflammation. Schreiber et al. reported no difference in concentrations of IL-10 in patients with CD vs those with UC but noted that the addition of IL-10 to either peripheral monocytes or intestinal macrophages from IBD patients restored the IL-1 : IL-1ra ratio to that found in normal subjects *(91)*. This suggested that there was not an absolute, rather than relative deficiency of IL-4 or IL-10 in IBD, with levels of IL-10 being inappropriately low relative to the degree of inflammation found.

Th1 lymphocytes produce IL-2, interferon-γ (IFN-γ), and TGF-β and are associated with cell mediated immune responses and increased IgG2 production. Th2 lymphocytes produce IL-4, IL-5, IL-6, and IL-10 and are associated with enhanced antibody synthesis by B cells, hypersensitivity reactions and increased IgG1 production. CD appears to be associated with activation of Th1 lymphocytes, whereas UC is associated with activation of Th2 lymphocytes as demonstrated by increased IL-4, IL-10, and IgG1 *(92)*.

Some cytokines, known as chemokines, are capable of attracting effector cells to sites of inflammation. The best characterized chemokine is IL-8, which is a potent chemoattractant of polymorphonuclear cells. In the intestinal mucosa, IL-8 can be produced by epithelial cells and is likely to be important in the initiation of an inflammatory response to pathogenic bacteria or their products. Another important source of IL-8 is the monocyte/macrophage. Studies in IBD suggest that macrophages are the major source of IL-8 in the inflamed mucosa, implying that the epithelial cell-derived IL-8 may be important in initiating inflammation (and disease) at the onset of relapse, but that macrophage activation is responsible for disease perpetuation. Another chemokine, IL-5, is a highly potent chemotactic factor for recruiting eosinophils, which have been implicated as important effector cells in the pathogenesis of CD. Using *in situ* hybridization techniques, Dubucquoi et al, showed that IL-5 mRNA expression was increased in areas of early relapse in patients who had undergone bowel resections for CD *(93–95)*.

The major cell source of proinflammatory cytokines are activated macrophages in the lamina propria, although other cell types may make important contributions. Cytokines, particularly IL-1, TNF, and IFN-γ stimulate epithelial, endothelial, and mesenchymal cells and activated immune cells. They are also involved in the regulation of wound healing and fibrosis. Cytokines may be useful as markers of disease activity, especially tissue IL-1 levels in UC and serum IL-2 receptor levels in CD.

Individual cytokines have been targeted for therapeutic purposes. For predominantly proinflammatory cytokines, attempts at neutralizing TNF and IL-1 have been particularly fruitful. Antiinflammatory cytokines such as IL-10 and IL-11, may also prove useful as new therapies for IBD.

SOLUBLE MEDIATORS AND CELL ADHESION MOLECULES

Immune and nonimmune cells can also exchange signals through secretion of various soluble mediators and expression of cell adhesion molecules. These interactions result in further cell activation and amplification of the production of antibodies, and additional cytokines and soluble mediators culminating in inflammation and tissue damage. Growth factors are a class of soluble mediators increasingly recognized as having a role in IBD pathogenesis. In addition to cytokines (peptide mediators), several nonpeptide mediators have been widely studied in IBD. These include lipid mediators (eicosanoids), oxygen radicals, nitric oxide, and short-chain fatty acids.

Growth factors are important in both prevention of mucosal injury, and healing after injury has occurred. TGF-β is a dominant mediator of mucosal restitution and defense. Trefoil peptide, which is produced in large amounts by epithelial cells in IBD, has a unique molecular structure conferring protection against injury. Increased expression of keratinocyte growth factor, a stromal cell-derived mitogen specific for epithelial cells, is also observed in areas actively involved by IBD, implicating mesenchymal cells in the modulation of epithelial cell renewal during inflammation. The exact role of each growth factor in IBD is still being established, but clearly, individual factors have distinct functions in different phases of IBD. In active CD and UC lesions, TGF-α is produced in quantities comparable to those present in normal mucosa, but TGF-β synthesis is increased. In contrast, when IBD activity enters in a quiescent phase, TGF-α levels increase, whereas TGF-β levels normalize. Thus, enhanced TGF-β synthesis may represent an effort to promote healing, but augmented TGF-α production may cause epithelial hyperproliferation and increase the risk of malignancy in IBD *(96)*.

Eicosanoids are products of arachidonic acid derived from membrane phospholipids. Prostaglandins and leukotrienes are products of the cyclooxygenase and 5-lipoxygenase enzymes respectively. There are two isoforms of the cyclooxygenase (COX) enzyme: COX-1 and COX-2. COX-1 is the constitutive form expressed by many different cell types whereas COX-2 is the inducible form, the expression of which can be induced by proinflammatory mediators such as the cytokines IL-1 and TNF. Enhanced prostaglandin synthesis in active IBD was demonstrated before the recognition of the two different COX isoenzymes. Recent studies suggest that this increase is derived from COX-2, the expression of which is induced in active IBD. This induction occurs predominantly in epithelial cells and lamina propria mononuclear cells. While mucosal expression of COX-2 is induced in an animal model of colitis, treatment with a selective COX-2 inhibitor led to worsening of the colonic inflammation. Thus, COX-2 may have a protective role in the inflamed mucosa and its inhibition by NSAIDS may explain previous reports of relapse in patients treated with these drugs *(97,98)*.

Enhanced mucosal synthesis of leukotrienes in active IBD has also been demonstrated. Leukotriene B4 (LTB4) has been of particular interest as it is a potent chemoattractant and activator of polymorphonuclear cells. However, studies with the orally active 5-lipoxygenase inhibitor, zileuton, in the treatment of active UC, or maintenance of remission have been disappointing *(99,100)*.

Enhanced release of reactive metabolites of oxygen (e.g., superoxide and hypochlorite), derived largely from polymorphonuclear cells and macrophages, has been demonstrated in IBD. Although capable of mediating antimicrobial activity, these oxygen radicals have also been implicated in tissue damage. Recent studies have provided direct evidence of an in vivo oxidant injury in colonic epithelial cells in IBD. Such studies support the investigation of compounds with antioxidant activity as new treatments for IBD *(101)*.

Nitric oxide (NO) is a molecule of considerable biological importance. It is derived from the amino acid L-arginine in a reaction that is catalyzed by the enzyme nitric oxide synthase (NOS). Three isoforms of NOS have been identified. Two of these, neuronal NOS (NOS1) and endothelial NOS (NOS3) are constitutively expressed and are calcium dependent. The third isoform is inducible NOS (iNOS; NOS2), which is calcium independent and can be induced by proinflammatory cytokines (IL-1 and TNF) and bacterial products. A number of cell types can express inducible NOS. Mucosa from patients with active UC has been shown to express calcium-independent NOS activity, consistent with iNOS. Recent studies have confirmed this and demonstrated that iNOS in the inflamed mucosa is expressed in the epithelium and lamina propria mononuclear cells and neutrophils. Nitric oxide can interact with superoxide to produce peroxynitrite, which is toxic to cells. The action of NO on smooth muscle cells may also be responsible for colonic dilatation in severe colitis. However, because NO also expresses anti-microbial activity, the question of whether iNOS is an appropriate target for therapy remains to be demonstrated (102,103).

Colonic epithelium in UC may inadequately oxidize butyrate (a short-chain fatty acid) perhaps resulting in an energy-depleted condition of the mucosa. This has been supported by the clinical observations that irrigation of diversion colitis with short-chain fatty acids results in marked improvement, and that butyrate enemas may induce clinical improvement in distal UC (104,105).

Adhesion molecules represent a large family of molecules essential for cell communication, activation, and homing. In view of the gut infiltration by inflammatory cells, a fundamental role of these adhesion molecules is expected in IBD. Whereas recruitment of leucocytes into the mucosa occurs during active IBD, aberrant expression of cell adhesion molecules in areas of inflammation is confirmed by several reports. In active IBD, mucosal macrophages show a dramatic increase in the expression of intercellular adhesion molecule-1 (ICAM-1). In addition, marked increase of ICAM-1 and leucocyte functional antigen 1 (LFA-1) expression by mononuclear cells and E-selectin by venules has also been demonstrated. Surprisingly, the expression of vascular cell adhesion molecule 1 (VCAM-1) by immune and endothelial cells is not increased in IBD when compared to control mucosa. Although these changes could be nonspecific consequences of inflammation, there is also evidence that an aberrant display of adhesion molecules differs in the two major forms of IBD. Increased expression of CD44 v6 and CD44 v3 has been demonstrated in UC but not CD colonic crypt cells. Furthermore, CD, UC, and normal intestinal T and B cells show variable integrin patterns, perhaps representing different homing properties in each type of bowel inflammation. To some degree, the dysregulation of adhesion molecule expression in the gut is reflected in the peripheral circulation, where circulating levels of soluble adhesion molecules, such as ICAM-1, are found during active disease. A recent randomized, controlled trial of the remission inducing and steroid-sparing properties of ICAM-1 antisense oligonucleotides, ISIS 2302, in active steroid-dependent patients with CD failed to show efficacy (106,107).

ANIMAL MODELS

Numerous excellent animal models have now been described for IBD, including both spontaneous and induced systems (Table 2) *(108)*. Nongenetic models have been known for some time and include Freund's adjuvant, immune complexes, indomethacin, dextran sulphate sodium, acetic acid, trinitrobenzene sulphonic acid (TNBS), peptidogly-can-polysaccharide, and carrageenan. Experimental colitis induced by topical exposure to the contact allergen TNBS has aroused considerable interest. In this model, a chronic granulomatous colitis is believed to occur via a classic hapten-induced delayed-type hypersensitivity response, mediated by Th1 cells. However, the animal models that have generated the greatest interest in recent years include genetically manipulated mice involving either gene inactivation (knock-out) or the overexpression of genes (transgenic). Gene inactivation models include deletion of IL-2, IL-2 receptor, IL-10, TGF-β1, MHC class II, or their T-cell receptor. Transgenic animals with dominant expression of HLA-B27 and IL-7 have also been described.

Models employing immune system reconstitution have also been shown to induce gut inflammation, as with the transfer of CD45RB[high] (T effector) subpopulation of T cells into mice with severe combined immune deficiency (SCID), which lack functional T or B cells or bone marrow cells into cyclosporine-treated mice. The spontaneous models of colitis include the cotton top tamarin and C3H/HeJ Bir mice. The only spontaneous model of experimental CD is the SAMP1/Yit mouse model characterized by a terminal ileitis that spontaneously manifests itself after 30 wk of age, and is significantly ameliorated by TNF blockade.

Investigations in animal models of colitis have highlighted the permissive effect of the intestinal flora in the pathogenesis of colitis. For example injection of bacterial cell wall components causes chronic granulomatous inflammation with both intestinal and extraintestinal manifestations in a rat model. HLA-B27 transgenic rats develop inflammation in multiple organs, but small and large bowel are spared when these rats are kept in a germ-free environment. Similar results are observed in IL-2 and IL-10 and T-cell receptor-(TCR[1])-knockout mice. The reverse is also true, e.g., reconstitution of germ-free HLAB27 transgenic rats with normal luminal bacteria, especially *Bacteroides* species, reinstates gut inflammation. It is possible that certain species or combinations of flora may be especially colitogenic, whereas others may be protective.

Experimental animal models of chronic intestinal inflammation illustrate the importance of CD4[+] T cells as the major mediators of IBD,

Table 2
Animal Models of Inflammatory Bowel Disease

Models	Site of disease	Primary Abnormality	Characteristics of disease phenotype
Chemical induced			
Acetic acid	Colon	Exogenous	UC
Oxazolone	Colon	Exogenous	UC
Formalin immune complex	Colon	Exogenous	UC
Indomethacin	Colon	Exogenous	UC
Carageenan	Colon	Exogenous	UC
2,4,6-Trinitro- benzene sulfonic acid	Colon	Exogenous	UC
Dextran sodium sulfate	Colon	Epithelial barrier	UC
Cyclosporin	Colon	Exogenous	UC
Peptidoglycan-polysaccharide	Colon	Exogenous	UC
Transgenic/gene targeted			
IL-2$^{-/-}$	Colon	Immunoregulation	UC
IL-2 R$\alpha^{-/-}$	Colon	Immunoregulation	UC
IL-10$^{-/-}$	Small intestine, colon	Immunoregulation	CD/UC
TGF$\beta^{-/-}$	Colon	Immunoregulation	UC
Gαi2$^{-/-}$	Colon	Signal transduction	UC
TCR$\alpha^{-/-}$	Colon	Immunoregulation	UC

Model	Location	Function	Disease
TCRβ$^{-/-}$	Colon	Immunoregulation	UC
CRFB4$^{-/-}$	Colon	Immunoregulation	UC
MHC Class II$^{-/-}$	Colon	Antigen presentation	UC
mdr1a$^{-/-}$	Colon	Epithelial barrier	CD
TNFδARE$^{-/-}$	Small intestine	Immunoregulation	UC
Stat4-transgenic	Colon	Immunoregulation	UC
IL-7 transgenic	Colon	Immunoregulation	UC
HLA-B27 transgenic rats	Small intestine, colon	Antigen presentation	UC
N-cadherin dominant negative$^{-/-}$	Small intestine	Epithelial barrier	UC
Intestinal Trefoil Factor$^{-/-}$	Colon	Epithelial barrier	UC
Immunologic			
CD4^{+}CD45RB^{hi}/mice SCID or Rag$^{-/-}$	Colon	T-cell regulation	CD/UC
Bone marrow Tge26 mice	Colon	T- and NK cell regulation	UC
Spontaneous			
Cotton-top tamarin	Colon	Unknown	UC
C3HeJBir mouse	Colon	Unknown	UC
SAMP1/Yit mouse	Small intestine	Unknown	CD

CD, Crohn's disease; IL, interleukin; MHC, major histocompatibility complex; TCR, T-cell receptor; TGF, transforming growth factor; TNF, tumor necrosis factor; UC, ulcerative colitis; mdr, multidrug resistance; ARE, AU rich elements; SCID, severe combined immune deficiency

Adapted from: Arsenau KO, et al. Discovering the causes of inflammatory bowel disease: lessons from animal models. *Curr Opin Gastroenterol* 2000, 16:310–317.

and consequently the potential therapeutic implications of T-cell manipulation. Breeding experiments with IL-2 deficient mice show that the animals still develop colitis when crossed with B-cell (JH$^{-/-}$) deficient mice, but not when crossed with mice lacking T and B cells (RAG2$^{-/-}$). Elson et al. have recently proposed two broad therapeutic strategies for T-cell manipulation that could be effective in IBD: 1) inhibition of the effector CD4$^+$ T cells (Th1 or Th2); or 2) stimulation of the regulatory CD4$^+$ T cell subsets, which, in turn, would inhibit these effectors. There are experimental data from animal models supporting both of these strategies (109,110).

Inhibition of the Th1 subset is an example of inhibition of effector CD4$^+$ T cells. CD4$^+$ Th1 cells may preferentially express an isoform of the cell surface antigen CD44. Monoclonal antibodies to this CD44 v7 isoform have recently been shown to be effective in downregulating experimental colitis, although the exact mechanism is unclear. CD4$^+$ T cells are stimulated along the Th1 pathway by IL-12, a cytokine produced by antigen-presenting cells (APC), i.e., dendritic cells, and macrophages. In turn, Th1 cells produce IFNγ, which stimulates production of more IL-12, creating a self-reinforcing feedback loop. These Th1: APC interactions also require cell-to-cell contact via CD40L on Th1 cells and its receptor, CD40, on APCs. Neutralization of IL-12 by a specific monoclonal antibody has both prevented and treated active colitis in two different experimental models, while anti-CD40L has prevented colitis in another animal model (111).

Feeding mice the contact allergen TNBS prior to induction of TNBS/ethanol colitis has been shown to be protective for colitis by causing immune unresponsiveness (tolerance). In one study this protection was blocked by the administration of anti-TGFβ, suggesting that the mechanism was mediated by Th3 regulatory cells induced by antigen feeding. In the CD4$^+$CD45RB^{high} transfer model of colitis, cotransfer of T-regulatory-1 (Tr1) CD$^+$ T cells along with pathogenic CD4$^+$CD45RB^{high} T cells prevents colitis when the Tr1 cells are appropriately triggered by their specific antigen. This strategy may have therapeutic implications, because if specific as yet unidentified environmental agents are proven to cause human IBD through an antigen-specific sensitization process, then the oral intake of these antigens could theoretically induce tolerance and resolution of gut inflammation by stimulating Th3 regulatory cells or Tr1 cells specific for these antigens. This could reset the regulator-effector T-cell balance.

Genetic manipulation of molecules related to intestinal epithelium also causes colitis in mice, suggesting a defect of intestinal barrier function, alone or in association with other triggers may be an additional etiology of IBD. Such models include mice deficient in the multidrug resistance gene (MDR-1), and keratin 8, and transgenic mice dominant negative for N-cadherin. In the latter model, mice develops adenomas and carcinoma against a background of colitis. The abnormality is considered to be primarily in epithelial cells rather than in the immune system, presumably leading to exaggerated immune response to luminal (bacterial) antigens. Ablation of enteric glia by creation of herpes simplex virus tyrosine kinase (astroglial cell targeted) transgenic mice, has also been reported to lead to the development of small intestinal inflammation. Partial defects of mucosal protective mechanisms result in inflammation, as well. Mice lacking intestinal trefoil factor are normal until a mild epithelial injury occurs, after which extensive colitis ensues. Thus, it is reasonable to assume that both single or combined defects, either of primary or secondary nature, may underlie the pathogenesis of chronic intestinal inflammation.

Recently, observations in experimental models have demonstrated the important role played by proinflammatory cytokines and neuropeptides in perpetuating mucosal inflammation. Kontoyiannis et al., have provided the first direct evidence that TNF, in fact, mediates chronic intestinal inflammation *(112)*. Their model, a specific deregulation of TNF synthesis in mice, i.e., targeted deletion of TNF AU-rich elements (ARE), results in systemic TNF overexpression and triggers a CD-like intestinal phenotype, characterized by transmural chronic ileitis, mucosal and submucosal granulomas, and intense infiltration of T cell and macrophages. Mice lacking the cell-surface enzyme neutral endopeptidase (NEP), which degrades and inactivates substance P develop severe colitis, which is suppressed by the administration of NEP or neurokinin 1 receptor (NK1R) antagonists. These results further raise the possibility that neuropeptides may be targeted in the treatment of IBD. In addition to genetic manipulation, animal models have also shed light on poorly understood but often-mentioned factors in association with the development and course of IBD, such as stress and environmental agents. The involvement of stress has been explored in cotton-top tamarins that develop spontaneous colitis only when kept in long-term captivity. The appearance of chronic colitis in these primates has been reported to correlate with stressful conditions *(113)*.

Animal models of colitis illustrate that the mechanisms responsible for IBD in animals and humans are diverse. Despite the ever expanding number of models, the fundamental question remains of whether imbalances of immunoregulatory, proinflammatory, and immunosuppressive cytokines can be manipulated in humans as effectively as in animal models.

REFERENCES

1. Fiocchi C. Inflammatory bowel disease: etiology and pathogenesis. Gastroenterology 1998;115(1):182–205.
2. Thomas GA, Rhodes J, Green JT. Inflammatory bowel disease and smoking—a review. Am J Gastroenterol 1998;93(2):144–149.
3. Harries AD, Baird A, Rhodes J. Non-smoking: a feature of ulcerative colitis. Br Med J (Clin Res Ed) 1982;284(6317):706.
4. Silverstein MD, Lashner BA, Hanauer SB, Evans AA, Kirsner JB. Cigarette smoking in Crohn's disease. Am J Gastroenterol 1989;84(1):31–33.
5. Franceschi S, Panza E, La Vecchia C, Parazzini F, Decarli A, Bianchi Porro G. Nonspecific inflammatory bowel disease and smoking. Am J Epidemiol 1987;125(3):445–452.
6. Sutherland LR, Ramcharan S, Bryant H, Fick G. Effect of cigarette smoking on recurrence of Crohn's disease. Gastroenterology 1990;98(5 Pt 1):1123–1128.
7. Timmer A, Sutherland LR, Martin F. Oral contraceptive use and smoking are risk factors for relapse in Crohn's disease. The Canadian Mesalamine for Remission of Crohn's Disease Study Group. Gastroenterology 1998;114(6):1143–1150.
8. Podolsky DK, Isselbacher KJ. Composition of human colonic mucin. Selective alteration in inflammatory bowel disease. J Clin Invest 1983;72(1):142–153.
9. Cope GF, Heatley RV, Kelleher JK. Smoking and colonic mucus in ulcerative colitis. Br Med J (Clin Res Ed) 1986;293(6545):481.
10. Raouf A, Parker N, Iddon D, et al. Ion exchange chromatography of purified colonic mucus glycoproteins in inflammatory bowel disease: absence of a selective subclass defect. Gut 1991;32(10):1139–1145.
11. Sher ME, Bank S, Greenberg R, et al. The influence of cigarette smoking on cytokine levels in patients with inflammatory bowel disease. Inflamm Bowel Dis 1999;5(2):73–78.
12. Madretsma S, Wolters LM, van Dijk JP, et al. In-vivo effect of nicotine on cytokine production by human non-adherent mononuclear cells. Eur J Gastroenterol Hepatol 1996;8(10):1017–1020.
13. Ainley C, Cason J, Slavin BM, Wolstencroft RA, Thompson RP. The influence of zinc status and malnutrition on immunological function in Crohn's disease. Gastroenterology 1991;100(6):1616–1625.
14. O'Morain C, Segal AW, Levi AJ. Elemental diet as primary treatment of acute Crohn's disease: a controlled trial. Br Med J (Clin Res Ed) 1984;288(6434): 1859–1862.
15. Lochs H, Steinhardt HJ, Klaus-Wentz B, et al. Comparison of enteral nutrition and drug treatment in active Crohn's disease. Results of the European Cooperative Crohn's Disease Study. IV. Gastroenterology 1991;101(4):881–888.
16. Griffiths AM, Ohlsson A, Sherman PM, Sutherland LR. Meta-analysis of enteral nutrition as a primary treatment of active Crohn's disease. Gastroenterology 1995;108(4):1056–1067.
17. Fernandez-Banares F, Cabre E, Esteve-Comas M, Gassull MA. How effective is enteral nutrition in inducing clinical remission in active Crohn's disease? A meta-analysis of the randomized clinical trials. JPEN J Parenter Enteral Nutr 1995;19(5):356–364.
18. Teahon K, Smethurst P, Pearson M, Levi AJ, Bjarnason I. The effect of elemental diet on intestinal permeability and inflammation in Crohn's disease. Gastroenterology 1991;101(1):84–89.
19. Lesko SM, Kaufman DW, Rosenberg L, et al. Evidence for an increased risk of Crohn's disease in oral contraceptive users. Gastroenterology 1985;89(5): 1046–1049.

20. Vessey M, Jewell D, Smith A, Yeates D, McPherson K. Chronic inflammatory bowel disease, cigarette smoking, and use of oral contraceptives: findings in a large cohort study of women of childbearing age. Br Med J (Clin Res Ed) 1986;292(6528):1101–1103.

21. Lashner BA, Kane SV, Hanauer SB. Lack of association between oral contraceptive use and ulcerative colitis. Gastroenterology 1990;99(4):1032–1036.

22. Kaufmann HJ, Taubin HL. Nonsteroidal anti-inflammatory drugs activate quiescent inflammatory bowel disease. Ann Intern Med 1987;107(4):513–516.

23. Arndt H, Palitzsch KD, Scholmerich J. Leucocyte endothelial cell adhesion in indomethacin induced intestinal inflammation is correlated with faecal pH. Gut 1998;42(3):380–386.

24. Demling L. Is Crohn's disease caused by antibiotics? Hepatogastroenterology 1994;41(6):549–551.

25. Wurzelmann JI, Lyles CM, Sandler RS. Childhood infections and the risk of inflammatory bowel disease. Dig Dis Sci 1994;39(3):555–560.

26. Rutgeerts P, D'Haens G, Hiele M, Geboes K, Vantrappen G. Appendectomy protects against ulcerative colitis. Gastroenterology 1994;106(5):1251–1253.

27. Herbert TB, Cohen S. Stress and immunity in humans: a meta-analytic review. Psychosom Med 1993;55(4):364–379.

28. Theis MK, Boyko EJ. Patient perceptions of causes of inflammatory bowel disease [letter]. Am J Gastroenterol 1994;89(10):1920.

29. Qiu BS, Vallance BA, Blennerhassett PA, Collins SM. The role of CD4+ lymphocytes in the susceptibility of mice to stress- induced reactivation of experimental colitis. Nat Med 1999;5(10):1178–1182.

30. Wakefield AJ, Sawyerr AM, Dhillon AP, et al. Pathogenesis of Crohn's disease: multifocal gastrointestinal infarction [see comments]. Lancet 1989;2(8671):1057–1062.

31. Wakefield AJ, Sankey EA, Dhillon AP, et al. Granulomatous vasculitis in Crohn's disease. Gastroenterology 1991;100(5 Pt 1):1279–1287.

32. Wakefield AJ, Sawyerr AM, Hudson M, Dhillon AP, Pounder RE. Smoking, the oral contraceptive pill, and Crohn's disease. Dig Dis Sci 1991;36(8):1147–1150.

33. Monsen U, Brostrom O, Nordenvall B, Sorstad J, Hellers G. Prevalence of inflammatory bowel disease among relatives of patients with ulcerative colitis. Scand J Gastroenterol 1987;22(2):214–218.

34. Tysk C, Lindberg E, Jarnerot G, Floderus-Myrhed B. Ulcerative colitis and Crohn's disease in an unselected population of monozygotic and dizygotic twins. A study of heritability and the influence of smoking. Gut 1988;29(7):990–996.

35. Bayless TM, Tokayer AZ, Polito JM, 2nd, Quaskey SA, Mellits ED, Harris ML. Crohn's disease: concordance for site and clinical type in affected family members—potential hereditary influences. Gastroenterology 1996;111(3):573–579.

36. Polito JMd, Rees RC, Childs B, Mendeloff AI, Harris ML, Bayless TM. Preliminary evidence for genetic anticipation in Crohn's disease. Lancet 1996; 347(9004):798–800.

37. Fiocchi C, Roche JK, Michener WM. High prevalence of antibodies to intestinal epithelial antigens in patients with inflammatory bowel disease and their relatives. Ann Intern Med 1989;110(10):786–794.

38. Hollander D, Vadheim CM, Brettholz E, Petersen GM, Delahunty T, Rotter JI. Increased intestinal permeability in patients with Crohn's disease and their relatives. A possible etiologic factor. Ann Intern Med 1986;105(6):883–885.

39. Koltun WA, Tilberg AF, Page MJ, Poritz LS. Bowel permeability is improved in Crohn's disease after ileocolectomy. Dis Colon Rectum 1998;41(6):687–690.

40. Gusella JF, Podolsky DK. Inflammatory bowel disease: is it in the genes?. Gastroenterology 1998;115(5):1286–1289.

41. Satsangi J, Welsh KI, Bunce M, et al. Contribution of genes of the major histo-compatibility complex to susceptibility and disease phenotype in inflammatory bowel disease. Lancet 1996;347(9010):1212–1217.

42. Asakura H, Tsuchiya M, Aiso S, et al. Association of the human lymphocyte-DR2 antigen with Japanese ulcerative colitis. Gastroenterology 1982;82(3):413–418.

43. Futami S, Aoyama N, Honsako Y, et al. HLA-DRB1*1502 allele, subtype of DR15, is associated with susceptibility to ulcerative colitis and its progression. Dig Dis Sci 1995;40(4):814–818.

44. Toyoda H, Wang SJ, Yang HY, et al. Distinct associations of HLA class II genes with inflammatory bowel disease. Gastroenterology 1993;104(3):741–748.

45. Roussomoustakaki M, Satsangi J, Welsh K, et al. Genetic markers may predict disease behavior in patients with ulcerative colitis. Gastroenterology 1997;112(6):1845–1853.

46. Orchard TR, Thiyagaraja S, Welsh KI, Wordsworth BP, Hill Gaston JS, Jewell DP. Clinical phenotype is related to HLA genotype in the peripheral arthropathies of inflammatory bowel disease. Gastroenterology 2000;118(2):274–278.

47. Satsangi J, Jewell DP. Are cytokine gene polymorphisms important in the pathogenesis of inflammatory bowel disease? [comment]. Eur J Gastroenterol Hepatol 1996;8(2):97–99.

48. Plevy SE, Targan SR, Yang H, Fernandez D, Rotter JI, Toyoda H. Tumor necrosis factor microsatellites define a Crohn's disease- associated haplotype on chromosome 6. Gastroenterology 1996;110(4):1053–1060.

49. Kyo K, Parkes M, Takei Y, et al. Association of ulcerative colitis with rare VNTR alleles of the human intestinal mucin gene, MUC3. Hum Mol Genet 1999; 8(2):307–311.

50. Yang H, Vora DK, Targan SR, Toyoda H, Beaudet AL, Rotter JI. Intercellular adhesion molecule 1 gene associations with immunologic subsets of inflammatory bowel disease. Gastroenterology 1995;109(2):440–448.

51. Hugot JP, Laurent–Puig P, Gower-Rousseau C, et al. Mapping of a susceptibility locus for Crohn's disease on chromosome 16. Nature 1996;379(6568):821–823.

52. Cavanaugh JA, Callen DF, Wilson SR, et al. Analysis of Australian Crohn's disease pedigrees refines the localization for susceptibility to inflammatory bowel disease on chromosome 16. Ann Hum Genet 1998;62(Pt 4):291–298.

53. Ohmen JD, Yang HY, Yamamoto KK, et al. Susceptibility locus for inflammatory bowel disease on chromosome 16 has a role in Crohn's disease, but not in ulcerative colitis. Hum Mol Genet 1996;5(10):1679–1683.

54. Satsangi J, Parkes M, Louis E, et al. Two stage genome-wide search in inflammatory bowel disease provides evidence for susceptibility loci on chromosomes 3, 7 and 12. Nat Genet 1996;14(2):199–202.

55. Rioux JD, Daly MJ, Green T, et al. Absence of linkage between inflammatory bowel disease and selected loci on chromosomes 3, 7, 12, and 16. Gastroenterology 1998;115(5):1062–1065.

56. Levine J, Ellis CJ, Furne JK, Springfield J, Levitt MD. Fecal hydrogen sulfide production in ulcerative colitis. Am J Gastroenterol 1998;93(1):83–87.

57. Turunen UM, Farkkila MA, Hakala K, et al. Long-term treatment of ulcerative colitis with ciprofloxacin: a prospective, double-blind, placebo-controlled study. Gastroenterology 1998;115(5):1072–1078.

58. Rutgeerts P, Goboes K, Peeters M, et al. Effect of faecal stream diversion on recurrence of Crohn's disease in the neoterminal ileum. Lancet 1991;338(8770): 771–774.

59. D'Haens GR, Geboes K, Peeters M, Baert F, Penninckx F, Rutgeerts P. Early lesions of recurrent Crohn's disease caused by infusion of intestinal contents in excluded ileum. Gastroenterology 1998;114(2):262–267.

60. Sartor RB. Review article: Role of the enteric microflora in the pathogenesis of intestinal inflammation and arthritis. Aliment Pharmacol Ther 1997;11 Suppl 3:17–22.

61. Afdhal NH, Long A, Lennon J, Crowe J, O'Donoghue DP. Controlled trial of antimycobacterial therapy in Crohn's disease. Clofazimine versus placebo. Dig Dis Sci 1991;36(4):449–453.

62. Thomas GA, Swift GL, Green JT, et al. Controlled trial of antituberculous chemotherapy in Crohn's disease: a five year follow up study. Gut 1998;42(4):497–500.

63. Liu Y, van Kruiningen HJ, West AB, Cartun RW, Cortot A, Colombel JF. Immunocytochemical evidence of Listeria, Escherichia coli, and Streptococcus antigens in Crohn's disease [see comments]. Gastroenterology 1995;108 (5):1396–1404.

64. Fukushima Y, Kawata Y, Hara H, Terada A, Mitsuoka T. Effect of a probiotic formula on intestinal immunoglobulin A production in healthy children. Int J Food Microbiol 1998;42(1–2):39–44.

65. Venturi A, Gionchetti P, Rizzello F, et al. Impact on the composition of the faecal flora by a new probiotic preparation: preliminary data on maintenance treatment of patients with ulcerative colitis. Aliment Pharmacol Ther 1999;13(8): 1103–1108.

66. Duerr RH, Targan SR, Landers CJ, et al. Neutrophil cytoplasmic antibodies: a link between primary sclerosing cholangitis and ulcerative colitis. Gastroenterology 1991;100(5 Pt 1):1385–1391.

67. Shanahan F, Duerr RH, Rotter JI, et al. Neutrophil autoantibodies in ulcerative colitis: familial aggregation and genetic heterogeneity. Gastroenterology 1992;103(2):456–461.

68. Vecchi M, Bianchi MB, Sinico RA, et al. Antibodies to neutrophil cytoplasm in Italian patients with ulcerative colitis: sensitivity, specificity and recognition of putative antigens. Digestion 1994;55(1):34–39.

69. Sandborn WJ, Landers CJ, Tremaine WJ, Targan SR. Antineutrophil cytoplasmic antibody correlates with chronic pouchitis after ileal pouch-anal anastomosis. Am J Gastroenterol 1995;90(5):740–747.

70. Das KM, Dasgupta A, Mandal A, Geng X. Autoimmunity to cytoskeletal protein tropomyosin. A clue to the pathogenetic mechanism for ulcerative colitis. J Immunol 1993;150(6):2487–2493.

71. Pirzer U, Schonhaar A, Fleischer B, Hermann E, Meyer zum Buschenfelde KH. Reactivity of infiltrating T lymphocytes with microbial antigens in Crohn's disease. Lancet 1991;338(8777):1238–1239.

72. Ueyama H, Kiyohara T, Sawada N, et al. High Fas ligand expression on lymphocytes in lesions of ulcerative colitis. Gut 1998;43(1):48–55.

73. Lopez-Cubero SO, Sullivan KM, McDonald GB. Course of Crohn's disease after allogeneic marrow transplantation. Gastroenterology 1998;114(3):433–440.

74. MacDermott RP, Nash GS, Nahm MH. Antibody secretion by human intestinal mononuclear cells from normal controls and inflammatory bowel disease patients. Immunol Invest 1989;18(1–4):449–457.

75. MacDermott RP, Nash GS, Auer IO, et al. Alterations in serum immunoglobulin G subclasses in patients with ulcerative colitis and Crohn's disease. Gastroenterology 1989;96(3):764–768.

76. Kett K, Rognum TO, Brandtzaeg P. Mucosal subclass distribution of immunoglobulin G-producing cells is different in ulcerative colitis and Crohn's disease of the colon. Gastroenterology 1987;93(5):919–924.

77. Harries AD, Fitzsimons E, Fifield R, Dew MJ, Rhoades J. Platelet count: a simple measure of activity in Crohn's disease. Br Med J (Clin Res Ed) 1983;286(6376):1476.

78. Mahida YR, Wu KC, Jewell DP. Characterization of antigen-presenting activity of intestinal mononuclear cells isolated from normal and inflammatory bowel disease colon and ileum. Immunology 1988;65(4):543–549.

79. Mahida YR. Mechanisms of host protection and inflammation in the gastrointestinal tract. J R Coll Physicians Lond 1997;31(5):493–497.

80. Bocker U, Damiao A, Holt L, et al. Differential expression of interleukin 1 receptor antagonist isoforms in human intestinal epithelial cells. Gastroenterology 1998;115(6):1426–1438.

81. Meijssen MA, Brandwein SL, Reinecker HC, Bhan AK, Podolsky DK. Alteration of gene expression by intestinal epithelial cells precedes colitis in interleukin-2-deficient mice. Am J Physiol 1998;274(3 Pt 1):G472–G479.

82. Stallmach A, Schuppan D, Riese HH, Matthes H, Riecken EO. Increased collagen type III synthesis by fibroblasts isolated from strictures of patients with Crohn's disease. Gastroenterology 1992;102(6):1920–1929.

83. Pender SL, Breese EJ, Gunther U, et al. Suppression of T cell-mediated injury in human gut by interleukin 10: role of matrix metalloproteinases. Gastroenterology 1998;115(3):573–583.

84. Binion DG, West GA, Ina K, Ziats NP, Emancipator SN, Fiocchi C. Enhanced leukocyte binding by intestinal microvascular endothelial cells in inflammatory bowel disease. Gastroenterology 1997;112(6):1895–1907.

85. Binion DG, West GA, Volk EE, et al. Acquired increase in leucocyte binding by intestinal microvascular endothelium in inflammatory bowel disease. Lancet 1998;352(9142):1742–1746.

86. Strobach RS, Ross AH, Markin RS, Zetterman RK, Linder J. Neural patterns in inflammatory bowel disease: an immunohistochemical survey. Mod Pathol 1990;3(4):488–493.

87. Bernstein CN, Robert ME, Eysselein VE. Rectal substance P concentrations are increased in ulcerative colitis but not in Crohn's disease. Am J Gastroenterol 1993;88(6):908–913.

88. Mantyh CR, Vigna SR, Bollinger RR, Mantyh PW, Maggio JE, Pappas TN. Differential expression of substance P receptors in patients with Crohn's disease and ulcerative colitis. Gastroenterology 1995;109(3):850–860.

89. Casini-Raggi V, Kam L, Chong YJ, Fiocchi C, Pizarro TT, Cominelli F. Mucosal imbalance of IL-1 and IL-1 receptor antagonist in inflammatory bowel disease. A novel mechanism of chronic intestinal inflammation. J Immunol 1995;154(5):2434–2440.

90. Cominelli F, Nast CC, Duchini A, Lee M. Recombinant interleukin-1 receptor antagonist blocks the proinflammatory activity of endogenous interleukin-1 in rabbit immune colitis. Gastroenterology 1992;103(1):65–71.

91. Schreiber S, Heinig T, Thiele HG, Raedler A. Immunoregulatory role of interleukin 10 in patients with inflammatory bowel disease. Gastroenterology 1995;108(5):1434–1444.

92. Sartor RB. Current concepts of the etiology and pathogenesis of ulcerative colitis and Crohn's disease. Gastroenterol Clin North Am 1995;24(3):475–507.

93. Mazzucchelli L, Hauser C, Zgraggen K, et al. Expression of interleukin-8 gene in inflammatory bowel disease is related to the histological grade of active inflammation. Am J Pathol 1994;144(5):997–1007.

94. Daig R, Andus T, Aschenbrenner E, Falk W, Scholmerich J, Gross V. Increased interleukin 8 expression in the colon mucosa of patients with inflammatory bowel disease. Gut 1996;38(2):216–222.

95. Dubucquoi S, Janin A, Klein O, et al. Activated eosinophils and interleukin 5 expression in early recurrence of Crohn's disease. Gut 1995;37(2):242–246.

96. Dignass AU, Podolsky DK. Cytokine modulation of intestinal epithelial cell restitution: central role of transforming growth factor beta. Gastroenterology 1993;105(5):1323–1332.

97. Rampton DS, Hawkey CJ. Prostaglandins and ulcerative colitis. Gut 1984;25(12): 1399–1413.

98. Singer, II, Kawka DW, Schloemann S, Tessner T, Riehl T, Stenson WF. Cyclooxygenase 2 is induced in colonic epithelial cells in inflammatory bowel disease. Gastroenterology 1998;115(2):297–306.

99. Laursen LS, Naesdal J, Bukhave K, Lauritsen K, Rask-Madsen J. Selective 5-lipoxygenase inhibition in ulcerative colitis. Lancet 1990;335(8691): 683–685.

100. Roberts WG, Simon TJ, Berlin RG, et al. Leukotrienes in ulcerative colitis: results of a multicenter trial of a leukotriene biosynthesis inhibitor, MK-591. Gastroenterology 1997;112(3):725–732.

101. McKenzie SJ, Baker MS, Buffinton GD, Doe WF. Evidence of oxidant-induced injury to epithelial cells during inflammatory bowel disease. J Clin Invest 1996;98(1):136–11.

102. Boughton-Smith NK, Evans SM, Hawkey CJ, et al. Nitric oxide synthase activity in ulcerative colitis and Crohn's disease. Lancet 1993;342(8867):338–340.

103. Middleton SJ, Shorthouse M, Hunter JO. Increased nitric oxide synthesis in ulcerative colitis. Lancet 1993;341(8843):465–466.

104. Harig JM, Soergel KH, Komorowski RA, Wood CM. Treatment of diversion colitis with short-chain-fatty acid irrigation. N Engl J Med 1989;320(1):23–8.

105. Breuer RI, Buto SK, Christ ML, et al. Rectal irrigation with short-chain fatty acids for distal ulcerative colitis. Preliminary report. Dig Dis Sci 1991; 36(2):185–187.

106. Burgio VL, Fais S, Boirivant M, Perrone A, Pallone F. Peripheral monocyte and naive T-cell recruitment and activation in Crohn's disease. Gastroenterology 1995;109(4):1029–1038.

107. Yacyshyn BC, W Goff, B et al. Double-blinded, randomized, placebo-controlled trial of the remission inducing and steroid sparing properties of two schedules of ISIS 2302 (ICAM-1 antisense) in active, steroid-dependent Crohn's disease. Gastroenterology 2000;118:A570.

108. Arseneau KP, TT Cominelli, F. Discovering the cause of inflammatory bowel disease: lessons from animal models. Curr Opin Gastroenterology 2000;16: 310–317.

109. Elson CO, Beagley KW, Sharmanov AT, et al. Hapten-induced model of murine inflammatory bowel disease: mucosa immune responses and protection by tolerance. J Immunol 1996;157(5):2174–2185.

110. Ma A, Datta M, Margosian E, Chen J, Horak I. T cells, but not B cells, are required for bowel inflammation in interleukin 2-deficient mice. J Exp Med 1995;182 (5):1567–1572.

111. Wittig B, Schwarzler C, Fohr N, Gunthert U, Zoller M. Curative treatment of an experimentally induced colitis by a CD44 variant V7-specific antibody. J Immunol 1998;161(3):1069–1073.

112. Kontoyiannis D, Pasparakis M, Pizarro TT, Cominelli F, Kollias G. Impaired on/ off regulation of TNF biosynthesis in mice lacking TNF AU- rich elements: implications for joint and gut-associated immunopathologies. Immunity 1999;10(3):387–398.

113. Stonerook MJ, Weiss HS, Rodriguez MA, et al. Temperature-metabolism relations in the cotton-top tamarin (Saguinus oedipus) model for ulcerative colitis. J Med Primatol 1994;23(1):16–22.

4 Genetics of Inflammatory Bowel Disease

Judy Cho, MD

CONTENTS

INTRODUCTION

The inflammatory bowel diseases (IBD) (Crohn's disease [CD] and ulcerative colitis [UC]) are defined by chronic, intermittent inflammation of the intestines, resulting in abdominal pain, diarrhea, and rectal bleeding. These diseases have a peak incidence between 15–30 yr of age, and a combined prevalence of 200–300/100,000 in the United States, therefore representing a major cause of morbidity in young adults *(1–3)*. The earliest steps in the pathogenesis of IBD are currently undefined. Development of significantly better medical therapies for IBD is

From: *Clinical Gastroenterology:*
Inflammatory Bowel Disease: Diagnosis and Therapeutics
Edited by: R. D. Cohen © Humana Press Inc., Totowa, NJ

dependent on developing a more specific understanding of the earliest stages of pathogenesis. Furthermore, reclassification of these disorders based on identification of molecular mechanisms of pathogenesis holds the promise of tailoring medical therapies to individual patients.

EPIDEMIOLOGIC EVIDENCE THAT IBD IS A COMPLEX GENETIC DISORDER

Several studies have compared the risk of developing inflammatory bowel disease in relatives of patients with IBD compared to relatives of controls. It is estimated that 5–10% of patients have a first degree relative also affected by IBD. IBD is found 15 times more frequently in relatives of CD and UC patients then relatives of normal controls (4). That familial aggregation is primarily genetic rather than caused by shared environmental etiology such as an infectious agent is suggested by a lack of increased risk to spouses and aggregation occurring among relatives raised separately. The strongest epidemiological evidence for a genetic risk comes from twin studies. In the Swedish twin registry, proband pairwise concordance was 44% for Crohn's disease in identical twins and 3.9% in fraternal twins. The fraternal twin concordance is not much different than the nontwin sibling concordance, suggesting that within the same familial environment, the closer relationship of fraternal twins is not associated with a substantial increase disease risk. In comparison, the proband pairwise concordance for UC in identical twins was 6% as compared to 0% for paternal twins (5). Taken together, this indicates a more significant genetic component for CD compared to UC. These data also show, however that inflammatory bowel disease cannot be completely explained by genetics. The lack of complete concordance in identical twins is likely because the unaffected twin not exposed to an environmental trigger or risk factor. Alternatively the presence of a protective environmental affect be contributing. Finally, some IBD cases may be primarily a result of environmental factors that grossly mimic CD or UC. IBD (primarily UC) coexists with primary sclerosing cholangitis (PSC) so commonly that PSC patients should almost always be evaluated for UC. Furthermore, patients with PSC and UC are at an increased risk for colonic neoplasia (6).

DEFINING THE RISK OF IBD IN CHILDREN WITH ONE OR BOTH PARENTS WITH IBD

IBD is a multigenic genetic disorder as opposed to monogenic diseases with a defined mode of inheritance (i.e., autosomal dominant or recessive). It likely requires more than one susceptibility gene for an inherited risk of IBD. In a United States study, the lifetime risk to IBD in a first degree relative (parent, sibling, or child) was 5.2 to a relative of a non-Jewish Caucasian with CD, 1.6 to a relative of a non-Jewish Caucasian with UC, 7.8 to a relative of a Jew with CD, and 4.5 to a relative of a Jew with UC. The risk to siblings tended to be greater than the risk to parents. The data for the risk to offspring is more difficult to define, most likely because of the size of the study and ascertainment issues. The corrected lifetime risk to offsprings was 7.8% of a Jewish parent with either CD or UC, and the risk to offspring of a non-Jewish parent was zero if the parent had CD and 11.0 if the parent had UC. Similar to most other studies, the empiric risk to offspring was approx 2% *(7)*. There are no established guidelines for IBD risk to offspring of affected parents. The lifetime risk to children of a parent with IBD ranges between 5–10%. It may tend to be in the higher range if the parent is Jewish, has a family history or developed IBD at an early age. The risk of IBD to a child of parents who both have IBD—whether or not it is CD or UC—may be as high as 50%; in a US study of 19 couples who both have IBD, IBD, usually CD, developed in 12 out of the 23 children (52%) who were 20 yr of age or older *(8)*.

LINKAGE STUDIES IN IBD

Genetic linkage studies type families with more than one affected member at genetic markers throughout the genome for the purpose of identifying genomic regions shared in excess of statistical expectation. This excess sharing among affected individuals within a family observed significantly across large numbers of families implies that a disease-associated gene resides within the chromosomal region of increased sharing. Genome-wide linkage searches have provided a broad overview of the landscape of most significant genes contributing to IBD pathogenesis.

Given the large number of statistical tests applied in a genome-wide screen, not all suggestive linkage regions reported will ultimately be found to contain a disease susceptibility gene. Conversely, because IBD likely results from the contribution of multiple genes of modest effect, genetic linkage approaches may not be sufficiently powerful to identify linkages for all important susceptibility genes. Given these caveats, several broad generalizations can be made. First, although IBD is an inflammatory disorder, in contrast to searches in other chronic inflammatory disorders, such as celiac sprue *(9)* and insulin-dependent diabetes mellitus *(10)*, the role of the major histocompatibility complex (MHC) is not dominant, implicating a major pathogenetic role for non-

MHC genes in IBD. Significant genetic linkages have been observed on chromosomes 16, 12, 14, 19, 6, and 1 *(11–17)* for either CD and/ or UC. A second common finding is that for many of the implicated regions, evidence for linkage is observed in both CD and UC, suggesting that many major pathogenetic genes will be common to both diseases. A notable exception to this is the observed linkage in the pericentromeric region of chromosome 16, which represents by far the most well-established linkage region in IBD and confers risk primarily for CD *(11)*. It is now established that Nod2 in this region increases susceptibility to CD.

Environmental factors such as smoking may determine whether a CD-like picture (positively associated with tobacco use) or a UC-like phenotype (negatively associated with tobacco use) is observed. These trends are observed in families with more than one affected member. In families with only CD, the percentage of smokers among affected individuals is 64% compared to 31% in families having only cases of UC. Interestingly, in those mixed families (having one member with CD, and another with UC) the trends are similar, with 64% and 23% smokers among individuals with CD and UC, respectively *(18)*.

Finally, clustering of non-MHC susceptibility loci between different chronic inflammatory diseases (Crohn's disease, multiple sclerosis, psoriasis, asthma, type-I diabetes) has been observed. This nonrandom clustering of loci supports the hypothesis that distinct, chronic inflammatory disorders may have some common susceptibility genes, or members of similar gene families *(19)*.

NOD2 ON CHROMOSOME 16, IBD1, INCREASES SUSCEPTIBILITY TO CD

It is now established that the CD susceptibility gene at IBD1 is a protein called Nod2 (nucleotide oligomerization domain) *(20–22)*. Nod2 is expressed in peripheral monocytes and is involved in activation of NF-kB, transcription factors that activate expression of a large array of genes, including genes mediating inflammatory cascades. It is similar in its structure to the plant *R* genes, which are well known to mediate resistance to microbial pathogens.

The last portion of Nod2 contains the leucine rich repeat (LRR) domain, which is required for LPS-induced NF-kB activation. In vitro studies demonstrate that *Nod2* signaling is mediated by exposure to LPS, suggesting that *Nod2* may serve as an intracellular LPS receptor. Multiple mutations have been identified in the *Nod2* gene among CD patients, with many clustered in the LRR domain. Most significant among these is a frameshift variant, *Leu1007fsinsC*, which truncates the last 3% of the protein. This frameshift variant results in decreased LPS-induced NF-κB activation, which is somewhat counterintuitive given the role of NF-κB in mediating inflammation. Two additional major variants, *Arg702Trp* and *Gly908Arg* have been identified, which confer similar genetic risks. Heterozygous carriage of any of the three major risk alleles increases susceptibility 1.5- to three-fold, whereas homozygotes or compound heterozygotes are at 18- to 44-fold increased risk. Taken together these three major variants conservatively confer a 15–20% population attributable risk among familial CD, with likely a lesser contribution among the more common, sporadic cases of CD. Much remains to be learned about what will likely be very complex cellular interactions of Nod2, which may provide insight into new therapeutic approaches. Further studies are required in order to determine whether Nod2 variants can predict clinical course and/or response to therapy.

PATHOPHYSIOLOGY OF IBD: GENETIC VARIATION IN INFLAMMATORY RESPONSES TO LUMINAL ANTIGENS

Genetic engineering in mice of a broad array of different genes (interleukin-10, interleukin-2/R, T-cell receptor, tumor necrosis factor, multi-drug resistance gene, *N*-cadherin, HLA-B27) can result in a stereotypic, IBD-like picture. Genetic heterogeneity may similarly exist in humans, where different subsets of genes in different patients result in similar disease expression. The importance of gene–gene interactions is underscored by the observation that severity of disease expression for a given targeted gene is highly strain-specific in these murine models of IBD. Furthermore, host-responses are affected by environmental factors, including specific characteristics of intraluminal bacteria.

Cytokine/Cytokine Receptor Association Studies in IBD

Given the chronic inflammatory features that define IBD, candidate gene studies with various proinflammatory cytokines and their receptors represent reasonable first attempts to establish disease associations. In particular, studies on the tumor necrosis factor (*TNF*) gene illustrate some of the associated issues and challenges The *TNF* gene is located on chromosome 6p within the MHC. Multiple linkage studies have demonstrated significant evidence for linkage in this region. Increased expression of TNF has been observed in human IBD, and anti-*TNF* antibodies comprise a major new means of treating Crohn's disease. A murine model of ileitis resulting from deletion of an AU-rich region in the 3' untranslated region of the *TNF* gene (increasing RNA and protein expression of TNF) has been reported *(23)*. Whether proinflammatory cytokines such as *TNF* merely execute the final inflammatory events that lead to disease or are of primary pathogenic importance has yet to be resolved. Promoter variants in humans of the TNF gene have been correlated with increased susceptibility to cerebral malaria *(24)* and with different regulation of *TNF* expression. However, association studies in IBD patients at selected *TNF* variants have demonstrated conflicting results, perhaps because of different populations and promoter variants studied. A Japanese study observed increased prevalence of TNF promoter variants associated with increased inducible expression of TNF in CD, but not UC patients *(25)*. Given the baseline population differences in allele frequencies in various genes among healthy controls, combined with environmental differences, it is quite likely that the magnitude of disease associations may vary between populations.

Population-specific differences have also been observed with respect to an intronic variant (IL-1ra*2, allele 2) in the interleukin-1 receptor antagonist associated with decreased IL-1ra production from peripheral blood mononuclear cells. Increased carriage of IL-1ra*2 was observed in Hispanic and Jewish patients with UC, but not in Italian or non-Jewish American Caucasians with UC *(26)*. The interleukin-4 RA is located in the observed linkage region on chromosome 16 and intragenic variants have been associated with asthma, but no association with Crohn's disease has been observed *(27)*.

HLA Associations and IBD

The role of imflammatory T cells in IBD suggests that genetic polymorphism in major histocompatibily complex (MHC) class II genes may be of pathogenetic importance in IBD. There have been a number of conflicting association studies for HLA and non-HA genes in this region The enormous genetic and immunologic complexity in the MHC region increases the difficulty of ultimately identifying specific alleles contributing to disease. Genetic linkage has been observed in both pure CD and pure UC families, and various association studies have demonstrated association with both CD and UC patients at different HLA class II loci. It is possible that class II associations will be highly dependent on environmental and population-specific factors. As with many candidate gene association studies for complex genetic disorders, most published studies have possessed limited power, with definitive conclusions regarding HLA class II loci awaiting the completion of much larger studies.

Perhaps the most significant HLA associations will be identified with specific extraintestinal manifestation of IBD, such as the association of anklyosing spondylitis with HLA-B*27. HLA associations have also been reported based on subtypes of peripheral arthropathies based on their natural history and articular distribution *(28)*. Significant HLA associations here most likely arise from the pathogenic roles of arthritic peptides and molecular mimicry. Furthermore, there is some evidence to support the concept that the subset of patients with IBD and primary sclerosing cholangitis may be more HLA-restricted.

INDIVIDUALIZATION OF MEDICAL APPROACHES BASED ON UNDERSTANDING OF GENETIC DIFFERENCES IN PATIENTS WITH IBD

The elucidation of critical proinflammatory mediators, such as TNF, involved in the final inflammatory events that lead to disease has resulted in the development of effective, though nonspecific, methods to control inflammation. The development of more effective and targeted approaches to treat IBD may ultimately be elucidated by understanding genetic differences in different individuals with similar clinical phenotypes. Pharmacogenetics deals with genetic differences in metabolism and action of specific pharmacological agents. Important differences in the metabolism of 6-mercaptopurine have been identified, which contribute to interindividual differences in both its efficacy and toxicity. A separate issue is whether, through understanding of the genetic predisposition, and associated with this, broad scale expression differences, patients with similar clinical phenotypes, can be reclassified on a more pathogenetic basis. This reclassification then would form the basis for individualizing both existing and novel therapies for IBD.

PHARMACOGENETIC FACTORS IN IBD

The effects of 6-mercaptopurine are mediated by its intracellular conversion to 6-thioguanine (6-TG) and 6-methylmercaptopurine (6-MMP), with the later reaction mediated by the enzyme, thiopurine methyltransferase (TMPT). 6-TG levels are greater than 235 pmol/8 $\times$ 10^8 erythrocytes (which correlate with leukocyte levels are significantly associated with improved clinical response *(29)*. Conversely, hepatotoxicity correlated with 6-MMP levels of >5700 pmol/8 $\times$ 10^8 erythrocytes. Individuals heterozygous for low activity of TMPT (approx 11% of Caucasians) have higher levels of 6-TG. One in 300 individuals are homozygous for low activity of TMPT. Severe bone marrow toxic effects of 6-MP may occur in individuals with deficient levels of TMPT activity as a result of intracellular accumulation of 6-TG. Conversely, individuals with high levels of TMPT develop increased levels of 6-MMP, associated with hepatotoxicity. Importantly, not all observed drug toxicity can be accounted for by TMPT genotypes; in fact, most cases of cytopenia are unassociated with TMPT polymorphisms. The combination of TMPT genotyping and monitoring of metabolite levels may provide a means of optimizing 6-MP dosing to maximize efficacy with minimal toxicity. Genetic differences in drug metabolism are complicated by multidrug therapy. Mesalamine and sulfasalazine mediate their effects, in part through inhibition of the NF-κ B pro-inflammatory transcriptional pathway *(30)*. Mesalamine has been shown to inhibit activity of TMPT as well, although concomitant use of mesalamine has not been shown to affect response or toxicity to 6-MP.

Genetic polymorphisms are increasingly being identified in a broad range of proteins involved in drug metabolism. The multidrug resistance-1 *(MDR-1)* gene is an ATP-dependent plasma membrane transport protein which was initially identified at high levels within tumors resistant to a broad range of chemotherapeutic agents due to their efflux from cells by *MDR-1*. *MDR-1* is normally expressed by intestinal epithelial cells and peripheral blood lymphocytes and genetic polymorphisms within the gene have been identified which affect transporter expression levels and activity. Corticosteroids are substrates of *MDR-1* and higher *MDR-1* activities were found in those IBD patients not responding to acute corticosteroid therapy, thus requiring surgical intervention *(31)*. As more pharmacogenetic polymorphisms are identified, characterization of them in the context of pharmacologic trials will provide a better understanding of individual response to therapy.

REFERENCES

1. Calkins BM, Mendeloff AI. Epidemiology of inflammatory bowel disease. Epidemiol Rev 1986;8:60–91.
2. Gollop JH, Phillips SF, Melton III LJ, Zinmeister AR. Epidemiologic aspects of Crohn's disease: a population based study in Olmsted County, Minnesota,1943–1982. Gut 1988;29:1943–1982.
3. Stonnington CM, Phillips SF, Melton III LF, Zinmeister AR. Chronic ulcerative colitis: incidence and prevalence in a community. Gut 1987;28:402–409.
4. Binder V. Genetic epidemiology in inflammatory bowel disease. Dig Dis 1998;16:351–355.
5. Tysk C, Linkberg E, Jarnerot G, Floderus-Myrhed B. Ulcerative colitis and Crohn's disease in an unselected population of monozygotic and dizygotic twins: a study of heritability and the influence of smoking. Gut 1988;29:990–996.
6. Brentnall TA, Haggitt RC, Rabinovitch PS, Kimmey MB, Bronner MP, Levine DS, et al. Risk and natural history of colonic neoplasia in patients with primary sclerosing cholangitis and ulcerative colitis. Gastroenterology 1996;110:331–338.
7. Yang H, McElree C, Roth MP, Shanahan F, Targan SR, Rotter JI. Familial empirical risks for inflammatory bowel disease: differences between Jews and non-Jews. Gut 1993;34:517–524.

8. Bennett RA, Rubin PH, Present DH. Frequency of inflammatory bowel disease in offspring of couples both presenting with inflammatory bowel disease: differences between Jews and non-Jews. Gastroenterology 1991;100:1638–1643.

9. Zhong F, McCombs CC, Olson JM, Elston RC, Stevens FM, McCarthy CF, et al. An autosomal screen for genes that predispose to celiac disease in the western counties of Ireland. Nat Genet 1996;14:329–333

10. Concannon P, Gogolin-Ewens KJ, Hinds DA, Wapelhorst B, Morrison VA, Stirling B, et al. A second-generation screen of the human genome for susceptibility to insulin-dependent diabetes mellitus. Nat Genet 1998;19:292–6.

11. Hugot JP, Laurent-Puig P,Gower-Rousseau C, Olson JM, Lee JC, Beaugerie L, et al. Mapping of a susceptibility locus for Crohn's disease on chromosome 16. Nature 1996;379,821–823.

12. Satsangi J, Parkes M, Louis E, Lathrop M, Bell J, Jewell DP. Two stage genome-wide search in inflammatory bowel disesae provides evidence for susceptibility loci on chromosomes 3, 7 and 12. Nat Genetics 1996;14:199–202.

13. Cho JH, Nicolae DL, Gold LH, Fields CT, LaBuda MC, Rohal PM, et al. Identification of susceptibility loci for inflammatory bowel disease on chromosomes 1p, 3q, and 4q: Evidence for epistasis between 1p and IBD1. Proc Natl Acad Sci USA 1998;95:7502–7507.

14. Hampe J, Schreiber S, Shaw SH, Lau KF, Bridger S, Macpherson AJ, et al. A genomewide analysis provides evidence for novel linkages in inflammatory bowel disease in a large European cohort. Am J Hum Genet 1999;64:808–816.

15. Ma Y, Ohmen JD, Li Z, Bentley LG, McElree C, Pressman S, et al. A genome-wide search identifies potential new susceptibility loci for Crohn's disease. Inflamm Bowel Dis 1999;5:271–278

16. Duerr RH, Barmada MM, Zhang L, Pfutzer R, Weeks DE. High-density genome scan in Crohn disease shows confirmed linkage to chromosome 14q11-12. Am J Hum Genet 2000;66:1857–1862.

17. Rioux JD, Silverberg MS, Daly MJ, Steinhart AH, McLeod RS, Griffiths AM, et al. Search in Canadian Families with Inflammatory Bowel Disease Reveals Two Novel Susceptibility Loci. Am J Hum Genet 2000;66:1863–1870.

18. Lee JCW, Lennard-Jones JE. Inflammatory bowel disease in 67 families each with three or more affected first-degree relatives. Gastroenterology 1996; 111: 587–596.

19. Becker KG, Simon RM, Bailey-Wilson JE, Freidlin B, Biddison WE, McFarland HF, et al. Clustering of non-major histocompatibility complex susceptibility candidate loci in human autoimmune diseases. Proc Natl Acad Sci 1998; 95: 9979–9984.

20. Ogura Y, Bonen DK, Inohara N, Nicolae DL, Chen FF, Ramos R, et al. A frameshift mutation in NOD2 associated with susceptibility to Crohn's disease. Nature 2001;411:603–606.

21. Hugot JP, Chamaillard M, Zouali H, Lesage S, Cezard JP, Belaiche J, et al. Association of NOD2 leucine-rich repeat variants with susceptibility to Crohn's disease. Nature 2001;411:599–603.

22. Hampe J, Cuthbert A, Croucher PJ, Mirza MM, Mascheretti S, Fisher S, et al. Association between insertion mutation in NOD2 gene and Crohn's disease in German and British populations. Lancet 2001;357(9272):1925–1928.

23. Kontoyiannis D, Pasparakis M, Pizarro TT, Cominelli F, Kollias G. Impaired on/off regulation of TNF biosynthesis in mice lacking TNF AU-rich elements: implications for joint and gut-associated immunopathologies. Immunity 1999; 10:387–398.

24. McGuire W, Hill AV, Allsopp CE, Greenwood BM, Kwiatkowski D. Variation in the TNF-alpha promoter region associated with susceptibility to cerebral malaria. Nature 1994;371:508–510.
25. Negoro K, Kinouchi Y, Hiwatashi N, Takahashi S, Takagi S, Satoh J, et al. Crohn's disease is associated with novel polymorphisms in the 5'-flanking region of the tumor necrosis factor gene. Gastroenterology 1999;117:1062–1068.
26. Tountas NA, Casini-Raggi V, Yang H, Di Giovine FS, Vecchi M, Kam L, et al. Functional and ethnic association of allele 2 of the interleukin-1 receptor antagonist gene in ulcerative colitis. Gastroenterology 1999;117:806–813.
27. Olavesen MG, Hampe J, Mirza MM, Saiz R, Lewis CM, Bridger S, et al. Analysis of single-nucleotide polymorphisms in the interleukin-4 receptor gene for association with inflammatory bowel disease. Immunogenetics 2000;51:1–7.
28. Orchard TR, Thiyagaraja S, Welsh KI, Wordsworth BP, Hill Gaston JS, Jewell DP. Clinical phenotype is related to HLA genotype in the peripheral arthropathies of inflammatory bowel disease. Gastroenterology 2000;118:274–278.
29. Dubinsky MC, Lamothe S, Yang HY, Targan SR, Sinnett D, Theoret Y, et al. Pharmacogenomics and metabolite measurement for 6-mercaptopurine therapy in inflammatory bowel disease. Gastroenterology 2000;118:705–713.
30. Liptay S, Bachem M, Hacker G, Adler G, Debatin KM, Schmid RM. Inhibition of nuclear factor kappa B and induction of apoptosis in T-lymphocytes by sulfasalazine. Br J Pharmacol 1999;128:1361–1369.
31. Farrell RJ, Murphy A, Long A, Donnelly S, Cherikuri A, O'Toole D, et al. High multidrug resistance (P-glycoprotein 170) expression in inflammatory bowel disease patients who fail medical therapy. Gastroenterology 2000;118:279–288.

5

Presentation and Diagnosis
of Inflammatory Bowel Disease

Themistocles Dassopoulos, MD
and Stephen Hanauer, MD

INTRODUCTION

Crohn's disease (CD) and ulcerative colitis (UC) are the two major idiopathic inflammatory bowel diseases (IBD). Because there is no pathognomonic, diagnostic feature of either UC or CD, and because of the nonspecific features of intestinal inflammation, these "classic" diagnoses probably represent a spectrum of clinicopathological entities with overlapping features, including a significant proportion of patients with colitis that is "indeterminate," i.e., colitis with features that defy distinct categorization as UC or CD. Although the pathogenesis of IBD remains obscure, it is believed that, in genetically susceptible hosts, antigens within the intestinal lumen trigger a dysregulated mucosal immune response leading to chronic inflammation *(1)*. Innate immune cells (macrophages, neutrophils), adaptive immune cells (T cells), and nonimmune cells (including epithelial and endothelial cells, cells of the enteric nervous system, and fibroblasts) engage in complex interactions, culminating in the elaboration of pro-inflammatory mediators that overwhelm the homeostatic defenses of the intestine and injure the

From: *Clinical Gastroenterology:*
Inflammatory Bowel Disease: Diagnosis and Therapeutics
Edited by: R. D. Cohen © Humana Press Inc., Totowa, NJ

intestinal epithelium *(1)*. Moreover, the pattern of injury (location along the gastrointestinal tract, severity and penetration of injury) and reparative processes (i.e., intestinal scarring with stricture formation) influence clinical presentation, as well as prognosis and therapeutic approach *(2)*.

The symptoms and signs of IBD are nonspecific, as different types of injury (infection, ischemia, radiation, medications, and vasculitis) can affect the intestinal mucosa in similar manner and intestinal bleeding can arise from either neoplasia or mucosal or vascular injury. A unique feature of CD and UC is the potential presence of "extra-intestinal" manifestations, demonstrating systemic aspects of an overactive mucosal immune system. Endoscopy, mucosal biopsies, radiography, stool microbiologic studies, and, recently, serologic assays are used to confirm IBD and exclude alternative diagnoses. In our current state of knowledge, there remains no single pathognomonic diagnostic test to rule-in or rule-out IBD. In the final analysis, the diagnosis of IBD remains clinical.

This chapter discusses the presentation and diagnosis of UC and CD, with particular emphasis on critical features of the clinical presentation and diagnostic test data that allow the distinction between these and potentially confounding disorders in the differential diagnosis.

ULCERATIVE COLITIS
Clinical Presentation

HISTORY

Patients with UC are typically young with a peak age of onset in the second and third decade, although any age group can be affected. In up to 20% of patients there may be a family history of IBD and up to 40% of children who present will have another family member with the disease. These illnesses are more common in first world countries where infectious diarrheas are less common, however, many patients present after an apparent bout of infectious or travelers' diarrhea. Usually, though, the onset of symptoms is insidious and, at first, symptoms are often intermittent.

Numerous studies have demonstrated a protective effect of cigarette smoking in reducing the risk of UC *(3)*. Compared to lifelong nonsmokers, current smokers have a lower risk, and former smokers a greater risk of developing UC. In clinical practice, intermittent smokers report milder symptoms during periods of smoking. Former smokers develop symptoms within months of smoking cessation, and often enter remission once they restart smoking.

Use of aspirin or other nonsteroidal antiinflammatory drugs (NSAIDs) *(4,5)*, intercurrent infection (travelers' diarrhea, viral respiratory illness) *(6)*, and smoking cessation *(7)* have all been associated with new onset or exacerbations of preexistent UC. In female patients, increased gastrointestinal symptoms are associated with the menstrual cycle *(8)* and, occasionally, UC presents during pregnancy or in the peripartum period. Usually, with preexistent UC, disease activity during pregnancy correlates with activity levels at conception: active UC at conception is likely to remain active during pregnancy and, similarly, quiescent disease before conception tends to remain quiescent *(9)*.

SYMPTOMS

Ulcerative colitis always affects the rectum, and extends proximally, in a diffuse, symmetrical, and contiguous pattern for a distance that varies between individuals. Patients may develop proctitis, proctosigmoiditis, left-sided colitis (inflammation up to the splenic flexure), extensive colitis (inflammation extending proximal to the splenic flexure), or pancolitis (inflammation involving the entire colon). The location of inflammation tends to remain constant throughout the course in patients and the combination of disease extent and mucosal severity influence disease presentation and prognosis.

Because the rectum is inflamed in virtually all patients with UC, the hallmark symptoms are rectal bleeding, passage of mucopus, and urgency to evacuate. Diarrhea, in contrast, is related to the extent of colonic inflammation such that many patients with proctitis present with constipation and hematochezia. Other symptoms include tenesmus (a sensation of needing to evacuate stool, or "dry heaves of the rectum," that often is nonproductive) and abdominal cramping. Abdominal pain, *per se*, is uncommon as UC most commonly is limited to the mucosa, whereas pain receptors in the gut are present on the serosa and peritoneum. More seriously ill patients can present with accompanying anorexia, nausea, emesis (typically associated with bowel movements), and possible toxic manifestations of orthostasis, tachycardia, and fevers. Disease severity is assessed by the clinical criteria of Truelove and Witts *(10)*, modified in Table 1.

Patients with fulminant UC present with fever and continuous bloody diarrhea, consisting of greater than 10 bowel movements daily. Toxic megacolon, defined by fulminant colitis and radiographic evidence of colonic dilatation, is not unique to UC, and can also occur with Crohn's colitis or infectious colitides *(11)*.

The clinician should elicit any extraintestinal manifestations (see later and Table 2), previous or concomitant medication history (Table 3), smoking history, and family history of IBD.

Table 1
Assesment of UC Activity[1]

Variable	Mild Disease	Severe Disease	Fulminant Disease
Stools (no./d)	<4	>6	>10
Blood in stool	Intermittent	Frequent	Continuous
Temperature (°C)	Normal	>37.5	>37.5
Pulse	Normal	<90	>90
Hemoglobin	Normal	<75% of normal	Transfusion required
ESR (mm/h)	<30	>30	>30
Radiographic features	Normal gas pattern	Edematous colon wall, thumbprinting	Dilated colon
Clinical examination	Normal bowel sounds, nontender abdomen	Tender abdomen, no rebound tenderness	Distended abdomen, decreased bowel sounds, ±rebound tenderness

[1]Modified from references (2,10).

PHYSICAL EXAMINATION

Patients with mild-moderate UC usually present with a normal physical examination aside from mild left lower quadrant tenderness and perhaps evidence of pallor related to iron deficiency anemia. More severely ill patients present with evidence of systemic toxicity (fever, tachycardia, hypotension), dehydration, anemia, and more prominent localized abdominal tenderness. Severe disease is characterized by abdominal tenderness and possible colonic dilatation (high-pitch bowel sounds, tympany), and fulminant disease by rebound tenderness and prostration. However, a quite ill patient may appear deceptively well, and concomitant steroid therapy may obscure peritoneal signs. Colonic perforation can occur with toxic megacolon, but also in severe colitis without colonic dilatation. Life-threatening hemorrhage is rare. Colonic strictures in UC are rare and should raise suspicion of an associated carcinoma.

The presence of perianal disease (with the exception of small hemorrhoids or a small skin tag) argues strongly against UC, and in favor of CD. There may be findings related to extraintestinal manifestations of UC (Table 2) or complications from therapy (see Table 3).

COMPLICATIONS AND EXTRAINTESTINAL MANIFESTATIONS

Extraintestinal manifestations of IBD (listed in Table 2) may coincide with the diagnosis, predate, or complicate long-standing UC. Extraintestinal symptoms also are associated with the extent of colitis,

Table 2
Extraintestinal Manifestations of IBD [1,2]

Joints	Peripheral arthritis (oligoarticular)
	Ankylosing spondylitis
	Sacroiliitis
	Osteomalacia/Osteoporosis
	(calcium and vitamin D malabsorption in CD, steroids)
Skin	Erythema nodosum
	Pyoderma gangrenosum
	Aphthous stomatitis
	"Metastatic" CD (skin, vulva)
Eye	Iritis
	Uveitis
	Episcleritis
Hepatobiliary	Primary sclerosing cholangitis (PSC)
	Fatty liver
	Gallstones (in CD)
Kidney	Calcium oxalate stones
	Hydronephrosis (from ureteral obstruction in CD)

[1]Peripheral arthritis, erythema nodosum, iritis, and uveitis are related to IBD activity. Ankylosing spondylitis, sacroiliitis, and PSC are independent of the IBD activity. Pyoderma gangrenosum may or may not be related to the activity of the IBD.
[2]Central and peripheral arthritis, skin disease, eye disease, and PSC usually occur in the setting of colitis. Osteoporosis, gallstones, and calcium oxalate stones are metabolic complications of small bowel CD.

Table 3
Adverse Effects of Medical Therapy for IBD

Therapy	Adverse Effects
Sulfasalazine	Nausea, vomiting, headache, pancreatitis, reversible sperm abormalities, folate deficiency
Mesalamine	Exacerbation of colitis, pancreatitis, secretory diarrhea (olsalazine)
Metronidazole	Peripheral neuropathy, metallic taste
Ciprofloxacin	Nausea, diarrhea
Steroids	Osteoporosis, avascular necrosis of the hip, hypertension, cataracts, glaucoma, glucose intolerance, mood disturbance, thrush, periodontal disease
6-MP and Azathioprine	Nausea, pancreatitis, myelosuppression, hepatitis, fever, arthralgias, macrocytosis
Methotrexate	Hepatitis, hepatic fibrosis, myelosuppression, pneumonitis
Cyclosporine	Opportunistic infection, nephrotoxicity, hypertension, hyperkalemia, hypomagnesemia, seizures (in patients with low cholesterol), hepatotoxicity, headache, tremor, hirsutism, lymphoma (with chronic administration)
Infliximab	Acute and delayed hypersensitivity reactions, tuberculosis

being more common in patients with more extensive disease. The most common extraintestinal manifestations are arthralgias, typically affecting larger joints in an asymmetric pattern without evidence of rheumatoid nodules or radiographic joint destruction. The peripheral arthropathies tend to correlate with disease activity and often subside with treatment of colitis. Skin lesions including erythema nodosum or pyoderma gangrenosum are less common and also tend to correlate with colitis activity, as do minor ocular disorders such as episcleritis. In contrast, a number of extraintestinal manifestations such as uveitis and anklylosing spondylitis/sacroiliitis are more common in patients who are HLA B27 positive, although there are is no direct association of HLA B27 and the risk of developing IBD. The HLA B27-associated manifestations tend to run an independent course from the colitis activity. Similarly, primary sclerosing cholangitis (PSC), which has a disease spectrum from mild inflammation of portal triads (pericholangitis) manifest only as elevated alkaline phosphatase and GGTP, to progressive stricturing of intra- and extra-hepatic biliary radicals leading to secondary biliary cirrhosis, also runs a course independent from the colitis activity. Rarely, PSC is complicated by cholangiocarcinoma.

A longstanding complication of UC greater than 10 yr duration is the development of colonic mucosal dysplasia and adenocarcinoma. Risk factors include the extent and duration of disease, as well as the presence of PSC. Patients with UC of greater than 8–10 yr duration and patients with PSC are recommended to undergo periodic surveillance colonoscopy *(12)*.

DIAGNOSIS

The diagnosis of UC is clinical and based on the combination of the clinical presentation, mucosal appearance at endoscopy or radiography, and histologic findings in mucosal biopsies.

The laboratory features of UC are nonspecific and reflect the severity of inflammation (i.e., increased erythrocyte sedimentation rate, leukocytosis with a "left shift"), complications of diarrhea (hypokalemia, alkalosis, other electrolyte disturbances), or complications of mucosal exudation (anemia from chronic blood loss and iron deficiency or hypoalbuminemia from protein exudation).

Recently, serologic tests have been evaluated for sensitivity and specificity in IBD. In UC there is a unique *perinuclear* antineutrophil cytoplasmic antibody (pANCA) that is present in approx 60% of confirmed cases. The specificity of pANCA is only approx 80% for UC. In contrast anti-*Saccharomyces cerevisiae* antibodies (ASCA) are more common in patients with CD. The combination of a positive pANCA and a negative ASCA supports, but does not confirm, the clinical diagnosis of UC. However, because of their limited sensitivity and specificity, these serologic tests do not generally alter the clinical impression as to the presence or absence of IBD *(13)*.

A hallmark of active colitis is the presence of fecal leukocytes on wet mount. Additional stool studies are necessary to rule out infectious colitis due to bacteria [including Clostridium difficile and enterohemorrhagic *E. coli* (E.coli O157:H7)] or parasites (especially amebiasis).

Plain abdominal radiography is mostly useful in excluding perforation or megacolon. Rarely, CT scans are used to rule out an abdominal abscess. However, for the most part, while air-contrast barium enemas can be used to confirm mucosal inflammation in UC, these studies have been supplanted by endoscopic examinations with flexible sigmoidoscopes or colonoscopes. Colonoscopy, including examination into the terminal ileum, is eventually performed in all patients to assess the extent of involvement, obtain biopsies and rule out ileitis. However, in the acute setting, flexible sigmoidoscopy is sufficient to assess severity and extent beyond proctosigmoiditis, and to obtain biopsies. Careful sigmoidoscopy is safe in patients with severe disease. The inflammatory changes are nearly always more severe distally, and range from mild (erythema, loss of vascular pattern and granularity), to moderate (friability, petechiae, nonconfluent ulcerations), or severe (confluent ulcerations, mucopus, spontaneous hemorrhage). Additional findings may include the presence of postinflammatory pseudopolyps.

Mucosal biopsies reflect the diffuse, continuous, superficial inflammation with acute and chronic inflammatory cells, cryptitis, and crypt abscesses. These changes are nonspecific and may be difficult to distinguish from changes secondary to infection. In contrast, distortion of intestinal crypts (irregular, elongated, or branched crypts) is a hallmark of idiopathic IBD and persists, not only in active UC (or CD) but also in quiescent UC. The diffuse, superficial mucosal changes in UC differentiate it from CD, where focal and transmural inflammation is more common. The colonic mucosa proximal to the demarcating margin of colitis is normal.

DIFFERENTIAL DIAGNOSIS

When a patient presents with chronic diarrhea or rectal bleeding, lower endoscopy helps differentiate between colitis and other colonic sources of bleeding, such as hemorrhoids and other anorectal pathology, large polyps, carcinoma, diverticular disease, and arteriovenous malformations. In the presence of rectal bleeding, microscopic colitis and irritable bowel syndrome (IBS) should not be part of the differential.

The most important considerations in the differential diagnosis of endoscopically verified colitis are, in addition to UC, CD, the infectious colitides, colitis related to NSAIDs, ischemia, and radiation injury (Table 4). In the general North American and European populations, exposure to NSAIDs is extremely common, is probably underdiagnosed, and accounts for a larger proportion of colitis than idiopathic IBD.

Most cases of acute colitis represent infection, and not IBD. Infectious colitis usually has an abrupt onset and colonic biopsies do not reveal crypt distortion. In *C. difficile* colitis, there is frequently history of antibiotic use or nosocomial exposure, and sigmoidoscopy may reveal pseudomembranes (yellowish plaques). *E.coli* O157:H7 can cause segmental colitis (mimicking ischemia) and, less frequently, diffuse colitis. Amebiasis should be suspected in patients who have traveled to endemic areas or engage in homosexual intercourse. In severe colitis, exclusion of amebiasis by serology, stool studies and/or biopsies, is extremely important, as treatment with steroids may lead to systemic amebiasis.

Ischemia and radiation injury should be suspected in the appropriate clinical setting. Ischemic colitis is seen in elderly patients with vascular disease, where endoscopy reveals patchy erythema, submucosal edema, and hemorrhage (corresponding to the "thumbprinting" seen radiographically), and, in more severe cases, ulcerations. The changes are segmental, occurring in watershed areas (splenic flexure and rectosigmoid junction), and rectal involvement is unusual. Radiation injury can occur acutely or years after the radiation treatment, and most commonly affects the rectosigmoid with characteristic telangiectatic vessels. Moreover, the terms ischemic "colitis" and radiation "colitis" are misnomers: in both conditions, biopsies do not reveal inflammation but, rather, vascular lesions.

It must be remembered that enteric infections, aspirin, and NSAIDs, can sometimes "trigger" the onset of IBD, or expose preexisting but silent IBD. Even in the patient with an established diagnosis of UC, any exacerbation of symptoms does not necessarily imply an UC flare. An intercurrent infection, medications (aspirin, NSAIDs, and even mesalamine) or an exacerbation of underlying IBS, can all mimic the symptoms and mucosal changes of UC. Frequently, the patient develops stereotypical symptoms with each flare. Careful evaluation is nevertheless necessary in order to determine the exact cause of the symptoms and institute appropriate treatment.

Table 4
Differential Diagnosis of Ulcerative Colitis or Crohn's Colitis

Proctitis (distal 15 cm)	Herpes simplex virus
	Lymphogranuloma venereum (LGV)
	Non-LGV Chlamydia trachomatis
	Syphilis
	Gonorrhea
	Lymphoid follicular proctitis
	Solitary Rectal Ulcer Syndrome
	Chemical injury (enemas, suppositories)
Proctosigmoiditis (inflammation extending above 15 cm)	Entamoeba histolytica
	Shigella
	Campylobacter jejuni
	Salmonella (in AIDS)
	LGV
	Radiation
	Protein allergy (in infants)
Colitis	Infectious colitis

	Bacterial	Mycobacterial
	Campylobacter jejuni	*M. tuberculosis*
	Salmonellosis	Viral
	Shigella	Cytomegalovirus
	Yersinia enterocolitica	Fungal
	E. coli	Histoplasmosis
	C. difficile	Parasitic
	Aeromonas hydrophila	*Entamoeba histolytica*
	Pleisiomonas shigelloides	*Schistosomiasis*

Crohn's colitis
Diverticulitis
Drug-induced (NSAIDs, gold, penicillamine)
Ischemic colitis
Radiation colitis
Vasculitis

CROHN'S DISEASE
Clinical Presentation

HISTORY

The predisposing factors are the same for UC and CD, with the exception of family history and cigarette exposure. There is a greater concordance within families for CD than UC, and adults with CD are far more likely to be cigarette smokers than patients with UC or the general public. In addition, the onset of CD is often more insidious and chronic than the symptomatic onset of UC.

SYMPTOMS

CD can affect the entire gastrointestinal tract, from mouth to anus, and presents with varied disease patterns according to the location and pattern of gastrointestinal tract inflammation.

Patients with *inflammatory* CD (mucosal inflammation without stricturing, abscess, or fistula) present with more systemic symptoms including fever, anorexia, and weight loss, as well as symptoms that depend on disease location along the gastrointestinal tract. Ileitis presents with right lower quadrant abdominal pain and diarrhea. Patients with ileocolitis or colitis tend to present with rectal bleeding and diarrhea. Weight loss, fevers, night sweats, arthralgias, and fatigue are common. Nocturnal diarrhea discriminates inflammatory disease from IBS.

Fibrostenotic CD causes more postprandial abdominal pain, distension, nausea, and vomiting that may present as intestinal obstruction. Sudden or complete intestinal obstruction is more characteristic of adhesions (related to prior surgeries), food impaction as a result of dietary indiscretion, and malignancy. Diarrhea secondary to small bowel bacterial overgrowth can also occur in the setting of chronic intestinal strictures.

Fistulizing CD represents an aggressive, transmural disease pattern, in which fistulae originating in the bowel penetrate the bowel wall to reach adjacent organs. Perianal abscesses or fistulae are most common. The bladder (resulting in pneumaturia and fecaluria), vagina (in women who have undergone hysterectomy, and resulting in dyspareunia and painful vaginal discharge), adjacent bowel (mostly asymptomatic), skin (with discharge at surgical scars and the umbilicus), and retroperitoneum (resulting in a psoas abscess, manifested by back pain and a new limp) may also be involved. A walled-off perforation results in abscess; free perforation with peritonitis is less common.

There are several, and often, coexistent mechanistic causes of diarrhea in CD. The most common cause is intestinal inflammation and is manifest by the presence of fecal leukocytes. Malabsorption may be caused by loss of healthy small bowel mucosal absorptive surface as a result of disease or surgical resections. With disease or resection of less than 100 cm of terminal ileum, bilt salts are poorly absorbed, enter the colon and cause a secretory diarrhea (choleretic diarrhea). Disease or resection of >100 cm of terminal ileum leads to bile salt deficiency and steatorrhea. In addition, small bowel bacterial overgrowth (with strictures or enteroenteric fistulas), rapid transit (with bowel resection or fistulas), medications (including NSAIDs), and dietary intake (poorly absorbable carbohydrates, excessive dietary fat) can all contribute to diarrhea. Weight loss reflects anorexia, malabsorption, and sitophobia. Coexistent IBS symptoms are not uncommon and are excluded by the presence of documented inflammation or malabsorption.

In children and adolescents, systemic symptoms including fever of unknown origin, anemia, arthritis, and/or delay of growth and sexual maturation often predominate over bowel-related findings.

In contrast to UC, smoking has a harmful effect on the course of CD, leading to disease exacerbations, refractoriness to medical therapy, and earlier postoperative recurrence *(3)*. As with UC, enteric infections and NSAIDs can precipitate CD flares.

In CD, as in UC, increased gastrointestinal symptoms are associated with the menstrual cycle *(8)*, and the activity of CD during pregnancy correlates with disease activity at conception *(9)*.

The clinician should elicit any history of complications of CD (see later), extra-intestinal manifestations (see later and Table 2), relation of disease to the menstrual cycle and pregnancy, adverse effects of medical therapy (Table 3), use of aspirin and NSAIDs, smoking history, and family history of IBD.

PHYSICAL EXAMINATION

The physical examination is often more revealing in CD than UC reflecting the transmural nature of the inflammatory process. Similar to UC the physical examination contributes to the assessment of disease severity and complications, including evidence of systemic toxicity, dehydration, anemia, malnutrition, and malabsorption. The abdominal examination may reveal an inflammatory mass, most often in the right lower quadrant, that represents thickening of the mesentery adjacent to inflamed ileocecal region. The abdomen is more often tender in CD than UC because of the transmural inflammation extending to the serosa. Examination of the abdomen is essential to assess for peritoneal signs or evidence of bowel obstruction. The psoas sign, in which extension of the right hip exacerbates pain in the right lower quadrant, indicates a localized ileal perforation extending to the retroperitoneum. Perianal examination is crucial to identify subtle changes of inflammatory skin tags that can be quite large ("elephant ears"), strictures within the anal canal or fistulae. Any of these findings differentiate CD from UC.

Patients with CD are more likely to develop clubbing of the fingers, particularly with more extensive small bowel disease. Oral aphthous ulcers are common in CD and are not expected in UC. In addition, cutaneous complications of vitamin or mineral deficiency include skin rashes or cheilosis. Osteoporosis is not rare at the time of CD diagnosis, but is usually not clinically apparent without more sophisticated diagnostic testing. Other signs of extraintestinal involvement (Table 2) or complications from therapy (Table 3) are similar to those in UC.

COMPLICATIONS AND EXTRAINTESTINAL MANIFESTATIONS

The most common complications of CD are related to malabsorption or intestinal bleeding. Anemia can be due to acute or chronic bleeding, or malabsorption of iron, vitamin B_{12}, or folic acid (according to the site of intestinal inflammation or resection). Fat malabsorption can result in hypocalcemia, metabolic bone disease, clotting abnormalities, and enteric hyperoxaluria. In the latter condition, malabsorbed fatty acids bind luminal calcium, which would otherwise bind to oxalate, leaving excessive free oxalate that is hyperabsorbed in the colon and excreted excessively in the urine as calcium oxalate.

An additional complication involving the urinary tract includes ureteral obstruction secondary to an inflammatory mass compressing the ureter and causing hydronephrosis. CD patients are also more susceptible to gallstones secondary to bile salt depletion in the setting of ileal disease or resection.

In both CD and UC, there is an increased risk of thromboembolic complications. Longstanding CD can be complicated by amyloidosis.

Extraintestinal manifestations of CD are listed in Table 2. Erythema nodosum and aphthous stomatitis are more common in CD than in UC.

Similar to UC, CD may be complicated by adenocarcinoma correlating with disease duration and anatomic extent. The risk extends, however, to involve the small intestine as well as the colon. Unfortunately, because of colonic strictures and the inaccessibility to the small bowel, surveillance recommendations are not as well established for CD. Additionally, there is an increased risk of intestinal and extraintestinal lymphoma, and squamous cancer of the anus and vulva.

DIAGNOSIS

Similar to UC, the diagnosis of CD is based upon a composite of clinical presentation, imaging studies (endoscopy and radiography), and histology.

The laboratory features of CD are nonspecific and reflect the severity of inflammation (i.e., increased erythrocyte sedimentation rate, leukocytosis with "left shift"), complications of diarrhea (electrolyte disturbances) or malabsorption, and anatomic complications such as strictures, abscesses or fistulae. A positive serologic test for ASCA is highly specific, but not sensitive, for CD.

In contrast to UC, radiographic studies are more commonly employed to assess the small intestine or complications related to extraluminal disease (fistula, abscess, or abdominal mass). Barium studies (small bowel series or enteroclysis) are useful in determining the nature, location, and extent of inflammatory changes or strictures, and in evaluating for obstruction or the presence of fistulizing disease. Skip lesions, aphthous ulcers, cobblestoning, and stellate sinus tracts are characteristic. Air-contrast barium enemas are also important for the assessment of potential colonic CD as the rectum may be spared at the initial proctoscopic or sigmoidoscopic exam. In addition, strictures in CD commonly prevent complete colonoscopic assessment of the colon.

Colonoscopy is useful in detecting colitis and ileitis, identifying strictures, and obtaining biopsies. Involvement is typically focal (segmental), with skip lesions and areas of normal intervening bowel. CD most often affects the ileocecal region and spares the rectum. Endoscopic findings range in severity from mild (erythema, friability, aphthoid erosions), to moderate (small or superficial ulcerations), to severe (deep, excavated ulcers, with a serpiginous or linear configuration). The mucosa surrounding the ulcers is normal in appearance, in contrast to UC where the surrounding mucosa is inflamed. Cobblestoning, a nodular mucosal pattern, usually caused by the interplay of parallel and transverse ulcerations, is characteristic of CD. Additional findings may include strictures, fistulae, and pseudopolyps. The ileocecal valve may be friable, ulcerated, fibrotic or stenotic. Findings in the ileum are similar to those in the colon.

Biopsies demonstrate inflammation in the mucosa, submucosa and muscularis propria, crypt distortion with foci of cryptitis and crypt abscesses, prominent lymphoid aggregates, and, occasionally, noncaseating granulomas (seen in approx 20% of patients). Crypt distortion favors IBD, and microscopic focality, submucosal inflammation or lymphoid aggregates, and granulomas favor CD.

Computed tomography of the abdomen and pelvis detects inflammatory masses and abscesses, and is useful in assessing perirectal involvement. Abdominal ultrasonography can assess bowel wall thickness (increased in CD) and MRI can be employed to visualize perianal fistulizing complications.

DIFFERENTIAL DIAGNOSIS

The differential diagnosis of CD depends upon the presentation and complications. The presentation of acute lower abdominal pain (usually right lower quadrant) requires consideration of diseases in organs adjacent to the ileum, including appendicitis, appendiceal abscess, cecal diverticulitis, tuboovarian abscess, pelvic inflammatory disease, endometriosis, and ovarian cysts and tumors. Other processes can

Table 5
Differential Diganosis of Crohn's Ileitis or Ileocolitis

Infectious
   ◆ Bacterial
     Salmonellosis
     Vibrio parahemolyticus
     Yersinia enterocolitica
   ◆ Mycobacterial
     M. tuberculosis
     M. avium intracellulare
   ◆ Parasitic
     Entamoeba histolytica
   ◆ Viral
     Cytomegalovirus
Drug-induced (NSAIDs)
Eosinophilic gastroenteritis
Lymphoma
Radiation enteritis
Ulcerative jejunoileitis
Vasculitis

directly involve the ileum and may mimic Crohn's ileitis: cecal carcinoma spreading proximally to the ileum, ileal carcinoid or lymphoma, metastatic cancer, vasculitis, radiation enteritis, intestinal infection (predominantly ileocecal tuberculosis, amebiasis, and Yersinia enterocolitis), ulcerative jejunoileitis (a refractory variant of celiac disease), and infiltrative disorders (eosinophilic gastroenteritis and amyloidosis). The differential diagnosis of endoscopically documented ileitis is presented in Table 5.

   In most circumstances, CD of the colon can be readily distinguished from UC. Features that point to CD include small bowel involvement, perianal disease, rectal sparing, fistulae, lack of rectal bleeding, focal, segmental or asymmentric colitis, and, on histology, microscopic focality and granulomas. In indeterminate colitis, the clinical, endoscopic and histologic features do not allow the differentiation between CD of the colon and UC, and the newer serologic tests (pANCA and ASCA) have not proven helpful in that regard. Ischemic colitis, diverticulitis, tuberculous colitis and amebiasis can cause a segmental colitis, mimicking CD. Again, intestinal ulceration secondary to NSAIDs must be considered as a mimicking or complicating factor.

SUMMARY

UC and CD are relatively uncommon disorders and can present with classic or nonspecific features. In every case, however, a systematic evaluation, consisting of a thorough history (including medication, smoking and family history), detailed physical examination (with attention to possible extraintestinal manifestations and complications), endoscopy with histology, and selective microbiologic and radiographic tests, can exclude alternative disorders and incriminate IBD as the culprit. Assessment of disease severity, location, and extent is critical in formulating the therapeutic plan.

REFERENCES

1. Fiocchi C. Inflammatory bowel disease: etiology and pathogenesis. Gastroenterology 1998;115(1):182–205.
2. Hanauer SB. Review Articles: Drug Therapy: Inflammatory bowel disease. N Engl J Med 1996;334(13):841–848.
3. Thomas GA, Rhodes J, Green JT. Inflammatory bowel disease and smoking—a review. Am J Gastroenterol 1998;93(2):144–149.
4. Bjarnason I, Hayllar J, MacPherson AJ, Russell AS. Side effects of nonsteroidal anti-inflammatory drugs on the small and large intestine in humans. Gastroenterology 1993;104(6):1832–1847.
5. Miner PB, Jr. Factors influencing the relapse of patients with inflammatory bowel disease. Am J Gastroenterol 1997;92(12 Suppl):1S–4S.
6. Koutroubakis I, Manousos ON, Meuwissen SG, Pena AS. Environmental risk factors in inflammatory bowel disease. Hepatogastroenterology 1996;43(8): 381–393.
7. Fraga XF, Vergara M, Medina C, Casellas F, Bermejo B, Malagelada JR. Effects of smoking on the presentation and clinical course of inflammatory bowel disease. Eur J Gastroenterol Hepatol 1997;9(7):683–687.
8. Kane SV, Sable K, Hanauer SB. The menstrual cycle and its effect on inflammatory bowel disease and irritable bowel syndrome: a prevalence study. Am J Gastroenterol 1998;93(10):1867–1872.
9. Korelitz BI. Inflammatory bowel disease and pregnancy. Gastroenterol Clin North Am 1998;27(1):213–24.
10. Truelove SC, Witts LJ. Cortisone in ulcerative colitis. Final report on a therapeutic trial. British Medical Journal 1955;4947:1041–1048.
11. Sheth SG, LaMont JT. Toxic megacolon. Lancet 1998;351(9101):509–513.
12. Kornbluth A, Sachar DB. Ulcerative colitis practice guidelines in adults. American College of Gastroenterology, Practice Parameters Committee. Am J Gastroenterol 1997;92(2):204–211.
13. MacDermott RP. Lack of current clinical value of serological testing in the evaluation of patients with IBD. Inflamm Bowel Dis 1999;5(1):64–65.

6 Radiological Findings in Inflammatory Bowel Disease

Peter M. MacEneaney, FRCR
and Arunas E. Gasparaitis, MD

INTRODUCTION

Radiology has evolved dramatically since the 1950s. At that time, plain film radiography and single-contrast barium studies were the only imaging techniques available. In the 1960s, two developments occurred that gave rise to the subspecialty of gastrointestinal radiology; the introduction of image intensifiers and of double-contrast techniques. The images produced redefined the radiological diagnosis of diseases of the gastrointestinal (GI) tract *(1)*. Double-contrast examinations are now the primary radiological modalities used in the investigation of inflammatory bowel disease (IBD).

In the 1980s, ultrasound (US), computerized tomography (CT), and magnetic resonance imaging (MRI) advanced, and over the next decade, became widely available. Initially, these were used more to identify complications of IBD and to stage-associated malignancies, rather than in the primary diagnosis of IBD. More recently, however, both CT and MRI have been combined with enteroclysis. These com-

From: *Clinical Gastroenterology:*
Inflammatory Bowel Disease: Diagnosis and Therapeutics
Edited by: R. D. Cohen © Humana Press Inc., Totowa, NJ

bined procedures are promising as they have the potential to anatomically delineate the extent of disease and, simultaneously, assess disease activity. Activity may also be assessed by various nuclear medicine scans. This chapter will discuss each imaging modality with respect to its role in assessing the extent, activity, and local complications of IBD.

RADIOLOGICAL FINDINGS AND COMPLICATIONS
Crohn's Disease

Crohn's disease (CD) is a transmural inflammatory process and is characterized by discontinuous and asymmetric involvement of the GI tract. Any location from mouth to anus may be involved, though the colon and terminal ileum are the most common sites. The patient's clinical condition does not always correlate well with radiological findings. Early disease begins in the submucosa and is characterized by lymphoid hyperplasia and mild lymphedema. This causes symmetric thickening of the valvulae conniventes. Shallow ulcerations develop in the affected segments. These 'apthous ulcers' are usually less than 5 mm in diameter and are surrounded by a rim of edema. Ulcerations typically occur on the mesenteric border of the small bowel. As the disease progresses, all layers of the bowel wall become inflamed. Mucosal features are obliterated by increasing edema and infiltrate. Apthous ulcers may extend through the submucosa to produce deep rose thorn ulcers, or they may undermine the mucosa to produce collar button ulcers. Both are typical of CD (Fig. 1).

In advanced disease, deep intersecting fissure ulcers are typical. These fissures separate islands of relatively normal mucosa. These islands are termed pseudopolyps. The net result is a "cobblestone pattern" of advanced CD seen on barium studies.

The bowel wall is thickened as inflammation and fibrosis extend through all its layers. The bowel wall is not directly visualized on small bowel serves (SBS) and enteroclysis. Rather, its thickness is inferred by measuring the separation of adjacent intraluminal barium columns. Fibrosis eventually causes strictures, which are a hallmark of advanced CD. Strictures are seen on barium studies as persistent areas of intestinal narrowing and shortening and may cause intestinal obstruction. They occur in 21% of cases of small bowel CD and are relatively rare in the colon (8%) (2). Enteroclysis is superior to SBS in identification and assessment of strictures by virtue of the pressure under which the barium is infused (vide infra). This serves to distend areas of spasm and so differentiates spasm from true fibrous strictures.

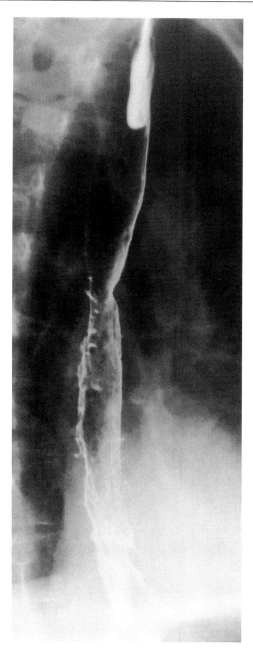

Fig. 1. Double contrast barium esophogram demonstrating multiple "rose thorn" ulcers typical of Crohn's disease.

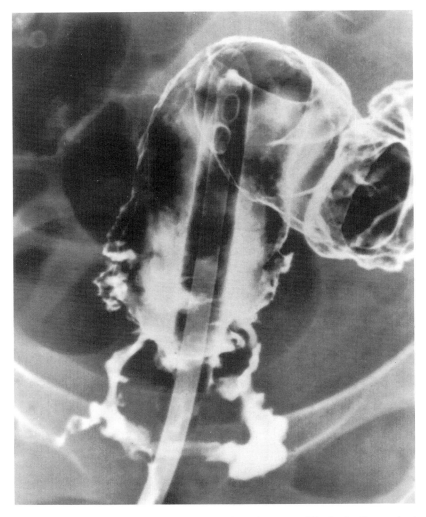

Fig. 2. Lower GI barium study demonstrating changes of Crohn's disease in the rectum. There is mucosal irregularity and ulceration. Two complex fistulas are opacified by barium.

Sinuses and fistulas occur in CD as a result of the transmural nature of inflammation and ulceration. Crohn's fistulae may arise at any point in the gastrointestinal tract and terminate in unusual locations. Ileo-cecal and entero-enteric fistulae are most common, though ileo-uterine, colo-bronchial, and colo-splenic fistulas have been reported *(3–7)*. Fistulas are better demonstrated on barium studies than endoscopy (Fig. 2). Sometimes the fistula is not opacified and secondary findings, such as

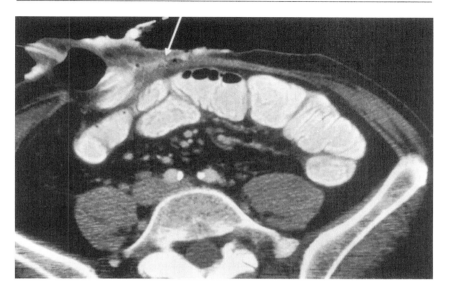

Fig. 3. CT enteroclysis examination demonstrating an enterocutaneous fistula (*arrow*) opacified by contrast at the site of an ileostomy.

air in the bladder, may help. CT and MRI are also valuable as they can better define the path of a fistula or sinus (Fig. 3).

MRI and US are established techniques for investigation of perianal fistulas. Inflammatory collections (phlegmons), abscesses, and lymphadenopathy are frequent additional findings in CD. These are best assessed by MRI or CT.

CD increases the risk of small bowel carcinoma *(8)*. These may arise in the bowel or in a fistula. Preoperative diagnosis may be very difficult as the bowel architecture is abnormal secondary to CD and the carcinomas have atypical features.

Ulcerative Colitis

In early acute ulcerative colitis (UC) mucosal edema and altered colonic mucus result in the appearance of mucosal granularity on double-contrast barium enema *(9,10)*. As the disease progresses, mucosal erosions and frank ulcerations develop. Ulcers extend through to the submucosa and undermine adjacent mucosa. This pattern is evident on barium studies as a collar-button ulcer. These enlarge and coalesce and cause large areas of colonic ulceration. Residual islands of mucosa are seen as 'pseudopolyps. In chronic disease, the colon is shortened and haustral folds are lost (Fig. 4). The mucosa is nodular and coarse.

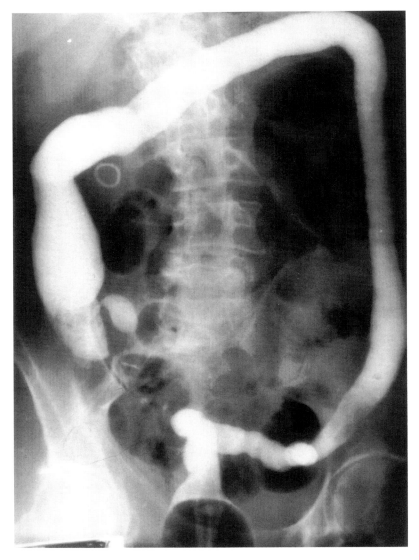

Fig. 4. Single-contrast lower GI study demonstrating a shortened featureless "lead pipe" colon typical of chronic UC. The whole colon is involved in this case.

In 15% to 20% of cases of pancolitis, the terminal ileum appears abnormal on barium studies and is termed backwash ileitis *(10)*. This is easily differentiated from CD in most cases.

The constant need to regenerate mucosa in UC leads to dysplasia and carcinoma. Colonic dysplasia is best diagnosed endoscopically, though it may be diagnosed on double-contrast barium studies in up to two-thirds of cases *(10)*. Carcinomas associated with UC are usually 'apple core lesions'; however, infiltrating tumors are more frequent in UC patients than in the general population *(10)*. Therefore, colonoscopy and biopsy are needed when any flattened, rigid, or strictured area is identified radiographically *(10)*.

DIFFERENTIAL DIAGNOSIS

UC differs in two fundamental ways from CD. The first is in the anatomic distribution of disease. UC almost always extends from the anorectal junction proximally and continuously to involve a length of colon, whereas CD can occur at any location in the GI tract and give rise to multiple discrete lesions (skip lesions). Crohn's disease usually spares the rectum.

The second difference between CD and UC is the depth of bowel wall involvement. Ulcerative colitis is limited to the mucosa and submucosa, whereas in CD, inflammation is transmural. Consequently, the degree of bowel wall thickening is greater in CD than UC, and fistulas, inflammatory collections, and fibro-fatty proliferation are not seen in UC (Fig. 5). The presence of a fistula in UC is strongly suggestive of a carcinoma.

IMAGING TECHNIQUES
Plain Radiography

Plain films are used in many settings in IBD. One is to assess for bowel obstruction. Gastric, small bowel, and/ or large bowel obstruction may be seen in CD, and large bowel obstruction in UC. Another is to assess for the presence and severity of colonic disease in either ulcerative or Crohn's colitis. Evidence of colitis may be seen, with "thumb printing" of the edematous mucosal lining. Severe colitis may result in the development of a megacolon, intramural air in the bowel wall, or even frank perforation, as evidenced by the finding of "free air." Sometimes a paucity of air may be reflective of severe colitis, or the apparent shifting of small bowel away from a region of the abdomen suspicious for phlegmon, abscess, or other mass effect. However, it is difficult to accurately assess the presence of less severe disease activity without the aid of a contrast study.

Plain film radiography also plays a role in the evaluation of common complications of inflammatory bowel disease, such as kidney stones, gallstones, sacroileitis, and even may suggest bone density loss and osteoporosis, as evidenced by demineralization of the pelvis or hips.

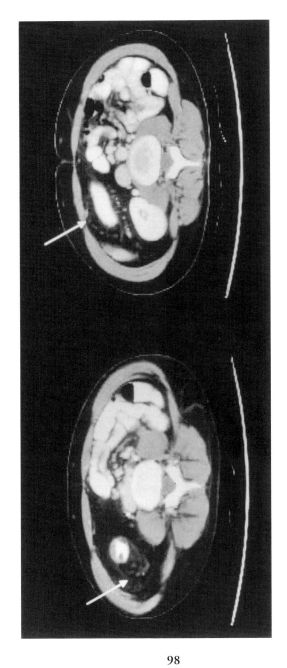

Fig. 5. Two nonsequential images from a CT study showing fibrofatty proliferation around the ascending and transverse colon typical of CD.

Barium Studies

Several varieties of small bowel contrast study exist. These primarily image the mucosa, and can, by inference, assess wall thickness. The oldest stems from the era of single-contrast exams of the stomach when one barium compound was used to investigate the stomach and small bowel. Barium compounds are now more sophisticated and those used for double-contrast exams of the stomach are not suitable for follow-through studies. Indeed, the upper GI and small bowel follow-through (UGI-SBFT) has been abandoned in most institutions. The choice for small bowel radiology currently lies between enteroclysis and a conventional small bowel series with or without peroral pneumocolon.

In a small bowel series, the patient drinks a relatively dense barium solution that passes through the bowel by peristalsis. Images are taken intermittently during transit. Peristalsis is occasionally augmented by properistaltic agents such as metoclopromide. This technique has two drawbacks. Multiple overlapping barium filled loops of small bowel can obscure pathology and the radiologist cannot sufficiently influence transit of contrast and so cannot distend the bowel to differentiate true bowel wall thickening from spasm.

The more accurate technique is enteroclysis *(11)*. Enteroclysis involves passing a catheter to the jejunum (beyond the Ligament of Treitz) and infusing contrast material through the small bowel. At the University of Chicago, we use a small volume of medium-density barium (positive contrast), and follow this with a solution of methylcellulose (negative contrast). This gives a double-contrast effect, which minimizes the problem of multiple overlapping loops of small bowel. The infusion of contrast material has the advantage of actively distending or stressing the small bowel and so helps differentiate inflammatory strictures from spasm. Exquisite mucosal detail can be obtained, hence, this is the ideal modality (allowing for its invasive nature) to identify early changes of small bowel CD. This is important because a delay of 2–4 yr is typical before a diagnosis of small bowel CD is made *(12)*. Enteroclysis has been recommended in the following situations *(13)*.

1. To demonstrate the early changes of CD and exclude small bowel disease.
2. To depict the full extent of involvement and to identify skip lesions.
3. To determine the cause of clinical deterioration in previously stable CD.
4. To distinguish between spasm, active stenotic disease, and fibrous strictures.
5. To investigate post-operative complications of CD.

In summary, the two main advantages enteroclysis has over small bowel series are increased mucosal detail afforded by a double-contrast exam, and the luminal distention achieved infusion of contrast, resulting in the improved accuracy of enteroclysis.

CT and CT enteroclysis (see later) are being used with increasing frequency for many of the indications aforementioned. Enteroclysis remains the primary modality for detection of early changes of disease.

The small bowel series with peroral pneumocolon involves taking barium orally and, when it reaches the terminal ileum, to insufflate air per rectum. This achieves a double-contrast (air / barium) examination of the terminal ileum, the primary site of small bowel CD. It is successful in more than 80% of cases *(14)*. It is particularly useful in post- surgical patients to investigate for disease recurrence in the neoterminal ileum. It is easier to get the double-contrast effect in these cases as there is no ileo-cecal value to resist retrograde flow of air. Standard small bowel series, without peroral pneumocolon, are adequate to follow-up known cases of CD.

The colon, like the small bowel, may be investigated using single- or double-contrast (barium–air) techniques. Double-contrast barium enema is preferred for demonstrating mucosal detail, whereas single-contrast exams are reserved for those who cannot tolerate a double-contrast study. Air-contrast barium enemas are relatively contraindicated in patients with severe colitis as the procedure may precipitate toxic megacolon or perforation.

Computerized Tomography

Computerized axial tomography ("CAT" or "CT" scan) has an intrinsic advantage over barium studies in that CT directly images the bowel wall and the extraintestinal complications of IBD. CT consequently plays a larger role in CD than in UC where inflammation is not classically transmural. CT is the examination of choice in suspected abscess formation and phlegmon. CT also demonstrates fistulas. Distal complications such as sclerosing cholangitis, urinary tract calculi, sacroilietis, and gallstones may also be identified. However, CT cannot equal the resolution of double-contrast barium studies. Accordingly, CT has a relatively poor yield in the setting of early mucosal disease. Therefore, CT and enteroclysis are often both performed to fully evaluate a new case of CD.

Recently, CT and enteroclysis have been combined into a single study: CT enteroclysis *(15,16)*. The jejunum is intubated and very dilute contrast is infused (2–3% barium solution). When contrast reaches the cecum, an intravenous (iv) contrast-enhanced CT study is performed. This has the advantage of thorough assessment of both luminal and extraintestinal disease. Multiplanar reconstructions of the CT data are helpful *(17)*. CT enteroclysis has not been fully validated in comparative trials, but is being used with increasing frequency in patients with known disease suffering an exacerbation, and in preoperative assessment. Standard enteroclysis is still preferred to establish in early CD.

CT, when performed with iv contrast, can estimate disease activity. Bowel wall enhancement can be assessed as a marker of active inflammation. A target appearance is seen in acute inflammation where the inner mucosa and outer muscularis and serosa enhance avidly and have the appearance of a target on cross section *(18)*.

MRI

The lungs and the bowel are the only organs not routinely imaged by MRI. Slow image acquisition allows time for movement artifact from respiratory motion and peristalsis. The presence of luminal air also causes susceptibility artifacts. However, rapid pulse sequences have been developed and now the abdomen can be imaged during a single breath hold, thereby removing respiratory motion. Some centers routinely administer glucagon to temporarily suspend peristalsis. Contrast agents are now available to opacify the GI tract *(19–21)*. These advances have made MRI of the bowel a reality. Now the excellent tissue characterization properties of MRI can be applied to the bowel.

MRI of the small bowel has been successfully employed in the investigation of small bowel CD disease *(22,23)*. Enhancement of the bowel wall by iv gadolinium and signal characteristics of the bowel wall and fibro-fatty proliferation on T2 weighted images were found to correlate well with disease activity *(23)*. This ability to noninvasively monitor the activity of CD within the small bowel represents a potentially powerful tool in following CD patients and an exciting surrogate end-point for clinical trials of therapeutic agents *(24)*. An additional benefit of MRI is the absence of ionizing radiation. The trials reported earlier *(22,23)* were performed without jejunal intubation. MRI enteroclysis has also been reported *(25,26)*. Complications such as fistulas and abscesses are readily identified. The roles of these new techniques in small bowel and colon imaging are yet to be defined, however, MRI is recognized as the likely future of bowel imaging *(27)*.

MRI is used extensively in the assessment of fistulous perianal CD *(28–33)*. Its accuracy for fistula-in-ano with surgical correlation is reported as 86% *(33)*. MRI using fat suppressed T1 weighted gadolinium enhanced sequences, or fat suppressed T2 weighted sequences are both effective in this setting *(31)*.

US

Transabdominal US, is an adjunctive imaging modality in IBD. It is useful in children and thin patients where there is relatively little body

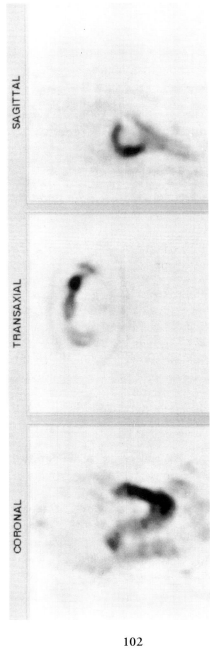

Fig. 6. PET scan of a patient with UC demonstrating abnormally increased activity throughout the colon. (Images courtesy of Dr. S. Skehan, St. Vincent's University Hospital, Dublin, Ireland).

wall fat to attenuate the ultrasound beam. Ultrasound has been used successfully to image the terminal ileum—the primary site of small bowel CD. Features such as wall thickening, fibro-fatty infiltration of the mesentery are readily identified in experienced hands. Doppler ultrasound can be used to assess vascularity of the bowel wall and mesentery, however, there is no consensus on the ability of Doppler ultrasound to differentiate active from inactive disease *(34)*.

In UC, transabdominal US may be used to evaluate colon wall thickening and may be useful in monitoring extension of disease. The degree of wall thickening, as evaluated by US, has been shown to correlate with the clinical, biochemical, and endoscopic activity of ulcerative colitis, both before and after treatment *(35)*. This suggests that ultrasound may be useful to evaluate the response of UC patients to medical therapy. However, of all the techniques described that address disease activity, US is the most operator-dependent and may not prove to be as reproducible as CT.

Trans-anal ultrasound is used in the setting of perianal CD where it accurately images fistulae, their relationship to the sphincter complex, and related abscesses *(36)*. Whether trans-anal ultrasound or MRI is used to assess complex fistulas depends on local availability and expertise.

Scintigraphy

Labeled white cell scanning is an adjunctive modality in assessment of IBD. Indium tropolonate and technetium HMPAO are the radioisotopes most frequently used, though because of radiation dose, image quality and availability technetium is preferred to indium *(37)*.

After harvesting and separating white cells from the patient, they are labeled and reintroduced to the circulation. They migrate to areas of inflammation and are then shed into the lumen of the bowel *(37)*. Areas of inflammation show abnormally increased activity on imaging. A trial assessing scintigraphy in a population of patients with CD and irritable bowel syndrome (IBS) reported sensitivity and specificity of 69% and 80%, respectively *(38)*. Better results have been reported in pediatric populations with active disease *(39,40)*.

These scintigraphic studies primarily image inflammation. Any cause of bowel inflammation may cause abnormally high activity on scintigraphic studies and so generate false-positive results. Conversely, quiescent disease may yield false-negative results. The degree of activity demonstrated on scintigraphic studies correlates weakly with the CD activity index and sedimentation rate *(41)*.

Positron emission tomography (PET) scanning is a form of metabolic imaging mainly used in oncology, although it may have a role in inflammatory bowel disease in the future *(42)* (Fig. 6).

SUMMARY

The vast array of imaging techniques available to today's physicians allows for "customization" of radiographic imaging for particular inflammatory bowel patients. Although standard radiographs are used to provide an initial "gestalt" in the evaluation of a patient with unknown or acute disease, contrast-based studies are invaluable in providing more details, especially in the evaluation of strictures, and of the small bowel (an area "out of the reach" of traditional endoscopy). More in-depth studies of the bowel wall and its environs or areas involved with fistulas by CT, MRI, or US provide a unique perspective, and radionucleotide studies may be helpful in locating areas of inflammation not seen by other approaches. New techniques combining technologies with CT or MRI and enteroclysis have provided stunning new insights into the evaluation of these elusive diseases, and will likely become more readily practiced and available in the future.

REFERENCES

1. Goldberg HI, Margulis AR. Gastrointestinal radiology in the United States: An overview of the past 50 years. Radiology 2000;216:1–7.
2. Bartram C, Laufer I. Inflammatory bowel disease., in: Double Contrast Intestinal Radiology. 2nd ed. Raven, New York, 1992;580–645.
3. Steinberg DM, Cooke WT, Alexander-Williams J. Abscess and fistulae in Crohn's disease. Gut 1973;14:865–869.
4. Wulfeck D, Williams T, Amin A, Huang TY. Crohn's disease with unusual enterouterine fistula in pregnancy. J Ky Med Assoc 1994;92:267–269.
5. Rowell DL, Longstreth GF. Colosplenic fistula and splenic abscess complicating Crohn's colitis. J Clin Gastroenterol 1995;21:74–75.
6. Mera A, Sugimoto M, Fukuda K, Tanaka F, Imamura F, Matsuda M, et al. Crohn's disease associated with colo-bronchial fistula. Intern Med 1996;35:957–960.
7. Karmy-Jones R, Chagpar A, Vallieres E, Hamilton S. Colobronchial fistula due to Crohn's disease. Ann Thorac Surg 1995;60:446–448.
8. Senay E, Sachar DB, Keohane M, Greenstein AJ. Small bowel carcinoma in Crohn's disease. Distinguishing features and risk factors. Cancer 1989;63:360–363.
9. Laufer I. The radiologic demonstration of early changes in ulcerative colitis by double contrast technique. J Can Assoc Radiol 1975;26:116–121.
10. Scotiniotis I, Rubesin SE, Ginsberg GG. Imaging modalities in inflammatory bowel disease. Gastroenterol Clin North Am 1999;28:391–421,ix.
11. Ekberg O. Crohn's disease of the small bowel examined by double contrast technique: a comparison with oral technique. Gastrointest Radiol 1977;1:355–359.
12. Steinhardt HJ, Loeschke K, Kasper H, Holtermuller KH, Schafer H. European Cooperative Crohn's Disease Study (ECCDS): clinical features and natural history. Digestion 1985;31:97–108.
13. Herlinger H, Caroline DF, Crohns disease of the small bowel, in: Textbook of Gastrointestinal Radiology. 2nd ed., W B Saunders, Philadelphia, PA, 2000; pp. 726–745.
14. Glick SN. Crohn's disease of the small intestine. Radiol Clin North Am 1987; 25:25–45.

15. Bender GN, Timmons JH, Williard WC, Carter J. Computed tomographic enteroclysis: one methodology. Invest Radiol 1996;31:43–49.
16. Bender GN, Maglinte DD, Kloppel VR, Timmons JH. CT enteroclysis: a superfluous diagnostic procedure or valuable when investigating small–bowel disease? AJR Am J Roentgenol 1999;172:373–378.
17. Raptopoulos V, Schwartz RK, McNicholas MM, Movson J, Pearlman J, Joffe N. Multiplanar helical CT enterography in patients with Crohn's disease. AJR Am J Roentgenol 1997;169:1545–1550.
18. Kelvin FM, Helinger H. Crohn's Disease, in: Clinical Imaging of the Small Intestine. 2nd ed. Springer-Verlag, New York, 1999; pp. 259–289.
19. Lomas DJ, Graves MJ. Small bowel MRI using water as a contrast medium. Br J Radiol 1999;72:994–997.
20. Low RN, Francis IR. MR imaging of the gastrointestinal tract with i.v., gadolinium and diluted barium oral contrast media compared with unenhanced MR imaging and CT. AJR Am J Roentgenol 1997;169:1051–1059.
21. Rubin DL, Muller HH, Young SW. Formulation of radiographically detectable gastrointestinal contrast agents for magnetic resonance imaging: effects of a barium sulfate additive on MR contrast agent effectiveness. Magn Reson Med 1992;23:154–165.
22. Rieber A, Wruk D, Nussle K, Potthast S, Reinshagen M, Brambs HJ. [Current imaging in Crohn's disease: value of MRI compared with conventional proceedings]. Rontgenpraxis 2000;52:378–383.
23. Maccioni F, Viscido A, Broglia L, Marrollo M, Masciangelo R, Caprilli R, Rossi P. Evaluation of Crohn disease activity with magnetic resonance imaging. Abdom Imaging 2000;25:219–228.
24. Lichtenstein GR, Schnall M, Herlinger H. MRI evaluation of Crohn disease activity. Abdom Imaging 2000;25:229.
25. Umschaden HW, Szolar D, Gasser J, Umschaden M, Haselbach H. Small-bowel disease: comparison of MR enteroclysis images with conventional enteroclysis and surgical findings. Radiology 2000;215:717–725.
26. Maglinte DD, Siegelman ES, Kelvin FM. MR enteroclysis: the future of small-bowel imaging? Radiology 2000;215:639–641.
27. Adamek HE, Breer H, Karschkes T, Albert J, Riemann JF. Magnetic resonance imaging in gastroenterology: time to say good-bye to all that endoscopy? [In Process Citation]. Endoscopy 2000;32:406–410.
28. O'Donovan AN, Somers S, Farrow R, Mernagh JR, Sridhar S. MR imaging of anorectal Crohn disease: a pictorial essay. Radiographics 1997;17:101–107.
29. Outwater E, Schiebler ML. Pelvic fistulas: findings on MR images. AJR Am J Roentgenol 1993;160:327–330.
30. Stoker J, Fa VE, Eijkemans MJ, Schouten WR, Lameris JS. Endoanal MRI of perianal fistulas: the optimal imaging planes. Eur Radiol 1998;8:7.
31. Semelka RC, Hricak H, Kim B, Forstner R, Bis KG, Ascher SM, et al. Pelvic fistulas: appearances on MR images. Abdom Imaging 1997;22:91–95.
32. Myhr GE, Myrvold HE, Nilsen G, Thoresen JE, Rinck PA. Perianal fistulas: use of MR imaging for diagnosis. Radiology 1994;191:545–549.
33. Barker PG, Lunniss PJ, Armstrong P, Reznek RH, Cottam K, Phillips RK. Magnetic resonance imaging of fistula-in-ano: technique, interpretation and accuracy. Clin Radiol 1994;49:7–13.
34. Rioux M, Sonography of the small bowel and related strutures, in Textbook of Gastrointestinal Radiology. 2nd ed. W B Saunders, Philadelphia, PA, 2000; pp. 125–152.

35. Maconi G, Ardizzone S, Parente F, Bianchi Porro G. Ultrasonography in the evaluation of extension, activity, and follow-up of ulcerative colitis. Scand J Gastroenterol 1999;34:1103–7.

36. Tio TL, Mulder CJ, Wijers OB, Sars PR, Tytgat GN. Endosonography of peri-anal and peri-colorectal fistula and/or abscess in Crohn's disease. Gastrointest Endosc 1990;36:331–6.

37. Giaffer MH. Labelled leucocyte scintigraphy in inflammatory bowel disease: clinical applications. Gut 1996;38:1–5.

38. Giaffer MH, Tindale WB, Holdsworth D. Value of technetium-99m HMPAO-labelled leucocyte scintigraphy as an initial screening test in patients suspected of having inflammatory bowel disease. Eur J Gastroenterol Hepatol 1996;8:1195–2000.

39. Shah DB, Cosgrove M, Rees JI, Jenkins HR. The technetium white cell scan as an initial imaging investigation for evaluating suspected childhood inflammatory bowel disease. J Pediatr Gastroenterol Nutr 1997;25:524–528.

40. Papos M, Varkonyi A, Lang J, Buga K, Timar E, Polgar M, et al. HM-PAO-labeled leukocyte scintigraphy in pediatric patients with inflammatory bowel disease. J Pediatr Gastroenterol Nutr 1996;23:547–552.

41. Scholmerich J, Schmidt E, Schumichen C, Billmann P, Schmidt H, Gerok W. Scintigraphic assessment of bowel involvement and disease activity in Crohn's disease using technetium 99m-hexamethyl propylene amine oxine as leukocyte label. Gastroenterology 1988;95:1287–1293.

42. Skehan SJ, Issenman R, Mernagh J, Nahmias C, Jacobson K. 18F-fluorodeoxyglucose positron tomography in diagnosis of paediatric inflammatory bowel disease . Lancet 1999;354:836–837.

7 Inflammatory Bowel Disease Markers

Marla C. Dubinsky, MD
and Stephan R. Targan, MD

CONTENTS

INTRODUCTION

For certain diseases that can only be diagnosed clinically, physicians rely heavily on the presence of disease markers to support or even at times modify their clinical impression. Typically, these markers play an important role in helping to establish a diagnosis and to evaluate the activity of a chronic disease over time. The diagnosis of inflammatory bowel disease (IBD), however, is not based solely on clinical grounds. Invasive endoscopic and radiological as well as histopathological criteria need to be met in order to make a correct diagnosis. The search for a noninvasive diagnostic marker that accurately distinguishes a group of patients with IBD from those unaffected by the disease has become an important focus in IBD research. The challenge lies in finding one marker or a combination thereof, that not only distinguishes IBD from non-IBD, or identifies at risk populations, but can also help clinicians distinguish between the IBD subtypes, ulcerative colitis (UC) or Crohn's

From: *Clinical Gastroenterology:*
Inflammatory Bowel Disease: Diagnosis and Therapeutics
Edited by: R. D. Cohen © Humana Press Inc., Totowa, NJ

disease (CD). Such diagnostic dilemmas occur as part of every day practice for clinicians caring for children and adults with suspicion of, or a diagnosis of, IBD. Efforts have also been focused on finding ideal evaluative markers that can be used to monitor disease activity and the effect of treatment over time. This search has taken a very exciting turn in the direction of finding markers that can assess the natural history and perhaps predict the course of individual's disease over time. This chapter highlights the recent advances in the area of IBD markers, discusses the utility and feasibility of these novel markers as well as provides a review of those currently employed in clinical practice.

DIFFERENTIATION OF IBD FROM NON-IBD PATIENTS

The recognition of IBD and subsequent diagnostic evaluation, in most cases, can be straightforward when the clinical presentation is unambiguous. However, a diagnostic challenge arises in patients who present with overlapping, nonspecific and indolent symptoms that are characteristic of both organic and nonorganic disorders. In the face of diagnostic uncertainly clinicians are often obligated to exclude IBD using invasive diagnostic testing, in particular contrast radiography and colonoscopy with biopsies. Suspicion of IBD commonly results in extensive diagnostic investigations of patients who are ultimately found to have a functional bowel disorder. In contrast, the diagnosis of IBD, particularly CD, can be missed or delayed owing to the nonspecific nature of both the intestinal and extraintestinal symptoms at presentation. Given these clinical challenges, the search has intensified for an accurate noninvasive diagnostic marker to aid clinicians in the prompt recognition of IBD and the differentiation of these disorders from mimickers.

Serological Markers

ANTIBODIES

The search for an etiologic agent responsible for triggering the immune mediated bowel injury characteristic of IBD, has lead to the discovery of immune markers present specifically in the sera of patients with Crohn's disease and/or ulcerative colitis. Antineutrophil cytoplasmic antibody (ANCA) was originally reported in IBD in the early 1980s *(1)*. Research and technological advancements subsequently led to the identification of a novel subset of ANCA, distinct from that observed in patients with Wegener's granulomatosis (WG) or systemic vasculitis with glomerulonephritis *(2)*. This IBD-specific ANCA displays a unique perinuclear highlighting (pANCA) on immunoflourence staining and is DNAse sensitive *(3)*. Although it remains undefined, it has been suggested that the antigen to which pANCA is directed is a nuclear histone (H1) *(4)*. This antigen is clearly distinct from the proteinase 3 or the myeloperoxidase reactivity observed in those patients with vasculitic disorders. pANCA is likely an autoantibody that is representative of a cross-reactivity with a luminal bacterial antigen *(5–7)*. Despite epidemiological and methodological differences, pANCA has been shown repeatedly to be prevalent in the sera of approx 60% and 20% of UC and CD patients, respectively (Table 1) *(8–14)*. Typically, <5% of non-IBD patients are pANCA positive.

Anti-*Saccharomyces cerevisiae (S. cerevisiae)* antibody (ASCA) was discovered in the course of studies designed to search for a putative dietary antigen involved in the pathogenesis of CD *(15–17)*. IgA and IgG antibodies are directed against a specific oligomannosidic epitope present on the cell wall of the yeast saccharomyces *(18)*. Studies in both the adult and pediatric IBD population have demonstrated that ASCA is expressed in the sera of approx 60% of CD, 10% of UC and <5% of non-IBD patients. (Table 1) *(12–14)*. It remains unclear whether the presence of ASCA represents an immune response to the antigens on the *S. cerevisiae* itself or to an unidentified antigen, perhaps on the cell wall of a luminal bacteria, which cross reacts with the yeast antigens.

Advances in technology have lead to the development of two novel serodiagnostic assays designed specifically to detect both pANCA and ASCA in the serum of patients with IBD (Prometheus Laboratories, 5739 Pacific Center Blvd., San Diego, CA; phone: 888-428-5227; fax: 958-824-0896; www.prometheus-labs.com) (Table 2). The traditional ASCA and pANCA assays are adjusted to maximize disease specificity (>90% specific for IBD) and accurately confirm a diagnosis of IBD when positive and differentiate UC from CD. However, these highly specific traditional assays are insufficiently sensitive to serve as diagnostic tools for populations with a lower prevalence of disease. Recently, assays have been modified to be more sensitive (>90% sensitive) and less expensive than the traditional assays.

To be clinically useful, a diagnostic marker must be both disease sensitive and specific in order to detect all patients with IBD and exclude all others. Neither the modified nor the traditional serodiagnostic assays are capable of achieving such high diagnostic standards on their own. However, recent research has focused on sequencing the sensitive modified assay with the specific traditional assay in order to improve the diagnostic accuracy of these noninvasive markers *(19,20)*. A similar strategy is currently used for the evaluation of patients with suspected systemic lupus erythromatosis (SLE), whereby first the sensitive antinuclear antibody (ANA) detection assay is followed by a second spe-

Table 1
Test Characteristics of pANCA and ASCA in Inflammatory Bowel Disease

Study	n	Antibody Marker	Test Population	Sensitivity (%)	Specificity (%)
Duerr, et al. (8)	209	pANCA	UC vs CD & controls	60	94
Proujansky, et al. (9)	122	pANCA	UC vs CD & controls	46	79
Winter, et al. (10)	215	pANCA	UC vs CD & controls	62	97
Oberstadt, et al. (11)	151	pANCA	UC vs CD & controls	68	93
Ruemmele, et al. (12)	209	ASCA	CD vs UC & controls	55	95
		pANCA	UC vs CD & controls	57	92
Quinton, et al. (13)	391	ASCA	CD vs UC	61	88
		pANCA	UC vs CD	65	85
Hoffenberg, et al. (14)	119	ASCA	CD vs UC	60	88
		pANCA	UC vs CD	60	65

Table 2
Novel Serodiagnostic Assays

Assay Name	Clinical Applications	Methodology	Assay Characteristics
Modified Assay	"Rule out" a diagnosis of IBD	ASCA ELISA; IgG & IgA sensitivity (>90%)	Titer cut-offs maximized for
"IBD First Step"	Objective: Distinguish IBD from non-IBD patients	ANCA ELISA	
Traditional Assay	1. "Rule in" a diagnosis of IBD	ASCA ELISA; IgG & IgA specificity (>90%)	Titer cut-offs maximized for
"IBD Diagnostic System"	Objective: differentiate inflammatory colitis from other colitides (infectious, ischemic)	ANCA ELISA + Indirect Immunoflouresence + DNase confirmation	
	2. IBD subtyping Objective: Distinguish UC from CD		

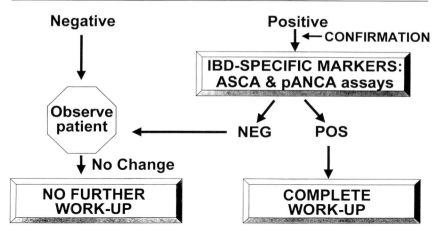

Fig. 1. Sensitive markers: ELISA-based ASCA and ANCA assays, hemoglobin platelets, ESR, CRP, and albumin. Proposed diagnostic strategy for individuals suspected of having IBD *(21)*.

cific confirmatory double-stranded DNA test. Studies in children showed that these paired tests were accurate in 84% of cases presenting with nonspecific symptoms suggestive of these IBD *(20)*. Based on the assay characteristics, a novel diagnostic strategy has been proposed to facilitate clinical decision making when the diagnosis of IBD is initially uncertain (Fig. 1). All patients undergo initial testing with the modified assay in addition to other sensitive routine laboratory tests (CBC and differential, ESR, CRP, and serum albumin). Only those patients with a positive modified assay result would undergo sequential confirmatory testing with the more specific traditional assay. Subsequently, only those patients with a positive confirmatory traditional assay would undergo a complete invasive work-up whereas all patients with a negative assay result, either the initial modified or the subsequent traditional after a positive modified assay, would be observed in follow-up. Patients with false negative serology will likely return with symptoms more compatible with IBD and should undergo a full work-up at that time. Although the diagnosis of IBD will be delayed in a proportion of patients, the advantage of this strategy really lies in its ability to avoid unnecessary and invasive investigations in the majority of patients who truly do not have IBD. Moreover, as new sensitive IBD markers are identified, fewer patients will be missed by this sequential testing strategy over time. Although promising, studies in larger adult and pediatric cohorts are needed to validate these initial findings.

CLASSIC LABORATORY MARKERS

Attempts have been made to differentiate IBD from functional bowel disorders using a panel of screening tools comprised of simple routine blood tests (e.g., complete blood count, platelet count, erythrocyte sedimentation rate [ESR], C reactive protein [CRP], and serum albumin) *(2–24)*. It has been demonstrated in children that when all of the results are normal, chronic inflammatory bowel disease is an unlikely diagnosis. Therefore, these screening lab tests may select from among patients with chronic gastrointestinal symptoms, those who require endoscopic assessment. These routine tests are very sensitive for inflammation, but lack the specificity for IBD. Thus, these tests need to be combined with other diagnostic markers that are diagnostic of patients with IBD and not other forms of inflammatory disorders.

Fecal Markers

Stool analysis has been proposed as a useful and inexpensive noninvasive test to help clinicians delineate the potential causes of chronic diarrhea. A simple latex agglutination test detecting the neutrophil protein, lactoferrin, has been shown to be potentially useful as a marker of colonic inflammation *(25)*. However, lactoferrin does not necessarily distinguish between the different forms of inflammatory colitis (e.g., ischemic vs microscopic vs ulcerative). Similarly, the distinction between inflammatory and infectious colitis may prove to be a challenge given that both forms of colitis give rise to fecal leukocytes. Thus, fecal markers may serve as an adjunct to the other noninvasive markers used to distinguish IBD form non-IBD.

Genetic Markers

The search for susceptibility genes continues to be a major focus among IBD researchers. The human major compatibility complex (MHC) region located on chromosome 6 has been proposed to contain potential candidate genes (MHC IBD-3 locus) *(26–29)*. Previous studies have suggested that the susceptibility contributed by the HLA class II genes to CD and UC are quite different. For epidemiological and methodological reasons, conflicting and inconclusive results have been reported regarding these genetic associations, particularly among the CD population *(30–33)*. A genome-wide search has led to the identification of three other potential candidate loci situated on chromosome 16 (IBD-1 locus, recently identified as the Nod-2 gene), chromosome 12 (IBD-2 locus), and chromosome 14 (IBD-4 locus) *(34–36)*. Given their role as initiators and perpetuators of the inflammatory process characteristic of IBD, genes involved in the regulation of cytokine production may be candidate loci for IBD susceptibility. The gene encoding the interleukin 1 (IL-1) receptor antagonist (IL-1RA), a protein that modulates the inflammatory response of IL-1, has also been suggested, although not confirmed, as a susceptibility gene in UC *(37)*. The multifactorial etiology of IBD likely precludes the use of these genetic markers alone as confirmatory diagnostic tools in IBD. However, the presence of these candidate genes may identify at risk populations. As work goes ahead in identifying these, it is likely that some of this will become part of the diagnostic panel. As discussed below, candidate genes may regulate distinct immune processes, which, in turn, are manifested as specific disease behaviors in patients with IBD.

DISTINGUISHING IBD SUBTYPES: ULCERATIVE COLITIS VS CROHN'S DISEASE

Although UC and CD share may epidemiologic, immunologic, therapeutic and clinical features, they are currently considered to be two distinct subtypes of IBD. Clinical, endoscopic, histopathologic and radiographic criteria have been put forth to help clinicians differentiate between these two diseases. However, despite published criteria, this discrimination may still prove to be difficult in patients with disease limited to the large bowel. This entity referred to as indeterminate colitis (IC) occurs in approx 10–15% of IBD patients. Classically, this term had applied to those patients whose diagnosis remained unknown even after careful examination of resected surgical specimens. However, the modern definition of IC refers to all patients pre or postcolectomy whose categorization remains undefined. It must be emphasized that both surgical options and medical treatment rely on a correct diagnosis. Not all therapies, particularly the novel biologics, are indicated for both CD and UC. Similarly, surgical procedures, such as the ileal pouch-anal anastomosis, is intended specifically for patients with ulcerative colitis.

Serological Markers

ANTIBODIES

Given the CD-specificity of ASCA and the UC-specificity of pANCA, the antibodies have become more widely accepted as useful discriminatory markers that help clinicians differentiate UC from Crohn's colitis (Table 3). Recent reports have demonstrated that approx 2/3 of cases of IC were reclassified preoperatively as either UC or CD based on the pANCA and ASCA profile *(38)*. The presence of pANCA in up to 25% of CD patients limits its ability to distinguish UC form CD on its own. However, the discriminatory strength of these markers is

Table 3
Diagnostic Accuracy of ASCA and pANCA in Differentiating UC
from CD Colitis and Non-IBD Colitis in Children

Population	Assay	Sensitivity (%)	Specificity (%)	Positive predictive value	Negative predictive value
CD colitis vs UC & non- IBD colitis	ASGA IgG or IgA	47	96	73	87
CD colitis vs UC & non- IBD colitis	ASCA IgG & IgA	29	100	100	87
UC vs CD & non- IBD colitis	pANCA	57	97	91	79

Table 4
Diagnostic Accuracy of ASCA and pANCA
in Differentiating UC from CD in a European IBD Population

Assay	Ulcerative colitis N = 101	Crohn's disease N = 1000	Sensitivity (%)	Specificity (%)	Positive predictive value (%)
pANCA +	66	15	65	85	74
ASCA +	12	61	61	88	89
pANCA+/ASCA–	58	3	57	97	93 for UC
pANCA–/ASCA+	3	49	49	97	96 for CD

amplified when they are evaluated in combination *(13,14)*. (Table 4). A pANCA+/ASCA– serological profile was shown to be 19 times more likely to be present in the serum of a patient with UC than CD. Conversely, pANCA–/ASCA+ is 16 times more likely in CD than UC *(39)*. Although pANCA and ASCA have provided clinicians with an important diagnostic tool, the search for the ideal serological profile that could accurately discriminate CD for UC in all patients continues.

Pancreatic antibodies (PAB) have been shown to be present in approx 15–20% of CD patients *(40–43)*. Although not particularly sensitive,

Table 5
Potential Markers of Disease Activity, Disease Relapse
and Effects of Therapy

Serological markers	Fecal markers	Pereability ratios
Antibodies	*Cytokines*	*Urinary Assays*
ASCA & pANCA	TNF *(63,64)*	Lactulose/L-rhamnose
(9–13,42–44)	IL-6 *(64)*	*(72–74)*
Classic laboratory tests	IL-1*(65)*	Lactulose/mannitol *(75)*
ESR *(50)*	IL-1RA *(65)*	
CRP *(46)*	*Neutrophil products*	
Orosomucoid *(50)*	Myeloperoxidase *(66)*	
Platelet count *(48)*	Calprotectin *(67)*	
Cytokines	*Enteric proteins*	
TNFα *(63)*	α-1-antitrypsin *(70)*	
TNFα receptor *(46)*		
IL-1RA *(54)*		
IL-2R *(55)*		
IL-6 *(56-58)*		

these antibodies are specific for CD and hence are very predictive of CD. The antigen reacting with PAB as well as its pathogenic significance in IBD remains unknown. Perhaps pancreatic antibodies will serve as an additional noninvasive marker that clinicians can add to pANCA and ASCA to help discriminate CD from UC. Assays to detect PAB are not currently commercially available.

MONITOR DISEASE ACTIVITY AND EFFECT OF TREATMENT

CD and UC-specific clinical activity indices have been developed as indirect assessments of a patient's overall condition. Although used in clinical trials, indices such as the Crohn's disease activity index (CDAI) or the Truelove and Witt criteria are typically not used in everyday practice. Therapeutic efficacy criteria are typically based on appropriate changes in disease activity scores. Because of the subjective nature of these indices and inability to accurately assess inflammatory activity, their use for research purposes are at times questioned. Researchers continue to search for a simple noninvasive test that provides clinicians with an objective measure of intestinal function for the monitoring of disease activity and effect of treatment. Table 5 provides a list of potential markers if disease activity.

Serological Markers

ANTIBODIES

To date, an association between the presence and titer level of pANCA or ASCA and disease activity, IBD duration, patient gender or treatment has not been consistently demonstrated *(9,12,13,44,45)*. The presence of these markers has been shown to correlate with disease location in patients with CD. The presence of pANCA was associated with colonic involvement *(11,46)* and ASCA with small bowel involvement, alone or in combination with large bowel *(13,46)*. Unlike the ANCA associated vasculitides, IBD-specific antibodies do not become undetectable after initiating immunosuppressives nor does their persistence indicate frequent relapses. Titer level may correlate with age of onset of CD, as a recent study demonstrated that higher ASCA titers were observed in patients with early age of disease onset and high pANCA levels in patients with later age of onset *(46)*. Prospective studies are needed to determine if pANCA or ASCA expression changes in concordance with disease activity and monitor the effect of treatment.

The effect of intestinal surgery on antibody expression remains unknown. Future studies are needed to confirm whether pANCA persist postcolectomy as suggested and to determine the fate of ASCA expression post resection *(12,44)*.

CLASSIC LABORATORY MARKERS

Acute phase protein concentrations have classically been used as supplemental markers of clinical activity in IBD. The most common are the ESR, CRP and serum orosomucoid (α 1-acid glycoprotein). The latter protein has been shown to have similar sensitivity and specificity characteristics to the CRP. However, because of its long half-life, its ability to indicate improvement in disease activity is limited *(47)*. CRP has a significantly shorter half-life and thus rapidly decreases in response to a reduction in disease activity *(48)*. A prospective longitudinal study confirmed that CRP is also useful in monitoring the response to treatment *(49)*. Platelet counts, yet not white counts, have also been shown to be a useful measure of disease activity *(50)*. Few tools are available to help clinicians identify those IBD patients at risk for a disease relapse. This knowledge may be of value for determining which patients in remission would benefit from treatment. In prospective longitudinal studies, both the ESR and CRP have proven to be accurate in identifying those patients at high risk of disease relapse *(49,51,52)*. These markers may be of particular use in children with mild nonspecific symptoms in whom a diagnosis as well as an assessment of disease activity is difficult. Further studies are needed to determine which combination of classic laboratory markers forms the ideal prognostic index.

Cytokines. Concentrations of proinflammatory cytokines are increased in the intestinal mucosa in patients with active CD. The evaluation of serum concentrations on intestinally produced cytokines as surrogate markers of bowel inflammation has yielded inconsistent results. The theory being that in comparison to the classic laboratory markers, cytokines more accurately reflect the underlying immunopathogenic process. Although tumour necrosis factor-α (TNFα) production is increased in the mucosa of patients with active CD, serum levels of TNFα have not been consistently useful as markers of disease activity in these patients *(48,53–55)*. However, an association between disease activity and serum levels of soluble TNFα receptors in both CD and UC has been described (48). Further studies are needed to confirm this association.

It has been suggested that the production of IL-1 receptor antagonist (IL-1RA) may be a manner by which the host down regulates the inflammatory process perhaps amplified by IL-1. IL-1RA levels were found to be increased in patients with active CD and UC as compared to patients with inactive and infectious colitis *(56)*. Interestingly, these IL-1RA concentrations correlated with CRP and orosomucoid levels. IL-2 receptor is shed into the circulation by activated T cells along with IL-2. Levels of IL-2R have been suggested as a new measure of disease activity *(57)*. IL-6 possesses both anti- and proinflammatory properties. It has also been suggested that serum IL-6 levels correlate with disease activity in both CD and UC patients *(58–60)*. Interestingly, in the Reinish study, patients with primarily luminal inflammation displayed higher IL-6 levels than CD patients with fibrostenosis or those with extensive bowel resection. Vascular endothelial growth factor (VEGF) is a cytokine released by cells that potentiate vascular permeability and neovascularization. Significantly increased levels of VGEF have been observed in the serum of patients with active CD and UC *(61,62)*. The potential pathogenic role of VEGF induced vascular permeability in IBD remains unknown.

The role of cytokines as predictors of clinical relapse has also been a focus of investigation. In one study, serum IL-6 level proved to be the greatest predictor of time to relapse with a 17-fold risk over a 12-mo period when levels reached a specific cut point (20 pg/mL). Of the other variable tested, soluble TNF receptor, IL-2R and serum orosomucoid levels also appeared to be useful for predicting the course of disease in patients with quiescent CD *(63)*. Thus, the combination of classic biological markers with the novel cytokine markers may prove to be the ideal serological prognostic index. A recent study suggested that the capacity of intestinal lamina propria cells to secrete TNF and IL-1 may identify patients at risk of a relapse and that may benefit from appropriate anti-inflammatory therapy *(64)*. The practicality and feasibility of a tissue assay is limited compared to that of the serologic analysis.

Cytokine profiles exhibit interindividual variability and thus no one cytokine will necessarily correlate with disease activity in all IBD patients. Future association studies are needed to address this variability.

Fecal Markers

Inflammation of the gut is associated with leakage of cells, cellular products, such as cytokines, and serum proteins. Given that circulating cytokines may not accurately reflect mucosal production, researchers have questioned whether stool cytokine levels may more closely mirror the mucosal inflammation. Preliminary studies demonstrated that stool TNFα and IL-6 concentrations were elevated in children with active CD and UC *(65,66)*. A more recent study observed a significant correlation between stool concentrations of IL-1 and IL-1RA and disease activity in CD and UC patients *(67)*. TNFα was not increased in patients with active disease. As observed with serum cytokine levels, the associations are inconsistent and further studies are needed.

Leukocytes play an important role in initiating and amplifying the mucosal immune process characteristic of IBD. Myeloperoxidase, a constituent of neutrophil granules, has been shown to reflect the number of neutrophils. Stool levels of myeloperoxidase were found to be elevated in patients with active IBD and correlated well with classic laboratory parameters and endoscopic indices of inflammation. Although the presence of stool leukocytes is a sensitive marker of inflammation, these results suggest that the stool levels of myeloperoxidase may be more specific for IBD *(68)*. Levels of fecal calprotectin, a calcium-binding protein found in neutrophil granulocytes, have been shown to correlate with histologic and endoscopic assessment of disease activity in UC patients *(69)*. Additionally, its ability to predict clinical relapse has been recently demonstrated among CD and UC patients alike *(70)*. Enteric protein loss in the face of inflammation may be reflected in the measurement of serum proteins in the stool. Fecal α 1-antitrypsin has been shown to be a sensitive, yet nonspecific marker of enteric inflammation *(71)*. It has been shown to reflect disease activity in patients with CD, but not UC likely owing to the small bowel involvement *(72)*.

The results of these small studies bring forth the notion that fecal markers, like serological markers, may prove to be useful surrogate markers of gut inflammation and helpful in differentiating active from inactive disease. The true utility of these markers as predictors of relapse needs to be evaluated prospectively so to determine if early treatment based on subclinical marker changes will avert relapse and perhaps alter a patients clinical course. As with tissue markers, the practicality of fecal analysis is questionable and larger validation studies are needed.

Markers of Intestinal Permeability

Increased intestinal permeability is a well documented feature of CD. It is unclear whether this increased permeability plays a primary pathogenic role in IBD, perhaps genetically determined, or is secondary to the inflammation. A number of permeability tests have been evaluated over time. The urinary lactulose/L-rhamnose permeability ratio was increased in the majority of children with active CD irrespective of disease location *(73)*. However, among UC patients, only those with extensive colitis had similar abnormal changes in permeability. Despite these findings, the utility of permeability assays is typically limited for use in only CD patients whose disease is confined to the small bowel *(74–76)*. These ratios appeared to normalize in patients who completed an initial course of steroids suggesting perhaps a role for permeability assays for monitoring the effect of treatment. More attention has been given to the potential role of sugar permeability assays in predicting disease relapse. In one study, serial testing using a lactulose/mannitol permeability assay was predictive of CD relapse over the short term *(77)*. Over a 12-mo period, approx 50% of 5-ASA treated IBD patients relapsed after a disease-free interval of at least 1 mo. Intestinal permeability was significantly increased in the CD patients who relapsed. The sensitivity of these assays are high (>80%) but the specificity for disease relapse is sub-optimal (<65%) *(70)*. These assays are not widely used in clinical practice. Although interesting, further longitudinal studies are needed to determine whether prophylactic treatment in asymptomatic patients, with the goal of averting disease relapse, will significantly alter patient outcomes.

ASSESS NATURAL HISTORY

The more classic categorization of IBD into UC and CD was based partially on the differences in the expected natural history of these two perceived separate disease entities. However, over time, we have come to realize that within each subtype patients behave very differently and that the natural history has now become more difficult to predict at the time of diagnosis. This observed clinical heterogeneity has lead to the development of certain classification systems in order to help character-ize patients as specific disease phenotypes. In other words, attempting to classify patients into more homogeneous subgroups. For UC, typi-cally patients are classified based on disease location and according to the most recent Vienna Classification, patients with CD are to be catego-rized based on disease location, behavior, and age of disease onset. Immunologic and genetic contributions play critical roles in defining this clinical heterogeneity.

Serological Markers

ANTIBODIES

ASCA and pANCA may serve as surrogate markers for the genetic contributions to the clinical heterogeneity observed among IBD patients. The expression of these markers has been shown to reflect specific disease phenotypes. The first clinical phenotype was described for the pANCA positive subgroup of UC patients. A strong association was observed between pANCA and the occurrence of chronic pouchitis after Ileal Pouch Anal Anastomosis (IPAA) (78,79). To date, not all centers have reproduced these findings (80–83). However, a recent prospective study using second generation assays (Prometheus Laboratories) reported that high levels of pANCA (>100 EU/mL) in UC patients pre-dicted the development of chronic pouchitis with a high degree of cer-tainty (84). Future studies are underway to determine if prophylactic antibiotic treatment would decrease the incidence of chronic pouchitis in at risk (high pANCA) individuals.

Standard treatment regimens are typically employed in all UC patients at the time of diagnosis based on disease location and disease severity. More aggressive immunosuppressive agents like 6-MP or azathioprine are often reserved for patients who, over time, become unresponsive to standard medical therapy. Unfortunately, an ideal tool to help clinicians predict therapeutic response upon initial presentation has not been developed. In a retrospective pilot study, however, the presence of pANCA was found to be associated with resistance to standard medical therapy in UC patients with left-sided colitis (85). Other studies have suggested that pANCA expression is a possible marker of an aggressive disease phenotype (86–88). These findings further suggest that pANCA may serve as a surrogate for the genetic heterogeneity that determines an individual's clinical course.

Although pANCA has been established as a UC-specific marker, approx 25% of all CD patients also express pANCA. These CD patients have been found to have clinical features of left-sided colitis with endo-scopic and/or histopathologic features of UC. These CD patients are described as "UC-like" *(89)*. Vasiliauskas et al. established criteria to define a "UC-like" state in patients with established CD. These patients had to have had clinical features of left-sided colonic disease as well as endoscopic and/or histopathologic criteria as outlined in Table 6 in order to be defined as "UC-like". Interestingly, none of the pANCA positive CD patients had isolated small bowel disease and pANCA expression was not related solely to the presence of colonic inflammation. Thus, the presence of pANCA may represent a distinct, genetically conditioned mucosal inflammatory process common to both UC and "UC-like" CD patients. The shared clinical features suggest that the expression of pANCA may help restructure the categorization of UC and CD into more homogeneous phenotypic subgroups (Fig. 2).

ASCA expression may reflect another unique inflammatory process in patients with CD. The results of a recent study demonstrated that higher ASCA levels were associated with earlier age of disease onset and both fibrostenosing and internal penetrating disease behaviors *(46)*. In contrast, high pANCA levels were associated with the onset of "UC-like" CD at an older age. Thus, the qualitative (expression) as well as the quantitative (titer level) analysis of ASCA and pANCA may represent select clinical phenotypes in CD patients.

If indeed IBD-specific antibodies are biological markers of distinct disease behaviors, as suggested, these tools may help predict the natural history of an individual's disease. With this knowledge clinicians can create and implement appropriate therapeutic management regimes based on the aggressiveness of the IBD subtype so to alter and thus improve the long-term prognosis. Prospective studies are needed to confirm the utility of ascertaining ASCA and pANCA status at the time of diagnosis and to evaluate the impact of this information on patient outcomes.

Genetic Markers

The clinical heterogeneity within UC and CD likely has a genetic basis. The search for the genetic contributions to the various disease phenotypes has been of great interest. Besides their possible implication in the determination of UC susceptibility, HLA class II genes may also influence the pattern of disease behavior. Certain HLA haplotypes and alleles of IL-1RA have emerged in various studies as potential markers of extensive UC, perhaps even predicting the need for surgery in a select group of patients *(26,88)*. The link between genotype and clinical phenotype may indeed be the expression of pANCA and ASCA. Although the results have not been consistent, certain HLA class II genes have been linked to pANCA expression *(91)*. Further association studies are needed to confirm genetic linkage with disease susceptibility, disease behaviors and antibody expression.

Table 6
"UC-Like" Crohn's Disease

Clinical Features of Left-sided Folitis

Rectal bleeding
Urgency
Tenesmus
Treatment with topical therapies
Recommended or performed total or near-total colectomy

Endoscopic Appearance

Inflammation extending proximally from the rectum
Inflammation more severe distally than proximally
Continuous inflammation
Shallow ulceration/lack of deep ulcerations

Histopathological Features

Homogenous, continuous, predominantly superficial inflammation
Crypt abscesses
Lack of granulomas
Lack of "focality" in biopsy specimens

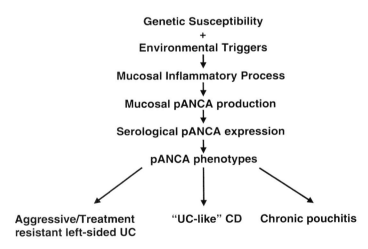

Fig. 2. Link between IBD genotypes and phenotypes based on pANCA expression.

IDENTIFY AT-RISK INDIVIDUALS

Both genetic and antibody markers may aid in the identification of individuals at risk of developing IBD in the future. The frequency of both ASCA and pANCA expression has been shown to be higher in the

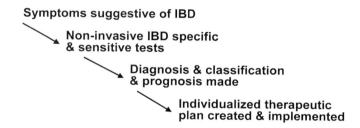

Symptoms suggestive of IBD

Non-invasive IBD specific & sensitive tests

Diagnosis & classification & prognosis made

Individualized therapeutic plan created & implemented

Fig. 3. Future of diagnostic and therapeutic management strategies for IBD patients.

nonaffected relatives of both CD and UC, respectively *(92,93)*. Not all centers have confirmed these findings. Studies in different population groups, using different methodologies may explain the discrepancies observed found between countries in Europe and North America *(94)*. It is unknown whether these patients will develop, or are at risk of developing, IBD over time. However, given the multifactorial etiology of IBD, the value of these antibodies alone as preclinical markers of disease is questionable. As hypothesized with other autoimmune diseases, the interaction between environmental and genetic factors is critical to the biologic onset of IBD. Prospective longitudinal studies are needed to document the outcome of patients identified as "high risk" based on the presence of subclinical markers, such as ASCA or pANCA. If these patients do develop IBD, then perhaps subclinical disease markers could help establish an early diagnosis and appropriate therapeutic decisions can then be made with the goal of improving patient outcomes in those who have the target disorder.

THE FUTURE OF IBD DISEASE MARKERS

The clinical utility and importance of IBD-specific markers has been reviewed in this chapter. Research and technological advancements have fostered a novel approach to understanding the intricate relationship between genetic and clinical expression of disease. Both genetic and serum antibody markers hold the most promise in helping researchers better comprehend disease heterogeneity and natural history. Although our current gold standard diagnostic tests do not possess this capability, exciting preliminary research suggests IBD-specific genetic and antibody markers may serve as predictors of an individual's disease course. Thus, the foundation has been laid upon which the discovery of novel IBD-specific and IBD-sensitive markers will enable researchers to identify at-risk individuals, as well as diagnose IBD and stratify patients into homogeneous subtypes with certainty (Fig. 3). Clinicians can then create and implement individual treatment plans designed to improve the long-term prognosis of these chronic diseases.

REFERENCES

1. Nielsen H, Wiik A, Elmgreen J. Granulocyte specific antinuclear antibodies in ulcerative colitis. Aid in differential diagnosis of inflammatory bowel disease. Acta Pathol Microbiol Immunol Scand [C] 1983;91:23–26.
2. Saxon A, Shanahan F, Landers C, Ganz T, Targan S. A distinct subset of antineutrophil cytoplasmic antibodies is associated with inflammatory bowel disease. J Allergy Clin Immunol 1990;86:202–210.
3. Vidrich A, Lee J, James E, Cobb L, Targan S. Segregation of pANCA antigenic recognition by DNase treatment of neutrophils: ulcerative colitis, type 1 autoimmune hepatitis, and primary sclerosing cholangitis. J Clin Immunol 1995;15:293–299.
4. Eggena M, Cohavy O, Parseghian MH, Hamkalo BA, Clemens D, Targan SR, Gordon LK, Braun J. Identification of histone H1 as a cognate antigen of the ulcerative colitis-associated marker antibody pANCA. J Autoimmun 2000;14:83–97.
5. Cohavy O, Harth G, Horwitz M, Eggena M, Landers C, Sutton C, et al. Identification of a novel mycobacterial histone H1 homologue (HupB) as an antigenic target of pANCA monoclonal antibody and serum immunoglobulin A from patients with Crohn's disease. Infect Immun 1999;67:6510–6517.
6. Cohavy O, Bruckner D, Gordon LK, Misra R, Wei B, Eggena ME, et al. Colonic bacteria express an ulcerative colitis pANCA-related protein epitope. Infect Immun 2000;68:1542–1548.
7. Seibold F, Brandwein S, Simpson S, Terhorst C, Elson CO. pANCA represents a cross-reactivity to enteric bacterial antigens. J Clin Immunol 1998;18:153–160.
8. Duerr RH, Targan SR, Landers CJ, Sutherland LR, Shanahan F. Anti-neutrophil cytoplasmic antibodies in ulcerative colitis. Comparison with other colitides/diarrheal illnesses. Gastroenterology 1991;100:1590–1596.
9. Proujansky R, Fawcett PT, Gibney KM, Treem WR, Hyams JS. Examination of anti-neutrophil cytoplasmic antibodies in childhood inflammatory bowel disease. J Pediatr Gastroenterol Nutr 1993;17:193–197.
10. Winter HS, Landers CJ, Winkelstein A, Vidrich A, Targan SR. Anti-neutrophil cytoplasmic antibodies in children with ulcerative colitis. J Pediatr 1994;125:707–711.
11. Oberstadt K, Schaedel W, Weber M, Classen M, Deusch K. P-ANCA as a differential diagnostic marker in inflammatory bowel disease. Adv Exp Med Biol 1995;371B:1313–1316.
12. Ruemmele FM, Targan SR, Levy G, Dubinsky M, Braun J, Seidman EG. Diagnostic accuracy of serological assays in pediatric inflammatory bowel disease Gastroenterology 1998;115:822–829.
13. Quinton JF, Sendid B, Reumaux D, Duthilleul P, Cortot A, Grandbastien B, et al. Anti-Saccharomyces cerevisiae mannan antibodies combined with antineutrophil cytoplasmic autoantibodies in inflammatory bowel disease: prevalence and diagnostic role. Gut 1998;42:788–791.
14. Hoffenberg EJ, Fidanza S, Sauaia A. Serologic testing for inflammatory bowel disease. J Pediatr 1999;134:447–452.
15. Main J, McKenzie H, Yeaman GR, Kerr MA, Robson D, Pennington CR, Parratt D. Antibody to Saccharomyces cerevisiae (bakers' yeast) in Crohn's disease. BMJ 1988;297:1105–1106.
16. McKenzie H, Main J, Pennington CR, Parratt D. Antibody to selected strains of Saccharomyces cerevisiae (baker's and brewer's yeast) and Candida albicans in Crohn's disease. Gut 1990;31:536–538.

17. Giaffer MH, Clark A, Holdsworth CD. Antibodies to Saccharomyces cerevisiae in patients with Crohn's disease and their possible pathogenic importance. Gut 1992;33:1071–1075.
18. Sendid B, Colombel JF, Jacquinot PM, Faille C, Fruit J, Cortot A, et al. Specific antibody response to oligomannosidic epitopes in Crohn's disease. Clin Diagn Lab Immunol 1996;3:219–226.
19. Dubinsky MC, Targan S, Braun J, Seidman EG. Predictive Value of Screening Tests in Pediatric Inflammatory Bowel Disease: A Prospective Comparative Study. AJG 1998;93:A585.
20. Dubinsky MC, Ofman J, Targan SR, FM Ruemmele, Seidman EG. ASCA and ANCA Testing: Important tools for clinical decision making in pediatric IBD. Gastroenterology 1999;114:A702
21. Seidman EG, Dubinsky M, Patriquin H, Marx G, Theoret Y. Recent developments in the diagnosis and Management of pediatric inflammatory bowel disease. In: Inflammatory bowel disease therapy 1999. Kluwer Academic Publishers, The Netherlands, 2000;87–95.
22. Shine B, Berghouse L, Jones JE, Landon J. C-reactive protein as an aid in the differentiation of functional and inflammatory bowel disorders. Clin Chim Acta 1985;148:105–109.
23. Thomas DW, Sinatra FR. Screening laboratory tests for Crohn's disease. West J Med 1989;150:163–164.
24. Beattie RM, Walker-Smith JA, Murch SH. Indications for investigation of chronic gastrointestinal symptoms. Arch Dis Child 1995;73:354–355.
25. Fine KD, Ogunji F, George J, Niehaus MD, Guerrant RL. Utility of a rapid fecal latex agglutination test detecting the neutrophil protein, lactoferrin, for diagnosing inflammatory causes of chronic diarrhea. Am J Gastroenterol 1998;93:1300–1305.
26. Toyoda H, Wang SJ, Yang HY, Redford A, Magalong D, Tyan D, et al. Distinct associations of HLA class II genes with inflammatory bowel disease. Gastroenterology 1993;104:741–748.
27. Satsangi J, Welsh KI, Bunce M, Julier C, Farrant JM, Bell JI, Jewell DP. Contribution of genes of the major histocompatibility complex to susceptibility and disease phenotype in inflammatory bowel disease. Lancet 1996;347:1212–1217.
28. Hampe J, Schreiber S, Shaw SH, Lau KF, Bridger S, MacPherson AJ, et al. A genomewide analysis provides evidence for novel linkages in inflammatory bowel disease in a large European cohort. Am J Hum Genet 1999;64:808–816.
29. Yang H, Plevy SE, Taylor K, Tyan D, Fischel-Ghodsian N, McElree C, et al. Linkage of Crohn's disease to the major histocompatibility complex region is detected by multiple non-parametric analyses. Gut 1999;44:519–526.
30. Smolen JS, Gangl A, Polterauer P, Menzel EJ, Mayr WR. HLA antigens in inflammatory bowel disease. Gastroenterology 1982;82:34–38.
31. Asakura H, Tsuchiya M, Aiso S, Watanabe M, Kobayashi K, Hibi T, et al. Association of the human lymphocyte-DR2 antigen with Japanese ulcerative colitis. Gastroenterology 1982;82:413–418.
32. Cottone M, Bunce M, Taylor CJ, Ting A, Jewell DP. Ulcerative colitis and HLA phenotype. Gut 1985;26:952–954.
33. Duerr RH, Neigut DA. Molecularly defined HLA-DR2 alleles in ulcerative colitis and an antineutrophil cytoplasmic antibody-positive subgroup. Gastroenterology 1995;108:423–442
34. Hugot JP, Laurent-Puig P, Gower-Rousseau C, Olson JM, Lee JC, Beaugerie L, et al. Mapping of a susceptibility locus for Crohn's disease on chromosome 16 Nature 1996;379:821–823.

35. Satsangi J, Parkes M, Louis E, Hashimoto L, Kato N, Welsh K, et al. Two stage genome-wide search in inflammatory bowel disease provides evidence for susceptibility loci on chromosomes 3, 7 and 12. Nat Genet 1996;14:199–202.
36. Ma Y, Ohmen JD, Li Z, Bentley LG, McElree C, Pressman S, et al. A genome-wide search identifies potential new susceptibility loci for Crohn's disease. Inflamm Bowel Dis 1999;5:271–278.
37. Mansfield JC, Holden H, Tarlow JK, Di Giovine FS, McDowell TL, Wilson AG, et al. Novel genetic association between ulcerative colitis and the anti- inflammatory cytokine interleukin-1 receptor antagonist. Gastroenterology 1994;106: 637–642.
38. Schwarz S, Ammirati, M, Korelitz B, Gleim G. Identification of Indeterminate Colitis using pANCA and ASCA. Gastroenterology 2000:118 (suppl 2):A1891
39. Panaccione R, Sandborn WJ. Is antibody testing for inflammatory bowel disease clinically useful? Gastroenterology 1999;116:1001–1002.
40. Stocker W, Otte M, Ulrich S, Normann D, Finkbeiner H, Stocker K, et alC. Autoimmunity to pancreatic juice in Crohn's disease. Results of an autoantibody screening in patients with chronic inflammatory bowel disease. Scand J Gastroenterol Suppl 1987;139:41–52.
41. Seibold F, Mork H, Tanza S, Muller A, Holzhuter C, Weber P, Scheurlen M. Pancreatic autoantibodies in Crohn's disease: a family study. Gut 1997;40: 481–484.
42. Folwaczny C, Noehl N, Endres SP, Loeschke K, Fricke H. Antineutrophil and pancreatic autoantibodies in first-degree relatives of patients with inflammatory bowel disease. Scand J Gastroenterol 1998;33:523–528.
43. Sandborn WJ, Loftus EV, Colombel JF, Fleming K, Seibold F, Homburger HA, et al. Utility of perinuclear anti-neutrophil cytoplasmic antibodies (pANCA), anti-saccharomyces antibody (ASCA), and anti-pancreatic antibodies (APA) as serologic markers in a population based cohort of patients with Crohn's disease (CD) and ulcerative colitis (UC). Gsatroeneterology 2000;118 (supplement 2):A696.
44. Pool MO, Ellerbroek PM, Ridwan BU, Goldschmeding R, von Blomberg BM, Pena AS, et al. Serum antineutrophil cytoplasmic autoantibodies in inflammatory bowel disease are mainly associated with ulcerative colitis. A correlation study between perinuclear antineutrophil cytoplasmic autoantibodies and clinical parameters, medical, and surgical treatment. Gut 1993;34:46–50.
45. Roozendaal C, Pogany K, Hummel EJ, Horst G, Dijkstra G, Nelis GF, et al. Titres of anti-neutrophil cytoplasmic antibodies in inflammatory bowel disease are not related to disease activity. QJM 1999;92:651–658.
46. Vasiliauskas EA, Kam LY, Karp LC, Gaiennie J, Yang H, Targan SR. Marker antibody expression stratifies Crohn's disease into immunologically homogeneous subgroups with distinct clinicial charracteristics. Gut 2000; 47(4): 487–496.
47. Chambers RE, Stross P, Barry RE, Whicher JT. Serum amyloid A protein compared with C-reactive protein, alpha 1- antichymotrypsin and alpha 1-acid glycoprotein as a monitor of inflammatory bowel disease. Eur J Clin Invest 1987; 17:460–467.
48. Nielsen OH, Vainer B, Madsen SM, Seidelin JB, Heegaard NH. Established and emerging biological activity markers of inflammatory bowel disease. Am J Gastroenterol 2000;95:359–367.
49. Boirivant M, Leoni M, Tariciotti D, Fais S, Squarcia O, Pallone F. The clinical significance of serum C reactive protein levels in Crohn's disease. Results of a prospective longitudinal study. J Clin Gastroenterol 1988;10:401–405.

50. Harries AD, Fitzsimons E, Fifield R, Dew MJ, Rhoades J. Platelet count: a simple measure of activity in Crohn's disease. Br Med J (Clin Res Ed) 1983;286:1476.
51. Campbell CA, Walker-Smith JA, Hindocha P, Adinolfi M. Acute phase proteins in chronic inflammatory bowel disease in childhood. J Pediatr Gastroenterol Nutr 1982;1:193–200.
52. Brignola C, Campieri M, Bazzocchi G, Farruggia P, Tragnone A, Lanfranchi GA. A laboratory index for predicting relapse in asymptomatic patients with Crohn's disease. Gastroenterology 1986;91:1490–1494.
53. Hyams JS, Treem WR, Eddy E, Wyzga N, Moore RE. Tumor necrosis factor-alpha is not elevated in children with inflammatory bowel disease. J Pediatr Gastroenterol Nutr 1991;12:233–236.
54. Murch SH, Lamkin VA, Savage MO, Walker-Smith JA, MacDonald TT. Serum concentrations of tumour necrosis factor alpha in childhood chronic inflammatory bowel disease. Gut 1991;32:913–917.
55. Gardiner KR, Halliday MI, Barclay GR, Milne L, Brown D, Stephens S, et al. Significance of systemic endotoxaemia in inflammatory bowel disease. Gut 1995;36:897–901.
56. Propst A, Propst T, Herold M, Vogel W, Judmaier G. Interleukin-1 receptor antagonist in differential diagnosis of inflammatory bowel diseases. Eur J Gastroenterol Hepatol 1995;7:1031–1036.
57. Williams AJ, Symons JA, Watchet K, Duff GW. Soluble interleukin-2 receptor and disease activity in Crohn's disease. J Autoimmun 1992;5:251–259.
58. Mahida YR, Kurlac L, Gallagher A, Hawkey CJ. High circulating concentrations of interleukin-6 in active Crohn's disease but not ulcerative colitis. Gut 1991;32:1531–1534.
59. Holtkamp W, Stollberg T, Reis HE. Serum interleukin-6 is related to disease activity but not disease specificity in inflammatory bowel disease. J Clin Gastroenterol 1995;20:123–126
60. Reinisch W, Gasche C, Tillinger W, Wyatt J, Lichtenberger C, Willheim M, et al. Clinical relevance of serum interleukin-6 in Crohn's disease: single point measurements, therapy monitoring, and prediction of clinical relapse. Am J Gastroenterol 1999;94:2156–2164.
61. Griga T, Tromm A, Spranger J, May B. Increased serum levels of vascular endothelial growth factor in patients with inflammatory bowel disease. Scand J Gastroenterol 1998;33:504–508.
62. Bousvaros A, Leichtner A, Zurakowski D, Kwon J, Law T, Keough K, Fishman S. Elevated serum vascular endothelial growth factor in children and young adults with Crohn's disease. Dig Dis Sci 1999;44:424–430.
63. Louis E, Belaiche J, van Kemseke C, Franchimont D, de Groote D, Gueenen V, Mary JY. A high serum concentration of interleukin-6 is predictive of relapse in quiescent Crohn's disease. Eur J Gastroenterol Hepatol 1997;9:939–944.
64. Schreiber S, Nikolaus S, Hampe J, Hamling J, Koop I, Groessner B, et al. Tumour necrosis factor alpha and interleukin 1beta in relapse of Crohn's disease. Lancet 1999;353:459–461.
65. Braegger CP, Nicholls S, Murch SH, Stephens S, MacDonald TT. Tumour necrosis factor alpha in stool as a marker of intestinal inflammation. Lancet 1992; 339:89–91.
66. Nicholls S, Stephens S, Braegger CP, Walker-Smith JA, MacDonald TT. Cytokines in stools of children with inflammatory bowel disease or infective diarrhoea. J Clin Pathol 1993;46:757–760.
67. Saiki T, Mitsuyama K, Toyonaga A, Ishida H, Tanikawa K. Detection of pro- and anti-inflammatory cytokines in stools of patients with inflammatory bowel disease. Scand J Gastroenterol 1998;33:616–622.

68. Saiki T. Myeloperoxidase concentrations in the stool as a new parameter of inflammatory bowel disease. Kurume Med J 1998;45:69–73.

69. Roseth AG, Aadland E, Jahnsen J, Raknerud N. Assessment of disease activity in ulcerative colitis by faecal calprotectin, a novel granulocyte marker protein. Digestion 1997;58:176–180.

70. Tibble JA, Sigthorsson G, Bridger S, Fagerhol MK, Bjarnason I. Surrogate markers of intestinal inflammation are predictive of relapse in patients with inflammatory bowel disease. Gastroenterology 2000;119:15–22.

71. Becker K, Frieling T, Haussinger D. Quantification of fecal alpha 1-antitrypsin excretion for assessment of inflammatory bowel diseases. Eur J Med Res 1998;3:65–70.

72. Becker K, Berger M, Niederau C, Frieling T. Individual fecal alpha 1-antitrypsin excretion reflects clinical activity in Crohn's disease but not in ulcerative colitis. Hepatogastroenterology 1999;46:2309–2314.

73. Miki K, Moore DJ, Butler RN, Southcott E, Couper RT, Davidson GP. The sugar permeability test reflects disease activity in children and adolescents with inflammatory bowel disease. J Pediatr 1998;133:750–754.

74. Wyatt J, Vogelsang H, Hubl W, Waldhoer T, Lochs H. Intestinal permeability and the prediction of relapse in Crohn's disease. Lancet 1993;341:1437–1439.

75. Teahon K, Smethurst P, Levi AJ, Menzies IS, Bjarnason I. Intestinal permeability in patients with Crohn's disease and their first degree relatives. Gut 1992;33: 320–323.

76. Bjarnason I, MacPherson A, Hollander D. Intestinal permeability: an overview. Gastroenterology 1995;108:1566–1581.

77. Hilsden RJ, Meddings JB, Hardin J, Gall DG, Sutherland LR. Intestinal permeability and postheparin plasma diamine oxidase activity in the prediction of Crohn's disease relapse. Inflamm Bowel Dis 1999;5:85–91.

78. Sandborn WJ, Landers CJ, Tremaine WJ, Targan SR. Antineutrophil cytoplasmic antibody correlates with chronic pouchitis after ileal pouch-anal anastomosis. Am J Gastroenterol 1995;90:740–747.

79. Vecchi M, Gionchetti P, Bianchi MB, Belluzzi A, Meucci G, Campieri M, de Franchis R. p-ANCA and development of pouchitis in ulcerative colitis patients after proctocolectomy and ileoanal pouch anastomosis. Lancet 1994;344: 886–887.

80. Esteve M, Mallolas J, Klaassen J, Abad-Lacruz A, Gonzalez-Huix F, Cabre E, et al. Antineutrophil cytoplasmic antibodies in sera from colectomised ulcerative colitis patients and its relation to the presence of pouchitis. Gut 1996;38:894–898.

81. Yang P, Oresland T, Jarnerot G, Hulten L, Danielsson D. Perinuclear antineutrophil cytoplasmic antibody in pouchitis after proctocolectomy with ileal pouch-anal anastomosis for ulcerative colitis. Scand J Gastroenterol 1996;31: 594–598.

82. Kaditis AG, Perrault J, Sandborn WJ, Landers CJ, Zinsmeister AR, Targan SR. Antineutrophil cytoplasmic antibody subtypes in children and adolescents after ileal pouch-anal anastomosis for ulcerative colitis. J Pediatr Gastroenterol Nutr 1998;26:386–392.

83. Yasuda N, Thomas P, Ellis H, Herbst F, Nicholls J, Ciclitira P. Perinuclear anti-neutrophil cytoplasmic antibodies in ulcerative colitis after restorative protocolectomy do not correlate with the presence of pouchitis. Scand J Gastroenterol 1998;33:509–513.

84. Fleshner PR, Vasiliauskas EA, Kam L, Abreu M, Targan SR. High level perinuclear antineutrophil cytoplasmic antibody (pANCA) in ulcerative colitis

patients before colectomy predicts the development of chronic pouchitis after ileal pouch anal anastomosis. Gastroenterology 1999;116(4):A716.

85. Sandborn WJ, Landers CJ, Tremaine WJ, Targan SR. Association of anti-neutrophil cytoplasmic antibodies with resistance to treatment of left-sided ulcerative colitis: results of a pilot study. Mayo Clin Proc 1996;71:431–436.

86. Vecchi M, Bianchi M, Torgano G, Meucci G, Omodei P, Levati M. Anti-neutrophil cytoplasmic antibodies (pANCA) are more prevalent in ulcerative colitis patients with clinically aggressive disease. Gastroenterology 1992; 102(Suppl):A708.

87. Vecchi M, Bianchi MB, Calabresi C, Meucci G, Tatarella M, de Franchis R. Long-term observation of the perinuclear anti-neutrophil cytoplasmic antibody status in ulcerative colitis patients. Scand J Gastroenterol 1998;33:170–173.

88. Boerr LA, Sambuelli AM, Katz S, Sole L, Gil A, Goncalves S. Clinical heterogeneity of ulcerative colitis in relation to frequency of pANCA reactivity. Gastroenterology 1994;108(suppl):A785.

89. Vasiliauskas EA, Plevy SE, Landers CJ, Binder SW, Ferguson DM, Yang H, et al. Perinuclear antineutrophil cytoplasmic antibodies in patients with Crohn's disease define a clinical subgroup. Gastroenterology 1996;110:1810–1819.

90. Roussomoustakaki M, Satsangi J, Welsh K, Louis E, Fanning G, Targan S, et al. Genetic markers may predict disease behavior in patients with ulcerative colitis. Gastroenterology 1997;112:1845–1853.

91. Yang H, Rotter JI, Toyoda H, Landers C, Tyran D, McElree CK, Targan SR. Ulcerative colitis: a genetically heterogeneous disorder defined by genetic (HLA class II) and subclinical (antineutrophil cytoplasmic antibodies) markers. J Clin Invest 1993;92:1080–1084.

92. Sendid B, Quinton JF, Charrier G, Goulet O, Cortot A, Grandbastien B, et al. Anti-Saccharomyces cerevisiae mannan antibodies in familial Crohn's disease. Am J Gastroenterol 1998;93:1306–1310.

93. Sutton CL, Yang H, Li Z, Rotter JI, Targan SR, Braun J. Familial expression of anti-Saccharomyces cerevisiae mannan antibodies in affected and unaffected relatives of patients with Crohn's disease. Gut 2000;46:58–63.

94. Lee JC, Lennard-Jones JE, Cambridge G. Antineutrophil antibodies in familial inflammatory bowel disease. Gastroenterology 1995;108:428–433.

8 Medical Therapy of Inflammatory Bowel Disease

Todd E. H. Hecht, MD, Chinyu G. Su, MD, and Gary R. Lichtenstein, MD

INTRODUCTION

Inflammatory bowel disease (IBD) comprises a family of idiopathic autoimmune disorders that affect multiple organ systems, particularly the gastrointestinal (GI) tract. Roughly half of all IBD patients have ulcerative colitis (UC), whereas the remainder have Crohn's disease (CD). These diseases afflict people of all age groups, ethnicities, and socioeconomic levels, with only a slight predominance in women as opposed to men. The purpose of this chapter is to explore the medical therapy of these challenging disorders.

AMINOSALICYLATES

Aminosalicylates are the most common drugs prescribed for the treatment and prevention of IBD *(1)*. Sulfasalazine, the first aminosalicylate

From: *Clinical Gastroenterology:*
Inflammatory Bowel Disease: Diagnosis and Therapeutics
Edited by: R. D. Cohen © Humana Press Inc., Totowa, NJ

used for IBD, is composed of an antibacterial, sulfapyridine, bound to 5-aminosalicylic acid (5-ASA, mesalamine). In the 1970s, it was discovered that the 5-ASA component of the molecule bears the antiinflammatory activity whereas the sulfa component functions solely as a carrier ensuring delivery to the colon, where sulfasalazine is broken down by colonic bacteria into its constituents *(2)*. This fact, along with the relatively high side effect profile of sulfasalazine and the ease of proximal absorption of mesalamine if not packaged, led to the creation of sulfa-free aminosalicylates that ensure more distal intestinal delivery of 5-ASA. These include various oral and topical mesalamine preparations, alternative azo-bonded carriers, and 5-ASA dimers (as shown in Table 1).

The exact mechanism of action of 5-ASA is not well understood though it has been shown to have numerous antiinflammatory properties in vitro. 5-ASA has been shown to have effects on the arachidonic acid (AA) pathway including the 5'-lipoxygenase pathway, prostaglandin and thromboxane synthesis, and inhibition of platelet activating factor synthase. Furthermore, 5-ASA inhibits the production of free oxygen radicals, impairs the function of lymphocytes and monocytes, and decreases the production of interleukin 1 (IL-1) and immunoglobulins *(3)*. Last, sulfasalazine has been demonstrated to block the activation and production of nuclear factor κ B (NF-κB), mitogen activated protein (MAP) kinase, and tumor necrosis factor α (TNF-α).

Oral Preparations

INDICATIONS

In UC patients with mild–moderate disease activity, oral aminosalicylates have been shown to be effective up to 80% of the time. Effective doses of these drugs are 4–6 g/d in four divided doses for sulfasalazine, 2–4 g/d for mesalamine, 2.0–6.75 g/d for balsalazide, and 1.5–3 g/d for olsalazine. In addition, these medications have been shown to prevent relapse in 50–75% of UC patients, usually at lower doses. There is little data regarding the effectiveness of aminosalicylates for more severe UC.

The effectiveness of some of these drugs for patients with CD is dependent on the site and stage of disease activity. Though sulfasalazine has some benefits for patients with active colonic or ileocolonic disease, it is not effective for those with isolated small bowel disease *(4,5)*. In addition, sulfasalazine has very little evidence to support its use in maintaining remission of CD *(4,5)*. On the other hand, newer mesalamine preparations that deliver 5-ASA to the small bowel (Table 1) may

Table 1
5-Aminosalicylic Acid Preparations

Generic name	Trade name	Components	Site of Release	Dosages
Sulfasalazine	Azulfidine®	Sulfapyradine	colon	4–6 g/d (active disease)
		+ 5-ASA		2–4 g/d (maintenance) divide dose 4 times daily
Mesalamine	Pentasa®	5-ASA	duodenum to colon	2–4 g/d
	Asacol®	5-ASA	distal ileum and colon	2.4–4.8 g/d
	Canasa®	5-ASA suppository	rectum	500 mg twice daily
	Rowasa®	5-ASA enema	distal colon	2–4 g/d
Olsalazine	Dipentum®	5-ASA dimer	distal ileum and colon	1.5–3 g/d
Balsalazide	Colazal®	5-ASA + 4-amino benzoyl beta alanine	colon	2–6.75 g/d

help CD patients with jejunal and ileal disease. A number of these agents, including Pentasa® and Asacol® at doses of up to 4.8 g/d, have demonstrated efficacy in the treatment of active Crohn's ileocolitis *(6,7)*. One study has indicated that Asacol®, given in 4 g/d doses, may be as effective as 40 mg/d of oral methylprednisolone for the treatment of active Crohn's ileitis *(8)*. Oral mesalamine preparations have been shown to be beneficial in maintaining remission of Crohn's disease, though this effect was most pronounced in patients with surgically induced remissions *(9)*. Mesalamine does not appear to be an effective steroid sparing agent once remission has been achieved with steroids *(10)*. All in all, oral mesalamine preparations seem to have some benefit in achieving and maintaining remission in CD patients, particularly in postoperative patients.

Side Effects

Sulfasalazine has a number of fairly common and dose-dependent side effects that lead to discontinuation in up to 10%–20% of patients with IBD. Adverse effects linked to plasma sulfapyridine levels include GI symptoms like nausea, vomiting, anorexia, and dyspepsia, as well as malaise and headaches *(3)*. There are also idiosyncratic reactions that include fever, rash, agranulocytosis, hepatitis, pancreatitis, and pneumonitis *(3)*. Folate supplementation is recommended for patients on sulfasalazine as it can impair folate absorption. The newer oral 5-ASA preparations generally have fewer side effects and have been tolerated by up to 80% of sulfasalazine-intolerant patients. The most common side effects are nausea, vomiting, dyspepsia, and headache. Olsalazine has the primary side effect of a dose-related diarrhea, which can decrease over time or with concurrent food ingestion.

Topical Preparations

Mesalamine is available topically in the form of enemas, suppositories, and foams (foams are not currently available in the United States). These agents are primarily indicated in patients with mild-moderate UC restricted to the colon distal to the splenic flexure. Mesalamine enemas (Rowasa®)at doses from 1–4 g/d have been shown to both induce and maintain remission in patients with distal UC of mild-moderate activity, often with fewer side effects than oral sulfasalazine. In addition, combination oral and topical mesalamine may be more effective than oral mesalamine alone for the induction and maintenance of remission of mild–moderate distal UC, although this may simply represent a dose-response curve. Mesalamine suppositories (Canasa® are efficacious for the induction and maintenance of remission in patients with proctitis.

CORTICOSTEROIDS

Corticosteroids have long been the mainstay of therapy for more severe IBD, particularly when requiring hospitalization. Despite their frequency of use, the exact mechanism of action in vivo in IBD is not fully understood. In vitro, corticosteroids block the arachidonic acid pathway through their inhibition of phospholipase A_2 *(3)*. Corticosteroids also interfere with the normal functions of neutrophils, monocytes, and eosinophils *(3)*. Other studies have shown that corticosteroids decrease production of cytokines and NF-κB. Corticosteroids can be given orally, parenterally, or topically, with topical steroids being reserved for the treatment of distal colitis. Owing to the extensive side effect profile of corticosteroids even when given topically *(3)*, newer oral and topical formulations (e.g., budesonide and fluticasone) that have less systemic absorption and/or more first-pass hepatic clearance have been developed *(11)*.

Corticosteroids, whether given orally or parenterally, are effective therapy in UC patients with moderate–severe disease activity *(12)*. Oral prednisone at doses of 40–60 mg/d has been shown to be superior to 20 mg/d for moderate UC, although the higher dosages were associated with more side effects. Parenteral corticosteroids are usually given in the form of methylprednisolone at 40–60 mg/d, although some physicians prefer adrenocorticotropic hormone (ACTH) for steroid-naïve patients. No benefit has been found in the addition of sulfasalazine to corticosteroids in patients with UC or CD of moderate–severe activity. Topical corticosteroids (Cortenema®, Cortifoam®) have been shown to be less effective than topical mesalamine for distal UC, though the combination may be superior to either alone. Studies of newer topical corticosteroid agents, particularly budesonide, have shown beneficial effects in patients with distal UC *(13)*. Despite the clear benefit of corticosteroids to induce remission in UC, there is a very little evidence to support the use of corticosteroids in the maintenance of UC remission *(14)*.

Corticosteroids, given orally or parenterally, are also indicated for the induction of remission of moderate–severe CD, with benefits seen regardless of site of intestinal involvement *(4,5)*. Effective doses of corticosteroids are equipotent to 0.5–0.75 mg/kg/d of prednisone *(14)*. A controlled ileal-release oral formulation of budesonide (Entocort-EC® has proven effective in ileal or ileocecal CD *(11,15)*. As with UC, there has been little data to support the use of steroids in CD patients to maintain remission, although there is conflicting evidence on the benefits of budesonide.

The potential side effects of corticosteroids are multiple and may be quite severe. They suppress intrinsic adrenal function and immune function. They may also induce hyperglycemia, truncal obesity, cataracts, acne, abdominal striae, myopathy, psychiatric disturbances, and avascular necrosis.

ANTIMICROBIALS

Enteric pathogens have long been suspected of playing a role in the cause of IBD, a fact that has led to the investigation of antimicrobial agents as a possible treatment option. Metronidazole (Flagyl®) and ciprofloxacin (Cipro®) are the two antibiotics with the most evidence to support their use. Although neither agent has been conclusively demonstrated to be of benefit in UC, they are used to treat pouchitis in patients status-postcolectomy with ileal-anal anastomosis *(16)* and one recent study *(17)* indicated a possible role for ciprofloxacin in UC.

In CD patients, metronidazole at doses of 10–20 mg/kg/d has been shown to be as effective as sulfasalazine and superior to placebo. Metronidazole has also been beneficial when used to treat perineal complications of CD *(18)* and when used to prevent recurrence for three months postoperatively *(19)*. There is no evidence to support the use of metronidazole for maintenance of nonsurgical remission. Side effects with metronida-zole are not uncommon and include nausea, vomiting, dysgeusia, a disulfuram-like reaction to alcohol, and peripheral neuropathy.

Ciprofloxacin has been shown in one study population to have simi-lar effects to mesalamine in CD patients (20). There has been one report of the beneficial use of ciprofloxacin for perianal CD and the combina-tion of ciprofloxacin and metronidazole has been used successfully to improve CD (1,21). Although one recent study (17) indicated a possible role for ciprofloxacin in UC, additional trials are necessary to clarify its utility. Ciprofloxacin is in general better tolerated than metronidazole with its most common side effects including nausea, vomiting, and diarrhea.

IMMUNOMODULATORS

Azathioprine and 6-mercaptopurine

The importance of immunologic mechanisms in the pathogenesis of IBD forms the basis of using immunomodulators for the treatment of IBD. Of the various immunomodulatory agents, the most widely used are azathioprine (Imuran®) and 6-mercaptopurine (6-MP; Purinethol®). These two agents are purine analogs that interfere with nucleic acid metabolism and cell growth. Azathioprine is nonenzymatically con-verted to 6-MP, which is then metabolized through a series of pathways to 3 metabolites, including the active product, 6-thioguanine (6-TG). In addition to cell-cycle inhibition, these agents also exert cytotoxic effects on lymphoid cells.

Azathioprine and 6-MP have been shown to be more efficacious than placebo in patients with active CD; in a meta-analysis of randomized controlled trials, the overall response rate was 55%, superior to the 33% response rate associated with patients receiving placebo drugs (22). In a similar meta-analysis, azathioprine was shown to maintain remission in approx 67% of patients compared to 53% of patients treated with placebo (22). The five-year relapse rate was 32% for patients main-tained on azathioprine/6-MP compared to 75% for patients who discon-tinue medications following induction of remission with these agents. In addition to inducing and maintaining remission, these agents have also demonstrated steroid-sparing effects. A reduction in steroid to a dose of <10 mg daily can be seen in 65% of the patients receiving induction therapy with azathioprine or 6-MP compared to 36% of those on placebo. Studies have also shown a positive effect of these agents in the treatment of perianal or fistulous Crohn's disease. In one early landmark study *(23)*, fistulas were closed in 31% of the patients treated with 6-MP as opposed to only 6% of the placebo patients.

Limited data from controlled studies have demonstrated efficacy of azathioprine both in the treatment of active UC and in the maintenance of remission. Treatment with azathioprine for at least 6 mo has been shown to lead to a significant reduction of steroid dosage and clinical improvement in steroid-dependent or chronic UC patients. The reported one-year relapse rate was 36% on azathioprine compared to 59% on placebo medication as maintenance therapy ($P = 0.04$) *(24)*. The relapse rate has been reported to be as high as 87% in one retrospective review of 105 patients treated with 6-MP for chronic refractory UC, where complete clinical remission was achieved in 65% of the patients *(25)*.

One major limitation in the use of these agents in the management of active disease is their delayed onset of action of 3–6 mo *(22)*. The initial enthusiasm for the administration of an intravenous loading dose to shorten the time to response was dampened by the negative result in a recent controlled trial *(26)*. Side effects of azathioprine and 6-MP may include nausea, vomiting, bone marrow toxicity, pancreatitis, allergic reactions, and increased liver associated chemistry tests. Patients who experience drug-related pancreatitis or hepatitis may be able tolerate thioguanine (Tabloid®), although the safety of this agent is of concern. Because of their potential suppressive effects on bone marrow, routine blood monitoring for leukopenia and thrombocytopenia is recommended. A complete blood count should be obtained routinely initially; for example, weekly for 4 wk, every other week for 4 wk, and then every 1–2 mo for the duration of time the patient is on azathioprine or 6-MP. The initial concern of an increased risk of lymphoma or leukemia as seen in patients with renal transplants treated with azathioprine or 6-MP has been refuted by recent studies showing a lack of an increased risk of lymphoma or leukemia in patients with IBD treated with these agents *(27,28)*.

The maximal doses for 6-MP and azathioprine are typically reported as 1.5 mg/kg/day and 2.5 mg/kg/d, respectively. However, some patients may respond to even higher doses. A retrospective study reported that the induction of leukopenia, defined by white blood cell count <5000 mm^3, is associated with therapeutic response. The only controlled trial, however, failed to demonstrate such a correlation *(26)*. Recent data have suggested that levels of the active metabolite 6-TG (greater than 235–250 pmol/8 × 10^8 erythrocytes) correlate with a clinical response. Furthermore, mesalamine derivatives may enhance the efficacy of azathioprine or 6-MP by inhibiting thiopurine methyltransferase (TPMT), an enzyme involved in the production of potentially toxic metabolites. At this time, there is no clear consensus on the use of metabolite levels and enzyme genotype/activity to determine the optimal treatment dosage. Additional data are still required to guide our therapeutic strategy in this area.

Methotrexate

Methotrexate (MTX) is a folic acid antagonist and has both immunomodulatory and antiinflammatory properties. It inhibits DNA synthesis and production of proinflammatory cytokines. In a randomized, multicenter, double-blind, placebo-controlled trial, intramuscular MTX at 25 mg/wk for 16 wk was effective in the induction of remission in CD *(29)*. Two controlled studies using oral MTX in a lower dose (12.5 mg/ wk and 15 mg/wk) failed to show a significant benefit for the treatment of active CD. In a more recent randomized controlled trial, intramuscular MTX at 15 mg/wk was shown to be effective as maintenance therapy for CD for the duration of this 40-wk study *(30)*. In the management of UC, unfortunately, oral MTX has not been shown to be effective. However, no study has given parenteral MTX to patients with UC.

Common side effects of MTX include nausea, vomiting, headache, and stomatitis. Bone marrow suppression may occur, but is less common than that with azathioprine or 6-MP *(3)*. Rare but potentially severe toxicities of MTX include hypersensitivity pneumonitis and hepatotoxicity. Hepatic fibrosis and even cirrhosis may result from prolonged MTX exposure, although limited data from the IBD population suggests a low incidence of severe hepatic toxicity even at cumulative doses beyond 1.5 g. A pretreatment liver biopsy should be performed in patients with abnormal liver associated chemistries; however, there is yet no consensus or controlled trial evaluating the utility of follow-up liver biopsy after a cumulative dose of 1.5 g of MTX.

Cyclosporine

Cyclosporine A (CyA) is a potent inhibitor of cell-mediated immunity. Its use in IBD is primarily in severe steroid-refractory UC. In the only placebo-controlled trial to date, the initial response rate to intravenous CyA 4 mg/kg/d was 82% in patients with severe UC unresponsive to 7 d of intravenous corticosteroids (equivalent to 300 mg hydrocortisone) *(31)*. With the addition of azathioprine or 6-MP, colectomy can be avoided in 80% of patients who initially responded to CyA. Thus, intravenous CyA can be viewed as a "bridge" until the azathioprine or 6-MP takes effect. Studies with oral cyclosporine have not demonstrated any beneficial clinical effect.

No controlled trials of parenteral CyA have been completed in patients with severe CD. However, fistulizing and refractory inflammatory CD may respond rapidly to intravenous CyA in uncontrolled reports *(32)*. Oral CyA has shown significant benefit in the treatment of active CD in one of four controlled trials. The dose in that study was a mean of 7.6 mg/kg/d compared to the mean dose of 5 mg/kg/d in the other three studies *(33–36)*. The new preparation of oral CyA (Neoral®), designed to minimize the variable absorption of the older preparation (Sandimmune®) may be as effective as parenteral CyA in the treatment of steroid-resistant UC based upon uncontrolled data.

When using CyA, whole blood trough CyA concentrations should be monitored daily with the goal between 200 and 400 ng/mL. Reversible side effects of CyA are hypertension, gingival hyperplasia, paresthesias, tremors, headache, electrolyte abnormalities, and increased liver-associated chemistries. Serious side effects include seizures, particularly in patients with serum cholesterol <120 mg/dL, anaphylaxis, opportunistic infections such as *Pneumocystis carinii* (*P. carinii*) pneumonia, and nephrotoxicity. Prophylaxis with Bactrim is now considered as a standard care. In addition to CyA concentrations, electrolytes (especially Mg and K) and renal function should be routinely monitored in patients treated with CyA.

Other Immunomodulatory Agents

Two other immunomodulatory agents commonly used in the post-organ transplantation to prevent rejection have also been used in IBD. These are mycophenolate mofetil (CellCept®) and tacrolimus (FK506, Prograf®).

Tacrolimus has a similar mode of action to CyA, but is significantly more potent than CyA. Preliminary uncontrolled data have suggested a beneficial effect of intravenous and oral tacrolimus in steroid-refractory IBD and fistulizing CD, although no controlled trials have been reported. Treatment with oral tacrolimus in combination with azathioprine or 6-MP also appears to have some clinical benefit in patients with refractory Crohn's disease complicated by fistulas. Side effects of tacrolimus include nausea, headache, paresthesias, tremors, hair loss, hypertension, and nephrotoxicity.

Mycophenolate mofetil is a purine synthesis inhibitor that also has a potent immunosuppressive profile. After preliminary studies suggesting efficacy in CD, a randomized trial comparing mycophenolate and azathioprine in patients with severely active disease requiring corticosteroids showed a greater and faster clinical improvement after 1 mo of treatment with mycophenolate than with azathioprine. Subsequent studies have questioned this agent's efficacy and safety record in patients with IBD. Side effects of mycophenolate are primarily gastrointestinal, with minimal nephrotoxicity, thus offering an attractive alternative in patients intolerant to CyA or tacrolimus secondary to nephrotoxicity. These agents represent alternative options in patients refractory to conventional medical therapy as well as other immunomodulators. However, more data is needed regarding the efficacy and safety of these agents in IBD before they can be more widely used.

BIOLOGICAL THERAPY

The past decade's research has led to an improved understanding regarding the pathogenesis of IBD and significant advances in molecular science. This has led to a recent interest in the use of novel therapeutic modalities, particularly biological therapies, in the treatment of inflammatory bowel disease. For many traditional therapies such as glucocorticoids or 5-ASA, their use in IBD derives from their known effects in other inflammatory conditions. The precise molecular mechanism of their antiinflammatory properties has been only partially elucidated despite decades of their widespread use. In contrast, these novel biological therapies have been designed to target specific aspects of the mechanism of IBD. These therapeutic targets include antigen presentation, specific and nonspecific inflammatory cytokines and mediators, cellular recruitment and adhesion, and wound repair and restitution.

Anti-Tumor Necrosis Factor (TNF) Therapy

INFLIXIMAB

Among the various biological therapies, infliximab has had the most research and is currently FDA-approved for clinical use. Infliximab (Remicade®) is a chimeric (75% human and 25% mouse) monoclonal antibody directed against human TNF-α. The hope that monotherapy with anti-TNF-α antibody can be effective in the treatment of IBD is based on the observation that TNF-α serves as a pivotal mediator in the cascade of mucosal inflammation. The mechanism of action of infliximab is not entirely understood, but is felt to be multifactorial, including transcriptional inhibition of the production of TNF-α, direct binding of soluble and membrane-bound TNF-α, and induction of T-cell apoptosis. In a randomized, double-blind, placebo-controlled study in patients with moderately to severely active CD, treatment with a single infusion of infliximab 5 mg/kg resulted in clinical improvement in 81% and remission in 48% of the patients after 4 wk *(37)*. This is significantly higher than the 4% remission rate and 17% response rate in patients receiving placebo. The subsequent large ACCENT I trial has shown that "induction" therapy with three 5 mg/kg infusions at 0,2, and 6 wk followed by maintenance infusions every 8 wk is effective in inducing and maintaining remission, is steroid-sparing, and heals the mucosa *(38)*. Dose escalation to 10 mg/kg in patients who initially responded, but then failed to improve with subsequent doses was also shown to be efficacious. The benefit of infliximab in chronic active CD, including endoscopic and histologic improvement, has also been confirmed by additional studies *(39)*.

Infliximab also appears to be effective for treating fistulas. Three doses of 5 mg/kg infliximab at 0, 2, and 6 wk resulted in a 50% or greater reduction in the number of draining fistulae in up to 68% of patients *(40)*. Complete fistula closure occurred in 55% of the patients, compared to only 13% of the patients receiving placebo. The median duration of response was nearly 3 mo *(40)*. The recently completed ACCENT II study suggests continued benefit with reinfusions every 8 wk, as well as efficacy with dose escalation to 10 mg/kg in those patients who stopped responding to the 5 mg dose. Uncontrolled data in small number suggest infliximab may be beneficial in UC, although large controlled studies are still ongoing. Currently, infliximab is approved by Food and Drug Administration for the use in patients with active enteric and fistulizing CD refractory to standard medical therapy.

Side effects of infliximab are numerous and include upper respiratory tract infections, abdominal pain, fatigue, myalgia, nausea, infusion reactions, and the development of human antichimeric antibodies (HACA) and antidouble-stranded DNA antibodies; the significance of the last complication is not known at this time. Rare instances of reactivation of tuberculosis has prompted the FDA to recommend PPD testing of all patients receiving infliximab, with appropriate therapy for possible carriers or patients with active TB infections. Though cases of lymphoma have been reported after infliximab infusion for CD *(41)*, the incidence is felt to be no higher than the baseline incidence in the general population. Further studies are still needed to evaluate the long-term efficacy and safety profile of infliximab.

CDP571 AND ETANERCEPT

CDP571 is a humanized (95% human and 5% murine) chimeric monoclonal antibody directed against TNF-α. In a small double-blind, placebo-controlled trial, 5 mg/kg of CDP571 demonstrated an initial benefit in patients with active CD, although remission rates were similar to those seen with placebo. In a larger randomized, double-blind, placebo-controlled trial in 71 patients with steroid-dependent CD, treatment with CDP571 (20 mg/kg at wk 0 followed by 10 mg/kg at wk 8) resulted in complete steroid withdrawal by 16 wk in 44% of the patients compared to 22% of the patients treated with placebo ($p = 0.049$) *(42)*. Once complete steroid withdrawal was achieved, an open-label extension of that trial showed an 87% success rate of maintaining steroid withdrawal after 6 mo. CDP571 appears to be effective in inducing clinical response, but not clinical remission, after 2 wk of treatment, and the optimal dose is 10 mg/kg. CDP571 also may be effective in the treatment of CD complicated by fistulas. No comparisons between this agent and infliximab have yet been undertaken. As an agent for ulcerative colitis, an uncontrolled trial of CDP571 in 15 patients with UC produced only modest improvement.

Etanercept (Enbrel®) is a human fusion protein combining the Fc portion of IgG with the ligand-binding portion of the TNF-α receptor, with the resultant effect of inactivating TNF-α. Although some promise was seen for this agent in a small pilot study of Crohn's patients, a subsequent larger placebo-controlled trial found no benefit of the drug when compared to placebo *(43)*.

THALIDOMIDE

Despite its notorious teratogenic effect in the 1950s, thalidomide has recently received revived attention as a therapeutic agent in CD because of its recently discovered inhibitory action on TNF-α production. Two recent small open-labeled trials suggest its possible benefit in CD. Treatment with thalidomide of variable doses (50 mg/d to 300 mg/d) for 12 wk resulted in a response rate ranging from 64% to 70% in steroid-dependent CD patients with moderately to severely active disease *(44,45)*. Thalidomide therapy also appears to have a favorable effect on fistulous diseases. A preliminary report of a small trial suggested this agent might be effective for patients with medically refractory UC. Other than its teratogenicity, thalidomide may cause sedation and peripheral neuropathy. Validation of these preliminary pilot studies still requires future randomized controlled trials.

Other Biological Therapy

Advances in molecule biologic techniques have further expanded the array of biologic therapies available to treat IBD. In addition to chimeric and humanized monoclonal antibodies as in the case of anti-TNF-α therapy, recombinant cytokines and antisense oligonucleotides all represent applications of molecular techniques.

It is known that cytokines play an important role in the pathogenesis of IBD by controlling the initiation and regulation of the inflammatory cascade. Certain cytokines, such as TNF-α, and interleukins (IL)-1, -2, -6, -8, and -12 are broadly categorized as "proinflammatory", while others, including IL-4, -5, -10, -11, -13, and transforming growth factor β (TGF-β) are considered "antiinflammatory." Consequently, it is not surprising that cytokines-directed therapies may be beneficial in IBD. In this regard, recombinant human IL-10 (rhIL-10) in both intravenous and subcutaneous forms has demonstrated clinical benefit in steroid-refractory or chronic active CD. Recombinant human IL-10 has also been investigated in patients with UC, with somewhat disappointing results. Another recombinant human cytokine, IL-11 (rhIL-11), has shown preliminary benefit in CD. In a larger trial comparing various dosing regimens in the treatment of active CD, the highest response rate was 42%, but the treatment required 5 subcutaneous infusions weekly.

In the hope to therapeutically target a different arm of intestinal inflammation, an antisense oligonucleotide that inhibits intercellular adhesion molecule 1 (ICAM-1) expression, ISIS 2302, was engineered. ICAM-1 is critical for the trafficking and activation of leukocytes. Circulating and tissue levels of ICAM-1 have been shown to be increased in active IBD. In a small pilot study, ISIS-2302 appears to be effective and steroid-sparing in the treatment of moderately active CD *(46)*. Unfortunately, the results of two more recent large randomized, placebo-controlled trials were disappointing, and did not support the use of ISIS 2302 in CD.

Another promising strategy utilizing the blockade of cellular interactions at the level of adhesion molecules involves the use humanized monoclonal antibodies directed against the lymphocyte adhesion molecules $\alpha4\beta1$(natalizumab; Antegren™) and $\alpha4\beta7$ (LDP-02). Their use in UC has also been investigated.

One biological agent that has recently received tremendous interest in the medical community, as well as the public at large, is human growth hormone. Although its precise effect in IBD is unknown, growth hormone has been shown to have multiple properties on the intestinal tract. Growth hormone improves net protein anabolism and stimulates wound healing; it exerts a trophic effect on the intestinal tract and is important in accelerating intestinal healing in animal models of small bowel ulceration. In a preliminary study of 37 patients with moderately to severely active CD, treatment with growth hormone (somatropin) (5 mg/d subcutaneously for 1 wk, followed by a maintenance dose of 1.5 mg/d) led to a mean decrease in Crohn's Disease Activity Index score of 143 points after 4 mo, compared to a decrease of 19 points in patients treated with placebo ($P = 0.004$) *(47)*. Whether these results can be translated into efficacy in inducing remission still awaits future large randomized controlled trials. Prospective studies attempting to better understand its mechanism of action are now ongoing.

Other biological therapies for IBD include monoclonal anti-CD4 antibodies for active CD and potentially the use of factors important for intestinal healing in IBD, including trefoil proteins and peptide growth factors (e.g.,, keratinocyte growth factor).

OTHER INVESTIGATIONAL THERAPY

Aside from the products of recent advances in molecular biology, two agents that are widely used for other medical conditions have been suggested to have a benefit in the treatment of IBD.

The first of these agents is heparin. The potential benefit of heparin in IBD was initially discovered as an incidental observation that patients with UC being treated with intravenous heparin for non-IBD-related indications (pulmonary embolus) had improvement in their gastrointestinal symptoms. Furthermore, unfractionated heparin has been shown to have potent immunomodulatory effects. The use of unfractionated heparin, usually involving intravenous (iv) administration followed by subcutaneous injections, has been reported to be beneficial in the treatment of highly active UC in both uncontrolled and controlled studies. A recent small randomized pilot study of 20 patients showed that unfractionated heparin is as effective as corticosteroids as a first-line therapy in the treatment of severe UC and Crohn's colitis. However, another study reported in abstract form comparing unfractionated heparin with steroid concluded that heparin as monotherapy is not effective in the treatment of severe UC. Future large, randomized trials are needed to answer these conflicting data, as well as to further evaluate the efficacy of low molecular weight heparin in the treatment of active UC.

Rosiglitazone (Avandia®) is another drug that may also have potential benefit in the treatment of IBD. This medication, currently on the market as an antidiabetic agent, is a ligand for peroxisome proliferator-activated receptor gamma (PPARγ). These ligands have recently been shown to have antiinflammatory properties in the intestinal tract both in vitro and in vivo. An open-label pilot study suggested that rosiglitazone may be effective in the treatment of UC *(48)*, although further randomized controlled trials are still needed to assess its efficacy.

MEDICAL THERAPY OF SPECIFIC
CLINICAL PRESENTATIONS
Ulcerative Colitis

PROCTITIS

Proctitis is defined as inflammation of the rectum. Topical therapy is often used initially, with mesalamine suppositories (Canasa® being preferred to corticosteroid enemas because of their higher remission rates and better efficacy in maintenance of remission. Clinical improvement frequently occurs within 2–4 wk and therapy should be continued at treatment doses until complete resolution of active disease. After completion of treatment, remission can be maintained with mesalamine suppositories or enemas (Rowasa®) two to three times weekly, although some patients can be followed without maintenance therapy. Topical steroid preparations (Cortenema®, Cortifoam®) are also effective, but long-term use may lead to steroid-related side effects. If topical therapy is poorly tolerated or not desired, oral aminosalicylate therapy can be tried. In severe or refractory cases, oral corticosteroid therapy or immunosuppressants may be required.

DISTAL UC

Distal UC is usually considered active disease limited to the distal 30–40 cm of colon *(21)*. In all but severe cases, topical therapy is frequently used as first-line. Agents are best selected based upon how far proximal the colitis extends: suppositories treat to 10 cm from the anal verge, and foam can cover to 15–20 cm, and enemas can extend to the splenic flexure *(12)*. Mesalamine enemas given nightly are preferred to corticosteroid enemas due to their higher efficacy at maintaining remission; once remission is attained, maintenance therapy should be undertaken with thrice weekly mesalamine enemas. If after 3–4 wk of therapy there is no remission, a corticosteroid enema or an additional mesalamine enema can be added in the morning *(21)*. Alternatively, oral aminosalicylates at moderate doses can be added or be used to supplant topical therapy. If moderate doses of oral aminosalicylates are ineffective, then high doses should be tried, although many patients will have difficulty with high-dose sulfasalazine. For patients with severe or refractory disease, treatment with oral corticosteroids equipotent to 40–60 mg/d of prednisone can be tried and then rapidly tapered over 10 d *(21)*.

PANCOLITIS

Pancolitis is defined as active disease extending to and beyond the hepatic flexure *(21)*. When disease extends beyond the mid-descending colon and especially the splenic flexure, topical therapy is usually inadequate. For patients with mild–moderate disease, oral aminosalicylates (Asacol®, Azulfidine®, Colazal®, Dipentum®, Pentasa®) should be tried, typically at higher doses *(12,21)*. Topical aminosalicylates can be added as patients have noted a quicker resolution with the combination *(12,21)*. Maintenance of remission may be attempted with lower doses of oral aminosalicylates. In patients refractory to the above treatments or with severe, but nontoxic pancolitis, oral prednisone at doses of 40–60 mg/d should be prescribed and continued until remission, followed by a slow taper over a few months *(12,21)*. In steroid-resistant or steroid-dependent UC patients, the immunomodulators azathioprine and 6-mercaptopurine have been useful both in achieving remission and in permitting steroid sparing; these drugs also have evidence to support their use in the maintenance of remission *(24)* (Figs. 1 and 2).

SEVERE AND FULMINANT UC

Severe colitis is defined as UC presenting with systemic signs such as fever, weight loss, bloody diarrhea, severe anemia, or volume depletion whereas fulminant UC is severe colitis in a patient that appears toxic. The first step in the management of these patients is immediate admission to a hospital and complete bowel rest. Parenteral corticosteroids at a doses equipotent to 48 mg/d of methylprednisolone are the first-line therapy, though some physicians recommend adenocorticotrophic hormone (ACTH) in steroid-naïve patients. Aminosalicylates are generally avoided in these patients. In patients with fever, leukocytosis, megacolon, or peritoneal signs, broad-spectrum antibiotics are frequently used empirically *(12)*, however, controlled trials of antibiotics have not shown improved outcomes. Given that the failure rate of medical therapy was found to be 38% in one review of severe UC, all patients should be followed carefully by an experienced surgeon *(12,21)*. Patients who fail to improve after 7–10 d of medical therapy are unlikely to respond to further medical management and should be treated either surgically or with therapy such as iv cyclosporine therapy. Studies have shown that iv cyclosporine can decrease disease activity and forestall surgery in the majority of patients with resistant UC *(31)*, however, many of these patients will ultimately require colectomy in the ensuing 6–12 mo, especially if they do not use an immunosuppressant such as 6-MP or AZA (Fig. 2).

Crohn's Disease

ACTIVE SMALL AND LARGE BOWEL DISEASE

Proper management of patients with active CD depends on the location and severity of disease (Figs. 3–5). For patients with mild–moder-

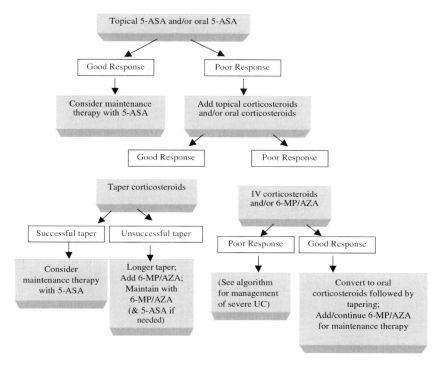

Fig. 1. Suggested guideline for management of mildly to moderately active ulcerative colitis (UC).

ate ileocolitis or colitis, oral aminosalicylate therapy can be tried first. Sulfasalazine *(4,5)* and mesalamine *(6,7)* have both been used successfully in these patients. If disease is more proximal or confined to the small bowel, then mesalamine preparations that can reach the site affected should be utilized *(see* Table 1) *(6–8)*. Dosages of aminosalicylates should be started at moderate doses and then increased gradually to maximal doses to improve patient tolerance *(6,7)*. If there is no improvement after 2–4 wk of aminosalicylates, antimicrobial therapy with metronidazole or ciprofloxacin can be tried.

If patients fail these regimens, present with more severe disease, or show systemic symptoms, then corticosteroids are typically the next treatment option. If patients appear well, oral corticosteroids at dosages equivalent to prednisone 40–60 mg/d can be prescribed *(4,5,14)* followed by a slow taper. A controlled-release form of budesonide (Entocort-EC™ has also been used successfully *(11,15)*. Severely ill patients with systemic symptoms should be hospitalized immediately,

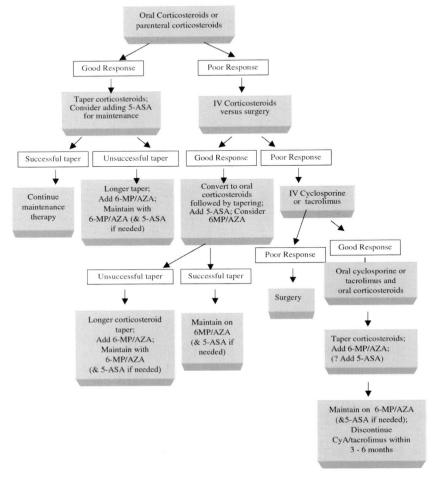

Fig. 2. Suggested guideline for management of severe UC.

placed on strict bowel rest, and given parenteral steroids. These patients are frequently administered empirical broad-spectrum antimicrobials and should be observed closely by an experienced surgeon. There is a growing trend to using the highly effective anti-TNF agent infliximab (Remicade®) sooner in patients who do not respond to the traditional agents, or who cannot wait for the multiple weeks to months for other immunosuppressants to become effective.

MAINTENANCE OF REMISSION

Until recently, there were few effective options available to maintain remission in CD. Sulfasalazine is ineffective at maintaining remission

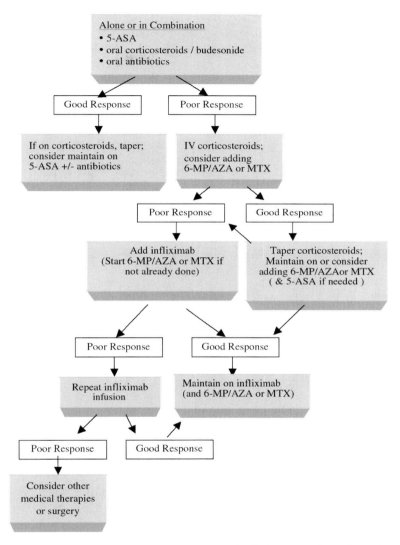

Fig. 3. Suggested guideline for management of mildly to moderately active Crohn's disease (CD).

of CD *(4,5)*. Oral mesalamine preparations have been shown to be beneficial in maintaining remission of CD, particularly postoperatively *(9)*, though they are less effective than in UC patients and relatively ineffective in patients with steroid-induced remission *(10)*. There is conflicting evidence on the effectiveness of corticosteroids including budesonide in preventing relapse in CD *(4,5)*, but most experts *(14)* caution against

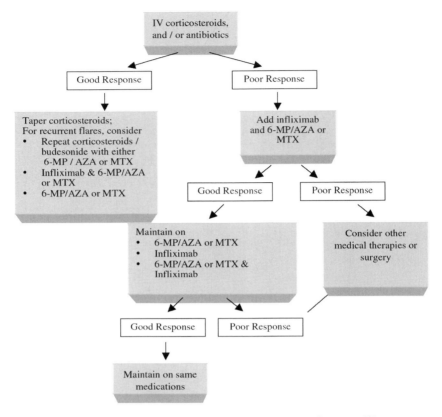

Fig. 4. Suggested guideline for management of severe CD.

the use of corticosteroids for maintenance of remission. Azathioprine and 6-mercaptopurine are useful in reducing steroid dependence of CD patients *(22,23)*. Antimicrobials play a limited role as metronidazole has been shown of benefit only to prevent postoperative recurrence *(19)* and they are needed for long periods of time at high doses, thereby resulting in side effects. Infliximab, however, appears to show promise as a maintenance therapy as the ACCENT I trial demonstrated significant reduction in relapse rates with infusions every 8 wk *(38)*. If this is borne out in future studies of TNF-α antagonists, these agents may become first-line therapy for the maintenance of CD remission.

FISTULAS AND PERIANAL DISEASE

Enteroenteric fistulas should be treated when symptomatic and, in general, medical therapy is preferred since recurrence after surgery is

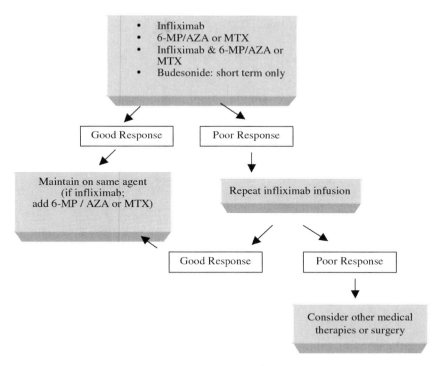

Fig. 5. Suggested guideline for management of CD in patients with intolerance or prior toxicity to steroids.

common *(21)*. Antimicrobial therapy with metronidazole and/or ciprofloxacin is the usual first-line therapy (Fig. 6). 6-mercaptopurine has been used effectively to treat fistulous disease *(23)*. Infliximab has demonstrated significant benefits in the treatment of fistulas and may become first-line therapy for fistulous disease in the future *(40)*. Other more experimental therapies include intravenous cyclosporine, tacrolimus, and oral thalidomide.

Perineal disease is also treated initially with antimicrobial agents, particularly metronidazole *(18)*. Lengthy courses of high-dose metronidazole (20 mg/kg/d) are frequently required and relapses are common. Failure of antimicrobial therapy usually leads to a trial of 6-MP or AZA *(23)*, although infliximab may come to play a larger role in this aspect of CD *(40)*.

POSTOPERATIVE RECURRENCE

By 4 yr, CD recurs in up to half of all patients who have achieved remission through surgery *(21)*. High-dose oral mesalamine *(9,49)* has

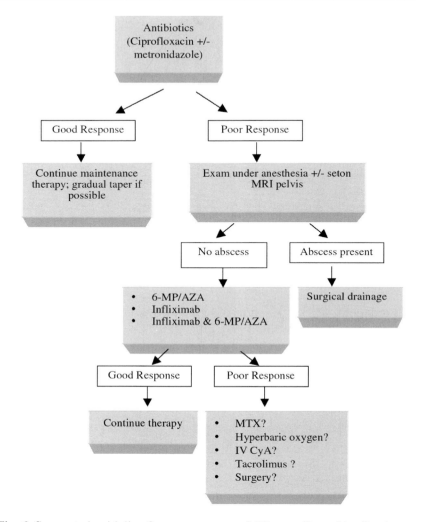

Fig. 6. Suggested guideline for management of CD complicated by fistulas or perianal disease.

shown limited benefits in reducing relapse rates in postoperative patients. Metronidazole has evidence to support its use, but the high doses required frequently cause side effects *(19)*. 6-Mercaptopurine was previously reserved for remission maintenance of more severe or highly recurrent disease *(21)*, although promising data has resulted in more widespread use of this agent. To date, infliximab has not been specifically studied for the maintenance of surgically-induced remissions, but is suspected to be effective.

Indications for Referral to a Subspecialist

Given the complexity of disease, the management of patients with IBD should be a joint venture between the non-subspecialist primary physicians (e.g., internists, family practitioners) and gastroenterologists. In general, all patients with IBD should be followed by gastroenterologists, while the systemic manifestations or complications of IBD such as osteoporosis are managed by their primary physicians. Perhaps the only exception is those UC patients with proctitis associated with infrequent mild exacerbations. This subgroup of IBD patients may be managed primarily by their primary physician, with episodic follow-up (e.g., yearly) by the gastroenterologists. Even in those patients, one should bear in mind that disease may extend beyond the initial presentation of proctitis and thus cannot be adequately assessed by office flexible sigmoidoscopy. Furthermore, this change in the extent of disease will impact the need for surveillance colonoscopy for colorectal cancer.

CONCLUSION

Treatment of IBD has historically been challenging both owing to the severity of the disease and the toxicity of the treatment in the United States. Aminosalicylates are first-line therapy for induction and maintenance of remission in mild–moderate IBD, with corticosteroids reserved for more severe cases. Antimicrobials, like metronidazole and ciprofloxacin, are useful for some CD patients whereas immunomodulators, like 6-mercaptopurine and azathioprine, have a role in the management of steroid-dependent or steroid-resistant disease. Promising new biologic therapies that have relatively few side effects, such as infliximab, are now emerging that appear to have benefit in the induction and maintenance of remission of IBD, even in circumstances previously refractory to medical therapy. In the coming years, the management of IBD, and CD in particular, may change dramatically with the initiation of these agents earlier in the course of treatment.

REFERENCES

1. Stein RB, Hanauer SB. Medical therapy for inflammatory bowel disease. Gastroenterol Clin North Am 1999;28(3):297–321.
2. Azad Khan AK, Piris J, Truelove SC. An experiment to determine the active therapeutic moiety sulphasalazine. Lancet 1977;2(8044):892–895.
3. Hanauer SB, Meyers S, Sachar DB. The pharmacology of antiinflammatory drugs in inflammatory bowel disease. In: Kirsner JB and Shorter RG, eds. Inflammatory Bowel Disease, 4th Edition. Williams & Wilkins, Baltimore, MD, 1995, pp. 643–663.
4. Malchow H, Ewe K, Brandes JW, et al. European cooperative Crohn's disease study (ECCDS): results of drug treatment. Gastroenterology 1984;86(2):249–266.

5. Summers RW, Switz DM, Sessions JT Jr, et al. National Cooperative Crohn's Disease Study (NCCDS): results of drug treatment. Gastroenterology 1979;77(4 Pt 2):847–869.

6. Singleton JW, Hanauer SB, Gitnick GL, et al. Mesalamine capsules for the treatment of active Crohn's disease: results of a 16-wk trial. The Pentasa Crohn's Disease Study Group. Gastroenterology 1993;104(5):1293–1301.

7. Tremaine WJ, Schroeder KW, Harrison JM, et al. A randomized, double-blind, placebo-controlled trial of the oral mesalamine (5-ASA) preparation, Asacol, in the treatment of symptomatic Crohn's colitis and ileocolitis. J Clin Gastroenterol 1994;19(4):278–282.

8. Prantera C, Cottone M, Pallone F, et al. Mesalamine in the treatment of mild to moderate active Crohn's ileitis: results of a randomized, multicenter trial. Gastroenterology 1999;116(3):521–526.

9. Camma C, Giunta M, Rosselli M, et al. Mesalamine in the maintenance treatment of Crohn's disease: a meta-analysis adjusted for confounding variables. Gastroenterology 1997;113(5):1465–1473.

10. Modigliani R, Colombel JF, Dupas JL, et al. Mesalamine in Crohn's disease with steroid-induced remission: effect on steroid withdrawal and remission maintenance. Groupe d'Etudes Therapeutiques des Affections Inflammatoires Digestives (GETAID). Gastroenterology 1996;110(3):688–693.

11. Greenberg GR, Feagan BG, Martin F, et al. Oral budesonide for active Crohn's disease. The Canadian Inflammatory Bowel Disease Study Group. N Engl J Med 1994;331(13):836–841.

12. Kornbluth A, Sachar DB. Ulcerative colitis practice guidelines in adults. Am J Gastroenterol 1997;92(2):204–211.

13. Danielsson A, Lofberg R, Persson T, et al. A steroid enema, budesonide, lacking systemic effects for the treatment of distal ulcerative colitis or proctitis. Scand J Gastroenterol 1992;27(1):9–12.

14. Hanauer SB, Meyers S. Management of Crohn's disease in adults. Am J Gastroenterol 1997;92(4):559–566.

15. Thomsen OO, Cortot A, Jewell D, et al. A comparison of budesonide and mesalamine for active Crohn's disease. International Budesonide-Mesalamine Study Group. N Engl J Med 1998;339(6):370–374.

16. Sandborn WJ. Pouchitis following ileal pouch-anal anastomosis: definition, pathogenesis, and treatment. Gastroenterology 1994;107(6):1856–1860.

17. Turunen UM, Farkkila MA, Hakala K, et al. Long-term treatment of ulcerative colitis with ciprofloxacin: a prospective, double-blind, placebo-controlled study. Gastroenterology 1998;115(5):1072–1078.

18. Bernstein LH, Frank MS, Brandt LJ, et al. Healing of perineal Crohn's disease with metronidazole. Gastroenterology 1980;79(2):357–365.

19. Rutgeerts P, Hiele M, Geboes K, et al. Controlled trial of metronidazole treatment for prevention of Crohn's recurrence after ileal resection. Gastroenterology 1995;108(6):1617–1621.

20. Colombel JF, Lemann M, Cassagnou M, et al. A controlled trial comparing ciprofloxacin with mesalazine for the treatment of active Crohn's disease. Groupe d'Etudes Therapeutiques des Affections Inflammatoires Digestives (GETAID). Ame J Gastroenterol 1999;94(3):674–678.

21. Michetti P, Peppercorn MA. Medical therapy of specific clinical presentations. Gastroenterol Clin North Am 1999;28(3):353–370.

22. Pearson DC, May GR, Fick GH, et al. Azathioprine and 6-mercaptopurine in Crohn's disease. A meta-analysis. Ann Intern Med 1995;123(2):132–142.

23. Present DH, Korelitz BI, Wisch N, et al. Treatment of Crohn's disease with 6-mercaptopurine: a long-term, randomized, double-blind study. N Engl J Med 1980;302(18):981–987.

24. Hawthorne AB, Logan RFA, Hawkey CJ, et al. Randomized controlled trial of azathioprine withdrawal in ulcerative colitis. Br Med J 1992;305(6844):20–22.

25. George J, Present DH, Pou R, et al. The long-term outcome of ulcerative colitis treated with 6-mercaptopurine. Am J Gastroenterol 1996;91(9):1711–1714.

26. Sandborn WJ, Tremaine WJ, Wolf DC, et al. Lack of effect of intravenous azathioprine on time to respond to azathioprine for steroid treated Crohn's disease. North American Azathioprine Study Group. Gastroenterology 1999;117(3): 527–535.

27. Lewis JD, Schwartz JS, Lichtenstein GR. Azathioprine for maintenance of remission in Crohn's disease: benefits outweigh the risk of lymphoma. Gastroenterology 2000;118(6):1018–1024.

28. Su CG, Stein RB, Lewis JD, Lichtenstein GR. Azathioprine or 6-mercaptopurine for inflammatory bowel disease: Do risks outweigh benefits? Dig Liver Dis 2000;32:518–531.

29. Feagan BG, Rochon J, Fedorak RN, et al. Methotrexate for the treatment of Crohn's disease. The North American Crohn's Study Group Investigators. N Engl J Med 1995;332(5):292–297.

30. Feagan BG, Fedorak RN, Irvine EJ, et al. A comparison of methotrexate with placebo for the maintenance of remission in Crohn's disease. North American Crohn's Study Group Investigators. N Engl J Med 2000;342(22):1627–1632.

31. Lichtiger S, Present DH, Kornbluth A, et al. Cyclosporine in severe ulcerative colitis refractory to steroid therapy. N Engl J Med 1994;330(26):1841–1845.

32. Egan LJ, Sandborn WJ, Tremaine WJ. Clinical outcome following treatment of refractory inflammatory and fistulizing Crohn's disease with intravenous cyclosporine. Am J Gastroenterol 1998;93(3):442–448.

33. Brynskov J, Freund L, Rasmussen SN, et al. A placebo-controlled, double-blind, randomized trial of cyclosporine therapy in active chronic Crohn's disease. N Engl J Med 1989;321(13):845–850.

34. Feagan BG, McDonald JW, Rochon J, et al. Low-dose cyclosporine for the treatment of Crohn's disease. The Canadian Crohn's Relapse Prevention Trial. N Engl J Med 1994;330(26):1846–1851.

35. Jewell DP, Lennard-Jones JE, et al. Oral cyclosporine for chronic active Crohn's disease: a multicentre controlled trial. Eur J Gastroenterol Hepatol 1994;6: 499–505.

36. Stange EF, Modigliani R, Pena AS, et al. European trial of cyclosporine in chronic active Crohn's disease: a 12-mo study. Gastroenterol 1995;109(3):774–782.

37. Targan SR, Hanauer SB, van Deventer SJ, et al. A short-term study of chimeric monoclonal antibody CA2 to tumor necrosis factor (α) for Crohn's disease. Crohn's Disease cA2 Study Group. N Engl J Med 1997;337(15):1029–1035.

38. Hanauer SB, Feagan BG, Lichtenstein GR, et al. Maintenance infliximab for Crohn's disease: the ACCENT I randomised trial. Lancet 2002;359(9317): 1541–49.

39. D'Haens G, van Deventer SJH, van Hogezand R, et al. Endoscopic and histological healing with infliximab anti-tumor necrosis factor antibodies in Crohn's disease: A European multicenter trial. Gastroenterology 1999;116(5): 1029–1034.

40. Present DH, Rutgeerts P, Targan S, et al. Infliximab for the treatment of fistulas in patients with Crohn's disease. N Engl J Med 1999;340(18):1398–1405.

41. Bickston SJ, Lichtenstein GR, Arseneau et al. The relationship between infliximab treatment and lymphoma in Crohn's disease. Gastroenterology 1999;117(6): 1433–1437.

42. Feagon BG, Sandborn WJ, Baker JP, et al. A randomized, double-blind, placebo, controlled multi-center trial of the engineered human antibody to TNF (CDP571) for steroid sparing and maintenance of remission in patients with steroid-dependent Crohn's disease [abstract]. Gastroenterology 2000;118:A665.

43. Sandborn WJ, Hanauer SB, Katz S, et al. Etanercept for active Crohn's disease: a randomized, double-blind, placebo-controlled trial. Gastro 2001;121(5): 1088–94.

44. Ehrenpreis ED, Kane SV, Cohen LB, et al. Thalidomide therapy for patients with refractory Crohn's disease: an open-label trial. Gastroenterology 1999;117(6): 1271–1277.

45. Vasiliauskas EA, Kam LY, Abreu-Martin MT, et al. An open-label pilot study of low-dose thalidomide in chronically active, steroid-dependent Crohn's disease. Gastroenterology 1999;117(6):1278–1287.

46. Yacyshyn BR, Bowen-Yacyshyn MB, Jewell L, et al. A placebo-controlled trial of ICAM-1 antisense oligonucleotide in the treatment of Crohn's disease. Gastroenterology 1998;114(6):1133–1142.

47. Slonim AE, Bulone L, Damore MB, et al. A preliminary study of growth hormone therapy for Crohn's disease. N Engl J Med 2000;342(22):1633–1637.

48. Lewis JD, Lichtenstein GR, Stein RB, et al. An open-label trial of the PPAR-gamma igand rosiglitazone for active ulcerative colitis. Am J Gastroenterol. 2001;96:3323–3328.

49. McLeod RS, Wolff BG, Steinhart AH. Prophylactic mesalamine treatment decreases postoperative recurrence of Crohn's disease. Gastroenterology 1995;109(2):404–413.

9

Surgical Management of Inflammatory Bowel Disease

Roger D. Hurst, MD

CONTENTS

INTRODUCTION

Approximately one-third of patients with ulcerative colitis (UC) and as high as 75% of patients with Crohn's disease (CD) will require surgery for the management of their disease. Surgery, however, is almost never performed as the sole therapy and thus operative intervention is employed as an integrated part of a mutidiciplinary approach to the management of inflammatory bowel disease (IBD). As such, surgical decision making, as part of the care of the IBD patient, requires close consultation and communication between the surgeon, the gastroenterologist, and the patient.

ULCERATIVE COLITIS

The surgical management of UC involves removal of the entire colon and rectum. This can be accomplished with either of two final results. Resection of the colon and rectum can be performed with removal of the anal sphincters and a permanent ileostomy; a total proctocolectomy (TPC). Alternatively, the anal sphincter mechanism can be preserved with creation of an ileal neo-rectum anastomosed to the anal canal; a

From: *Clinical Gastroenterology:*
Inflammatory Bowel Disease: Diagnosis and Therapeutics
Edited by: R. D. Cohen © Humana Press Inc., Totowa, NJ

Table I
Surgical Options for Ulcerative Colitis

Total Proctocolectomy
  With Brooke Ileostomy
  Or With Continent Ileostomy:
    Kock Pouch
    BCIR
Restorative Proctocolectomy with Ileal Pouch-Anal Anastomosis (IPAA)
  Stapled or Hand-Sutured Anastomosis
  J, W, or S Reservoir
  With or Without diverting loop ileostomy
Staged Colectomy with Brooke Ileostomy
and Hartmann's pouch (or Mucus Fistula)
  Followed by Delayed:
    Completion Proctectomy
    Or Restorative Proctectomy with IPAA

Table 2
Indications for Operation: UC

1. Failure of Medical Management
2. Cancer Risk
3. Recalcitrant Fulminate Colitis
4. Toxic Megacolon
5. Perforation
6. Hemorrhage

restorative proctocolectomy with ileal pouch anal anastomosis (IPAA) (Table 1). Because the IPAA avoids the need for a permanent stoma, it is the preferred option in a large majority of cases.

Indications for Operation

Failure of medical management is the most common indication for surgical treatment of UC *(1)* (Table 2). Medical therapy fails when significant symptoms are not adequately controlled or if medical therapy cannot be tolerated because of the development of side effects or complications. The inability to wean from steroid therapy without recurrent symptoms is also an indication for surgical therapy. Owing to the risk associated with long-term steroid therapy, steroids should not be used as maintenance or suppression therapy. Hence, if the patient cannot be maintained on alternative safer medications, the patient should be referred for surgical management.

Increased risk for adenocarcinoma is also a common indication for surgical treatment *(2)*. The precise circumstances that indicate a significant risk for cancer such that proctocolectomy would be required has been the subject of controversy. Most agree, however, that patients with a 10-yr history of colitis should at least undergo annual surveillance colonoscopies with multiple random biopsies. Should dysplasia be detected, then surgery is required. Additionally, patients with invasive adenocarcinoma obviously require surgical management.

Other indications for surgical treatment of UC include recalcitrant fulminant colitis, toxic megacolon, perforation, and hemorrhage *(3)*. Patients suffering from these acute complications are often too ill to undergo the extensive surgery of either a total proctocolectomy or an ileal pouch anal anastomosis and are, thus, treated with total abdominal colectomy with end ileostomy and rectal sparing *(4,5)*. The proctectomy, with or without an ileo-anal reconstruction, can then be performed several months later when the patient's overall condition is improved. (Table 1). Patients with significant rectal bleeding or severe tenesmus, however, will require proctectomy, even in the urgent setting.

Preoperative Preparation

Prior to operation, the surgeon should confer with the patient and family so that they understand the nature of the operation, the necessity for surgery, the treatment options including alternative therapies, operative hazards, possible complications, and potential benefits. Candidates for IPAA should have a thorough understanding of the realistic expectations of final bowel function. Both male and female patients should be counseled for possibility of impairment of sexual function. All appropriate candidates are given the opportunity for autologous blood donation. Additionally, male patients who may desire to father children in the future are advised to cryo-preserve a sample of their sperm prior to operation.

It is important that the patient understand the difficulty discerning UC from CD. They must also be aware of how this distinction would impact the surgical strategies. The surgeon should confirm that appropriate studies have been undertaken to support the diagnosis of UC, and colonoscopic biopsies should be reviewed by a pathologist experienced with IBD.

Most patients undergoing an IPAA will require a temporary ileostomy, hence, preoperative consultation with an enterostomal therapist should be obtained for IPAA and TPC patients. Selection of the optimal placement of the ileostomy should be determined preoperatively. Proper stoma location is of particular importance in the performance of total proctocolectomy as it will have a profound effect on the patient's adjustment to the ileostomy *(6)*. Ideally, the ileostomy site should be located over the right rectus abdominis muscle on a flat area away from deep skin folds and bony prominences. The surface of the abdomen should be evaluated in both the sitting and standing positions as this will often demonstrate skin folds and creases not evident in the supine position. Finally, the patient's belt line is determined and every effort is made to place the stoma below it. Once the optimal position of the stoma has been identified, it is marked in a manner that will not fade during the time interval prior to surgery. Marking the site with an indelible marker and then covering the mark with a clear adhesive dressing works well for this purpose.

The bowel is mechanically cleansed with a combination of a clear liquid diet beginning 48 h prior to operation. Oral polyethylene glycol solution or phospho soda prep is given the evening before surgery *(7)*. Patients recently treated with corticosteroids should be given intravenous (iv) stress dose hydrocortisone prior to induction of anesthesia and continued through the postoperative course. Intravenous prophylactic antibiotics should be administered 1 h prior to surgery so that maximal tissue antibiotic levels are achieved at the time of the skin incision *(8)*.

Operative Strategies

Because UC is limited to the colorectal mucosa, wide surgical dissection with radical mesenteric resection is not necessary. To minimize morbidity, the dissection should remain close to the bowel. This is particularly true for the pelvic dissection where close adherence to the wall of the rectum is necessary to avoid injury to the pelvic nerves *(9)*. In cases complicated by invasive adenocarcinoma, wide excision is of course undertaken as dictated by the oncologic requirements.

Total Proctocolectomy

Total proctocolectomy with permanent end-ileostomy (TPC) is indicated for those patients requiring surgical treatment of UC, yet are not candidates for IPAA. For the most part, this includes patients with preoperative anal incontinence and patients with rectal adenocarcinomas. In addition, a small number of patients will prefer to have TPC over IPAA. Concerns over functional results, risk of pouchitis, and need for multiple surgeries are commonly sighted reasons for patients to reject IPAA in favor of TPC with permanent ileostomy *(3,10)*. Some elderly patients and morbidly obese patients may be best served by TPC over IPAA.

Total proctocolectomy is best performed through either a vertical midline incision or an infraumbilical transverse incision. Both of these incisions provide adequate access to the recesses of the abdomen and pelvis.Upon entering the abdomen it is important to fully examine the viscera looking for possible manifestations of CD and synchronous pathology. The stomach, duodenum, and small bowel are closely examined. If clear evidence for CD is detected, then the need for TPC should be reassessed.

The abdominal colectomy is performed by first mobilizing the colon from its attachments. The right colon and cecum are first mobilized by incision the peritoneal reflection of the right gutter. The right ureter and the duodenum are identified. The transverse colon is mobilized to separating the attachments to the greater omentum. The greater omentum is preserved so that it can be used to fill the pelvic dead space after the rectum is removed. The splenocolic ligaments are divided and the descending colon is mobilized by incising its peritoneal reflection. The left ureter is then identified so that it remains free from harm. Once the colon is fully mobilized the terminal ileum is transected and the mesentery of the colon is divided. The transection of the mesentery of the cecum, ascending transverse and descending colon is undertaken at a convenient distance from the bowel wall (Fig. 1). To avoid injury, both ureters and the duodenum are visualized during the transection of the mesentery. To keep a safe distance from the sympathetic neural plexus, the division of the sigmoid mesentery is carried out close to the bowel, between the first and second vascular arcades. Once the division of the sigmoid mesentery has reached a level below the sacral promontory, the superior rectal vessels are ligated and divided.

With division of the superior rectal vessels at the level of the sacral promontory, access is gained to the space between the presacral fascia and the fascia propria of the rectum; the presacral space. It is along this plane that the posterior mobilization of the rectum is accomplished (Fig. 2). With posterior mobilization of the rectum, the pelvic sympathetic nerves can be seen dividing into two major trunks in the upper sacral area. These branching sympathetic trunks continue laterally to the right and left walls of the pelvis, passing through the tissue of the lateral rectal ligaments. To avoid injury to these nerves, the lateral rectal ligaments are divided as close as possible to the rectal wall (Fig. 3). Division of the lateral ligaments close to the rectum also avoids injury to the more caudal sacral parasympathetic nerves. For the dissection along the anterior rectal wall, the anterior peritoneum and underlying fatty tissue is incised to expose the longitudinal muscle fibers of the rectum. At this level (posterior to Denonvilliers' fascia), the anterior dissection is undertaken in an inferior direction. After the anterior dissection is complete, additional lateral dissection may be necessary so that the rectum is circumferentially mobilized to the level of the levator-ani muscles. With completion of the pelvic dissection, the distal rectum is stapled with a TA stapling device. The rectum is divided above the staple line leaving behind a short rectal pouch (Fig. 4).

To create the end ileostomy, a circular incision 2 cm in diameter is made over the previously marked ileostomy site. This incision is carried through the right rectus abdominis muscle to the peritoneal cavity. The cut end of the ileum is delivered through the ostomy incision with approx 6 cm of ileum extending above the surface of the skin. After the delivery of the ileum through the abdominal wall, the abdominal cavity is then irrigated and the abdominal incision is closed. The ileostomy is matured in a Brooke fashion by everting the distal 3 cm of ileum onto itself, resulting in a stoma that protrudes approx 2–3 cm above the abdominal wall *(11)* (Fig. 5).

Once the abdominal portion of the procedure is complete, the remaining rectal stump is removed by a perineal dissection in the lithotomy position. Removal of the rectal stump is best carried out along the plane between the internal and external sphincters *(12)*. The dissection is carried upward until the pelvic cavity is entered and the rectal stump is completely excised (Fig. 6). To complete the procedure, the perineal wound is closed by approximating the external sphincter mechanism in layers and the perineal skin is closed with simple sutures.

Complications

PERINEAL WOUND INFECTION

Perineal wound infection often manifests with fever, perineal pain, erythema, and purulent drainage. This complication is best avoided by proper bowel preparation, prophylactic antibiotics, and avoidance of fecal soilage. Intersphincteric perineal dissection as described earlier allows for effective closure of the perineal dead space and thus may also reduce the likelihood of this complication. When perineal wound infection occurs, the skin sutures are removed, purulent fluid is completely drained, necrotic tissue debrided, and the wound packed.

STOMAL COMPLICATIONS

Complications related to the ileostomy are common and include peristomal hernia, prolapse, and stricture. Approximately 25% of patients undergoing total proctocolectomy with end Brooke ileostomy will require surgical revision of their stoma to deal with one or more of these complications *(13)*.

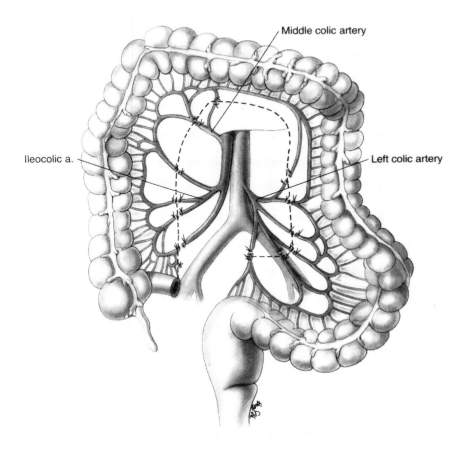

Fig. 1. The mesentery of the colon is divided at a convenient distance from the bowel wall. Radical mesenteric resections are not necessary and may increase the risk for complications. (Reprinted by permission from Hurst R. Procto-colectomy with ileostomy, abdominal colectomy with ileostomy and abdomi-nal colectomy with ileoproctostomy. Operative Strategies in Inflammatory Bowel Disease, Springer-Verlag, 1999.)

SMALL BOWEL OBSTRUCTION

Adhesive small bowel obstruction is not an uncommon complication following total proctocolectomy and appears to be more frequent than with other abdominal operations *(14)*. Approximately 10% of patients will experience some degree of small bowel obstruction with half of these cases requiring laparotomy to relieve the obstruction.

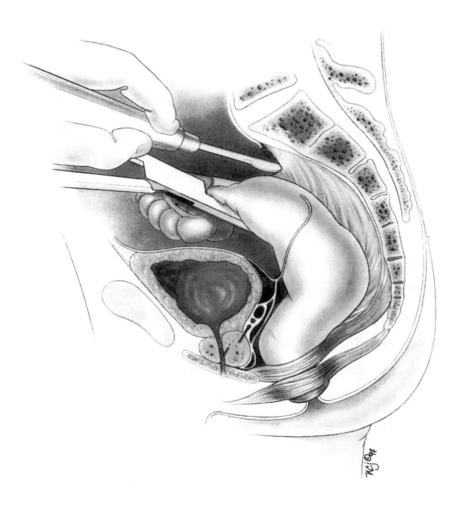

Fig. 2. The rectum is mobilized by separating the plane between the presacral
fascia and the fascia propria of the rectum. (Reprinted by permission from
Hurst R. Proctocolectomy with ileostomy, abdominal colectomy with ileostomy and abdominal colectomy with ileoproctostomy. Operative Strategies in
Inflammatory Bowel Disease, Springer-Verlag, 1999.)

URINARY RETENTION

Postoperative urinary retention is a common complication after proctectomy. Urinary retention may result from the use of opiates, anticholinergic medication, preexisting mechanical urinary obstruction, such

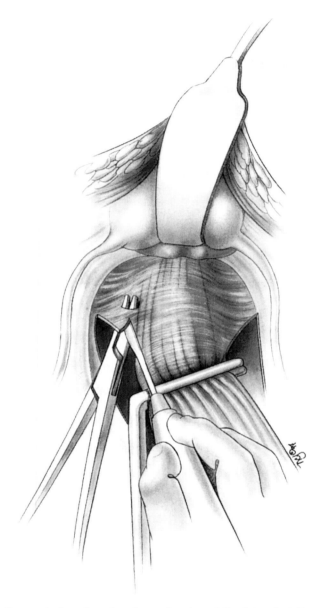

Fig. 3. After the posterior plane has been developed the lateral stalks of the rectum are divided close to the rectal wall. This dissection can be accomplished with the electrocautery as shown. (Reprinted by permission from Hurst R. Proctocolectomy with ileostomy, abdominal colectomy with ileostomy and abdominal colectomy with ileoproctostomy. Operative Strategies in Inflammatory Bowel Disease, Springer-Verlag, 1999.)

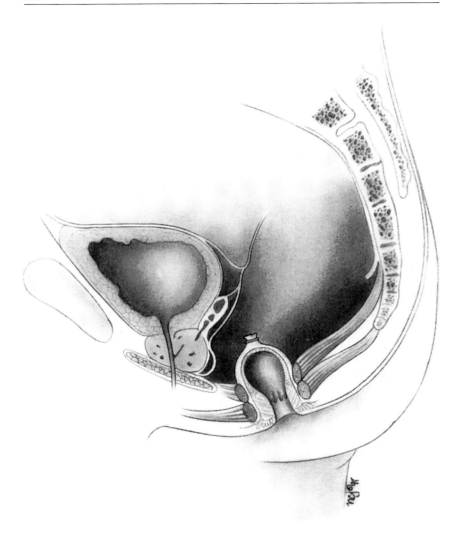

Fig. 4. Once the rectal mobilization is complete to the levator ani muscles, the rectal stump is stapled closed and the rectum is transected above the staple line. The resulting rectal stump is then removed through a perineal dissection if a TPC is to be performed. For a stapled IPAA the rectal staple line is placed as low as possible and an EEA stapler is inserted into the stump via the anus to create the anastomosis. (Reprinted by permission from Hurst R. Procto-colectomy with ileostomy, abdominal colectomy with ileostomy and abdominal colectomy with ileoproctostomy. Operative Strategies in Inflammatory Bowel Disease, Springer-Verlag, 1999.)

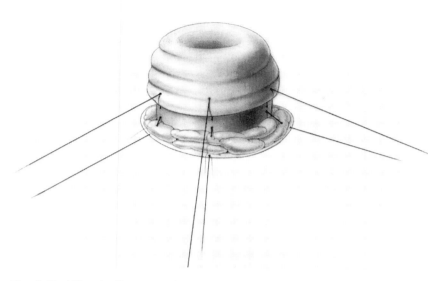

Fig. 5. End Brooke ileostomy is created by inverting the terminal 5 cm of the ileum onto itself. (Reprinted by permission from Hurst R. Proctocolectomy with ileostomy, abdominal colectomy with ileostomy and abdominal colectomy with ileoproctostomy. Operative Strategies in Inflammatory Bowel Disease, Springer-Verlag, 1999.)

as benign prostatic hypertrophy, or from intraoperative autonomic nerve injury. Overuse of opiates and the administration of anticholinergic medication should be avoided if the patient experiences difficulty voiding after urinary catheter removal. Patients with a history of symptoms consistent with urinary obstruction should be investigated prior to proctocolectomy.

SEXUAL DYSFUNCTION

Impotence is an uncommon complication following total proctocolectomy and occurs in approx 1–2% of male patients *(9)*. Retrograde ejaculation, however, is a little more common and has been reported to occur up to 5% of males. In women, mild dyspareunia is common, occurring in up to 30% of cases. When dyspareunia occurs after total proctocolectomy, it is often transient and is usually not severe enough to limit sexual activity. Female fertility is perhaps slightly diminished following total proctocolectomy, however, this procedure does not preclude full term pregnancy with normal vaginal delivery *(15)*.

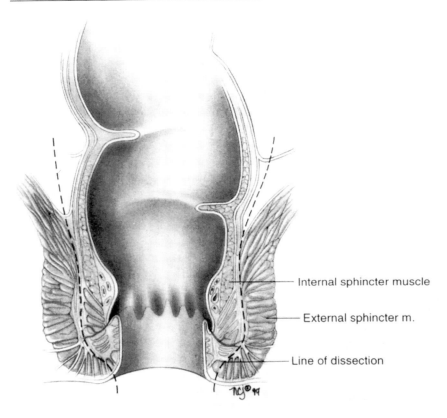

Internal sphincter muscle

External sphincter m.

Line of dissection

Fig. 6. The residual rectal stump is removed by a perineal dissection carried along the plane between the internal and external anal sphincters. (Reprinted by permission from Hurst R. Proctocolectomy with ileostomy, abdominal colectomy with ileostomy and abdominal colectomy with ileoproctostomy. Operative Strategies in Inflammatory Bowel Disease, Springer-Verlag, 1999).

Continent Ileostomy

Continent ileostomy (CI) is an alternative to the more common end Brooke ileostomy. Various techniques have been applied with a multitude of variations, but CIs are primarily categorized as a form of the Kock pouch *(16)* or the alternative Barnett continent ileal reservoir (BCIR) *(17)*. In each case, an internal ileal reservoir is fashioned to store intestinal content. The reservoir is emptied every few hours with manual insertion of a drainage catheter through a small stoma site on the abdominal wall. CIs do not require an external appliance and disfigurement of the abdominal wall is less than with a Brooke ileostomy.

CIs enjoyed a degree of popularity in the late 1970s and 1980s, but have now become uncommon procedures, supplanted in a vast majority of cases by the preferable IPAA. Currently, CIs for UC patients are limited to those who had undergone a total proctocolectomy without having had the option of IPAA, patients whose IPAA have failed (but not for patients with failures as a result of chronic pouchitis), and patients with anal incontinence such that IPAA is contraindicated. Elderly or frail patients who are not considered candidates for IPAA are also unlikely to do well with a CI, as these procedures entail prolonged recovery periods and high risk for reoperation. CIs are also difficult procedures to successfully perform in the obese patient.

CIs have been plagued with annoying complications and surgical revisions are commonly required (18). Potential complications include anastomotic dehiscence, intestinal fistula, pouchitis, valve disruption, and valve prolapse. In most cases with proper vigilance and intervention, these problems can be overcome and in appropriately selected patients a CI can be very gratifying (19).

Ileal Pouch-Anal Anastomosis

There are two main modifications of the IPAA procedure (20). In one method, the ileal reservoir is sutured to the anal canal at the level of the dentate line (Fig. 7). In the other, the reservoir is stapled to the top of the anal canal with the anal mucosa above the dentate line or the anal transition zone left intact (Fig. 8). When the anastomosis is made at the level of the dentate line, for technical reasons, this anastomosis must be hand sewn with needle and suture. For this reason, this modification is commonly referred to as the "hand-sutured" technique. When the anal transition zone is left intact and the anastomosis is performed at the top of the anal canal, the anastomosis cannot be sutured, but instead requires a stapling device. This modification is commonly referred to as the "stapled" ileoanal procedure. The key distinction between the hand-sutured and the stapled ileoanal procedures is not the method of anastomosis, but rather the level of the anastomosis. It was initially believed that leaving the anal transition zone intact with the stapled technique would allow for better long-term function of the pouch. However, randomized control studies comparing the hand-sutured and the stapled IPAA have failed to demonstrate any significant difference in the long-term results of the two techniques (21,22). The staple technique does put the patient at risk for inflammation of the small amount of retained mucosa. Inflammation of the anal transition zone (ATZ) is not often symptomatic, but when symptoms do occur, they are often readily controlled with mesalamine suppositories. Theoretically, the retained

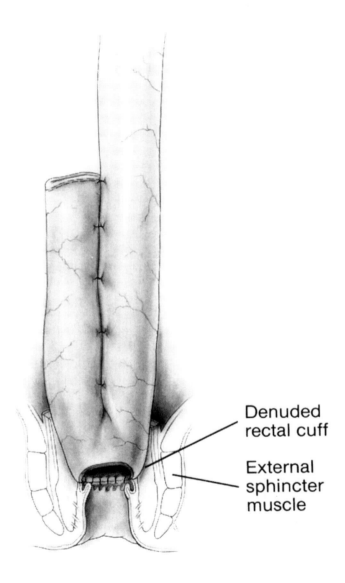

Denuded
rectal cuff

External
sphincter
muscle

Fig. 7. Hand-sutured IPAA is performed after trans-anal excision of the mucosa above the dentate line. (Reprinted by permission from Nivatvongs S. Ulcerative Colitis. In: Gordan PH, Nivatvongs S, eds. Principles and Practice of Surgery for the Colon, Rectum and Anus. Quality Medical Publishing, St Louis, MO, 1992.)

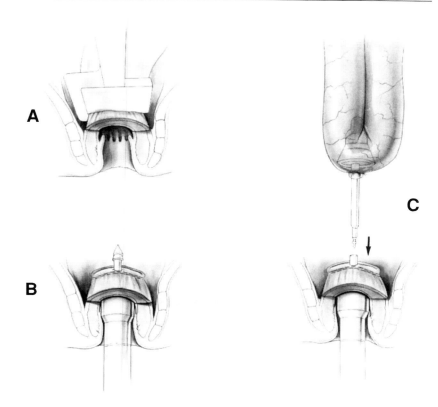

Fig. 8. Stapled IPAA performed with EEA stapler. The anal transition zone is left intact. (Reprinted by permission from Totally stapled abdominal restorative proctocolectomy, Kmiot WA and Keighley MRB, Br J Surg, 1989;79:961–964.)

mucosa of the ATZ may be at increased risk for malignancy, but the nature of this risk for malignant degeneration is not known *(23)*. Some surgeons recommend annual biopsy of the ATZ after stapled IPAA to rule out dysplasia. If any dysplasia is encountered, the mucosa of the ATZ can be excised and the ileal pouch advanced to the dentate line. This delayed conversion to hand-sutured IPAA is technically challenging, however, and may place the patient at risk for significant morbidity. The decision to perform a hand-sutured vs a stapled IPAA, in many cases, is a function of surgeon or institutional preference. Some data have been published indicating that the stapled technique may be associated with fewer short-term postoperative complications, yet the long-term risks of retained ATZ remain a concern *(23)*.

As with the total proctocolectomy, the IPAA is best performed through either a vertical midline incision or an infraumbilical transverse incision. At initial laparotomy, the abdominal viscera are closely examined. If clear evidence for CD is encountered, the IPAA procedure should not be performed. The abdominal colectomy for an IPAA is performed in the standard fashion by first fully mobilizing the colon from the cecum to the rectosigmoid junction. Care is given to avoid injury to the ureter, duodenum, and spleen. The greater omentum may or may not be resected with the specimen. Once the colon is fully mobilized from its peritoneal attachments, the terminal ileum is then divided with the GIA stapling device and the mesentery of the colon is transected at the convenient distance from the bowel wall (Fig. 1). It is important, however, to preserve the terminal branches of the ileocolic artery and the ileal branches of the ileocolic arcade so that the complete vascular supply to the ileum is left intact. To avoid injury to the hypogastric sympathetic neural plexus, the rectosigmoid mesentery is divided through the secondary arcades, preserving the main inferior mesenteric artery.

The pelvic dissection is performed in a manner designed to minimize the risk of pelvic autonomic nerve injury. The pelvic attachments to the rectum are divided close to the rectal wall in the same manner as described earlier for the total proctocolectomy. The pelvic dissection is carried down to the level of the levator ani muscles. If a stapled IPAA is planned, then the distal rectum is closed with a TA stapling device (Fig. 4). It is important that this staple line be placed as low as possible on the rectum as this staple line marks the ultimate level of the stapled anastomosis. The lower the TA staple line is placed, the shorter the amount of retained mucosal epithelium. The head of the TA stapling device is somewhat bulky as this is dictated by the engineering requirements of the instrument. The size of the stapler head can limit the ability to place the stapler in the most distal position. This is particularly true in the large male patient who has a narrow pelvis. In such cases, the length of retained mucosa above the dentate line may well exceed 3 cm.

If a hand-sutured anastomosis is planned, the retained rectum is simply transected at the level of the levator-ani muscles (25). This leaves an open rectal stump with about 2–3 cm of mucosa above the dentate line that is later excised during the perineal dissection of the hand-sutured IPAA.

Once the colon and rectum have been removed, the ileal reservoir is constructed. A variety of methods for creating the ileal reservoir have been described including the S, W, and J pouches. The S pouch was one of the earliest designs for the ileal reservoir. With the S pouch, the terminal ileum is folded onto itself twice and a long enterotomy is made (26,27).

The walls are then sutured together to create the reservoir (Fig. 9). The S pouch design has an afferent limb leading from the reservoir to the anal opening that consists of the terminal end of the ileum. It is important that this ileal afferent segment be 2 cm or less in length. Longer afferent limbs are known to result in significant problems with evacuation of the pouch and it is because of problems with efficient emptying that the S pouch is now rarely performed. The W pouch is formed by folding the ileum onto itself three times (Fig. 10). With the W pouch, the anastomosis is not formed at the terminal end of the ileum, but rather at the apex of the distal fold. This type of reservoir is favored by some surgeons who cite the good functional results of the W pouch *(28)*. The J pouch, however, is by far the most commonly performed ileal reservoir *(25,29)*. Construction of the J pouch is simple. Unlike the S or W pouches that require time-consuming suturing, the J pouch can be fashioned with a stapling device (Fig. 11). The long and short-term results of the J pouch are excellent.

Regardless of the type of ileal reservoir, if a stapled anastomosis is to be performed the anvil of the EEA stapling device should be placed in the pouch with its obturator protruding through the apex of the reservoir. Once the pouch construction is complete, the patient is placed in the lithotomy position so that the anastomosis can be fashioned. In the case of the stapled anastomosis, the EEA stapling device is inserted through the anus and its sharp obturator is advanced through the TA staple line of the short rectal stump. The anvil in the pouch is locked on to the obturator of the EEA stapler, the device is tightened and then fired to create the anastomosis (Fig. 8).

In the case of the hand-sutured IPAA, the perineum is prepped and draped in a sterile fashion. A retractor is then placed in the anal canal and the mucosa from the dentate line cephalad to the previous transection of the rectum; usually a distance of 1–3 cm is excised. This dissection is carried along the submucosal plane with care to avoid injury to the internal anal sphincter. Once the mucosectomy is complete, the ileal reservoir is delivered to the pelvis and a hand-sutured anastomosis between the ileal pouch and the anal canal is performed at the level of the dentate line through a transanal approach (Fig. 7) *(25)*.

One of the primary technical difficulties with the IPAA procedure relates to the tension that is often present at the anastomosis *(30)*. This tension is the result of the limitation of the length of the mesentery that supplies the pouch. The relative length and elasticity of the small bowel mesentery varies from individual to individual. In some cases, the mesentery is quite lengthy and no tension on the anastomosis is present. In other cases, the mesentery is short and considerable tension compli-

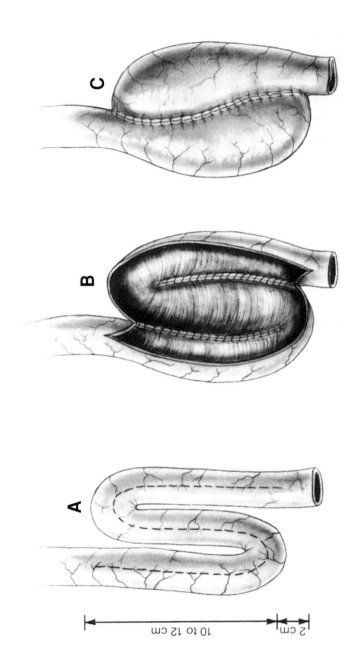

Fig. 9. S-pouch reservoir. (Reprinted by permission from Proctocolectomy with ileal reservoir and anal anastomosis, Parks AG, Nicholls RJ, Belliveau P, Br J Surg 1980;67:533–538.)

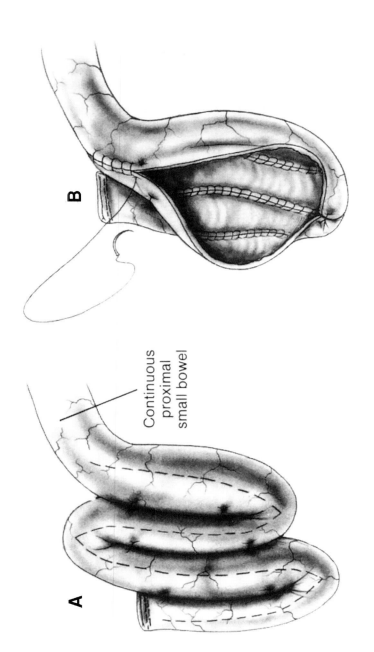

Fig. 10. W-pouch reservoir. (Reprinted by permission from Nivatvongs S. Ulcerative Colitis. In: Gordan PH, Nivatvongs S, eds. Principles and Practice of Surgery for the Colon, Rectum and Anus. Quality Medical Publishing, St. Louis, MO, 1992.)

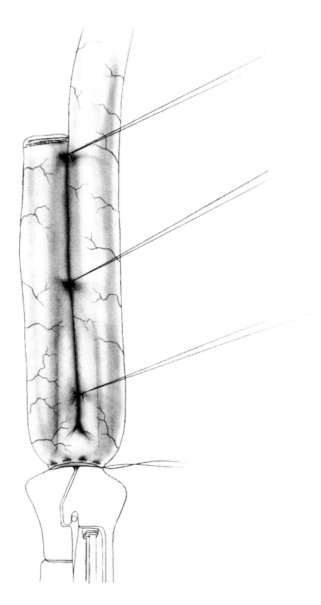

Fig. 11. J pouch reservoir. (Reprinted by permission from Nivatvongs S. Ulcerative Colitis. In: Gordan PH, Nivatvongs S, eds. Principles and Practice of Surgery for the Colon, Rectum and Anus. Quality Medical Publishing, St Louis, MO, 1992.)

cates the procedure. Tension on the anastomosis increases the risk for anastomotic dehiscence, pelvic sepsis and even runs the risk of complete pouch failure. Tension on the anastomosis is a likely contributing factor to the development of recurring anastomotic strictures. In rare instances, the mesentery may be so foreshortened that the anastomosis is not possible and a permanent ileostomy is required. It is very difficult to preoperatively predict which patients may be at risk for excessive tension. Obese patients, however, tend to have a thicker, less mobile mesentery, and thus, are a group of patients that can have difficulties. Obese patients should be counseled to attempt weight reduction prior to IPAA. Occasionally ileoanal procedures are staged with an initial total abdominal colectomy with a Hartmann's pouch and end ileostomy giving the patient the opportunity to lose weight prior to performing the ileoanal procedure.

At the time of operation and prior to the creation of the ileal reservoir, certain maneuvers can be undertaken to obtain some additional length from the mesentery. Some length is gained by full mobilization of the small bowel mesentery from the retroperitoneum to the point where the duodenum and pancreas are freed from these mesenteric attachments. Additionally, the peritoneum of the mesentery can be opened with small transverse incisions made in a direction perpendicular to the main superior mesenteric vessels. Mesenteric length can be assessed as adequate if the portion of the small bowel that is to form the apex of the planned pouch reaches to the lower level of the palpable pubic symphysis. If length is still a concern after mesenteric mobilization and incising the mesenteric peritoneum, the most distal branches of the superior mesenteric artery can be divided to lengthen the most distal arcades of the ileal mesentery (Fig. 12). This maneuver can add an additional 1–2 cm to the length of the mesentery. However, dividing mesenteric vessels for this purpose does run the risk of compromising the blood supply to the ileal pouch.

As a result of the concerns of anastomotic leak, the IPAA procedure is typically performed with a diverting loop ileostomy. The diverting stoma "protects" the anastomosis and lessens the likelihood of a symptomatic dehiscence and pelvic abscess. The universal need for this intestinal diversion has recently become a point of controversy (26,31–33). Some surgeons are now routinely omitting the diverting stoma. Others continue to use diversion in all cases. It would appear that a selective approach to the use of diverting ileostomies is a reasonable option. In those cases in which the patient is in general good health without sepsis or malnutrition, when the procedure is uneventful, the tissues are healthy and sturdy, and when there is no significant tension on the anastomosis, then a diverting stoma can be omitted, otherwise the temporary diversion should be performed.

Like the TPC procedure, potential complications with IPAA include adhesive small bowel obstruction, urinary retention, and sexual dysfunction in men and dyspareunia in women. Women undergoing IPAA may be at risk for infertility, but normal pregnancy with vaginal delivery is possible after IPAA. Vaginal delivery, however may weaken the anal sphincters and for this reason some surgeons recommend caesarian section for IPAA patients. The need for caesarian section, however, is controversial.

Complications specific to the IPAA include anastomotic dehiscence, pelvic sepsis, and anastomotic stricturing. Longer-term problems that can occur with IPAA include high stool frequency, incontinence, and pouchitis (24,34). Pouchitis is a nonspecific inflammation of the ileal reservoir that typically results in diarrhea, diminished continence, fever, malaise, and arthralgias. Although the etiology of pouchitis is unknown, standard treatment consists of oral antibiotics. Reports of the overall incidence of pouchitis vary from 20 to 50% (35). Recurrent pouchitis after successful treatment is about 66%. The incidence of chronic debilitating pouchitis has been reported to occur in 2 to 10% of patinents. The risk of pouchitis does not correlate with age, sex, or technique of IPAA (36). An increased risk of pouchitis has been observed in patients who manifest extra-intestinal manifestation of UC prior to colectomy. A very high incidence of pouchitis has been reported in patients with primary sclerosing cholangitis.

Initially, bowel function after IPAA can be erratic. However, at 6 to 12 mo after surgery patients can expect to have between three and six bowel movements per day (24,37–41). The majority of patients have fewer than six bowel movements per day, with three-fourths of them being pasty or formed. Fecal urgency is rare after IPAA and most patients can easily delay bowel movements for over 1 h. Up to 50% of patients do not feel compelled to engage in specific dietary restrictions and up to 80% do not take any drugs to alter stool frequency.

Fifty-five percent of patients are completely continent of stool and flatus after IPAA (25). An additional 25% have only occasional minor incontinence (less than once/wk, no stool lost). The remaining 20% experience stool incontinence fewer than once/d (12%) or more often than daily (8%). With time, the pouch matures and continence improves substantially during the first year, with improvement occurring all the way to 3 yr after surgery.

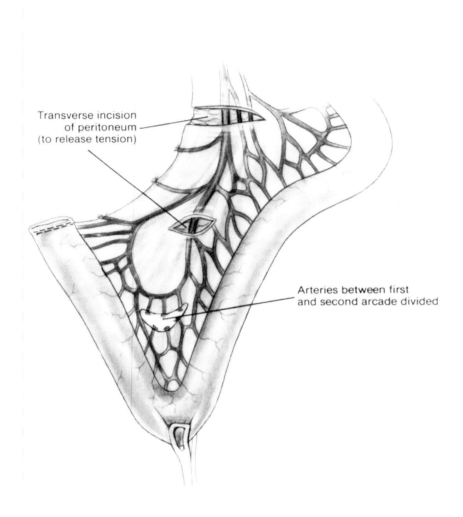

Fig. 12. To lengthen the ileal mesentery the mesenteric peritoneum is incised and the arcades of the mesenteric vessels can be divided. (Reprinted by permission from Nivatvongs S. Ulcerative Colitis. In: Gordan PH, Nivatvongs S, eds. Principles and Practice of Surgery for the Colon, Rectum and Anus. Quality Medical Publishing, St. Louis, MO, 1992.)

CROHN'S DISEASE

The clinical presentations and complications of Crohn's disease (CD) vary greatly and thus a wide range the surgical techniques are employed for the operative management of this disease (Table 3). CD is a recurring disorder that cannot be cured by simple surgical resection. Surgery, thus, is intended to provide palliation. When appropriately applied surgical therapy often provides significant and prolonged relief of debilitating symptoms and can resolve potentially life-threatening complications associated with CD. In each case, the surgeon must strive to alleviate symptoms as effectively as possible without exposing the patient to excessive morbidity. Optimal surgical management is accomplished only when the surgeon is mindful of the natural history of disease and the high risk for recurrence. This may require nonresectional techniques such as strictureplasty to avoid excessive loss of intestine or may even require surgical treatment of only portions of the gastrointestinal tract affected by severe disease while leaving segments with mild asymptomatic disease intact.

Indications for Operation

Failure of medical management to adequately control symptoms and disease activity is the most common indication for surgery *(2)* (Table 4). Medical treatment fails when symptoms of an acute flare do not improve or new complications of CD develop on optimal treatment. Some patients fail medical therapy because they develop significant side effects related to the medical therapy; others may experience resolution of symptoms with systemic steroid therapy only to recur with each attempt to wean the steroids. Because severe complications are inevitable with prolonged steroid use, surgery is indicated if the patient cannot be weaned off corticosteroids within 3–6 mo.

Partial or complete intestinal obstruction is a common indication for surgery for CD *(42)*. Chronic partial small bowel obstruction is much more common than acute complete obstruction. Luminal narrowing and partial small bowel obstruction from CD can result from acute inflammation with bowel wall thickening or chronic scarring with fixed stricture formation. Partial small bowel obstruction related to acute inflammation with bowel wall edema is best managed with a trial of medical therapy. Failure of medical treatment to relieve the obstructive symptoms in these patients obviously indicates the need for surgery. Patient's with obstructive symptoms that result from fibrotic fixed strictures will not benefit from attempts at medical therapy and are best treated with surgery.

Table 3
Surgical Options for the Treatment of Crohn's Disease

Resection and Anastomosis
    Ileocecectomy
    Ileocolectomy
    Hemicolectomy
    Segmental Colectomy
    Subtotal Colectomy
    Total Abdominal Colectomy with Ileal-Rectal Anastomosis
Resection and Stoma
    Proctectomy with Colostomy
    Total Proctocolectomy with Ileostomy
    Temporary diverting or Protecting Stoma
Strictureplasty
    Hieneke-Mikulicz
    Finney
    Side to Side Isoperistaltic Strictureplasty
Intestinal Bypass
    Gastrojejunostomy
Perianal Procedures
    Incision and Drainage
    Fistulotomy
    Seton Placement
    Rectal Advancement Flap
Other
    Closure of Intestinal Fistula
    Repair of Entero-vesical Fistula
    Drainage of Intra-Abdominal Abscess

Table 4
Indications for Operation: Crohn's Disease

Failure of Medical Management
Intestinal Obstruction
    Partial or Complete
Intestinal Fistulas
    Symptomatic Enteroenteric Fistula
    Enterocutaneous Fistula
    Enterovesical Fistula
    Enterovaginal Fistula
Intra-Abdominal Abscess
    IntraMestenteric Abscess
    Interloop Abscess
    Retroperitoneal Abscess
Inflammatory Mass
Hemorrhage
Perforation
Perineal Disease
    Perianal Abscess
    Superficial Fistula in Ano Unresponsive to Metronidazole
    Complex or Trans-sphincteric Fistula in Ano Unresponsive
      to Infliximab or 6-MP

Asymptomatic enteroenteric fistulas are not considered to be indications for operation in and of themselves. Only when they give rise to symptoms, or other complications develop, is surgery appropriate for enteroenteric fistulas. Surgery, however, is often indicated for the management of other types of enteric fistulas such as enterocutaneous fistulas, enterovesical fistulas, enterovaginal, and symptomatic enterocolonic fistulas.

Intraabdominal abscesses and inflammatory masses occur less frequently than fistulas, but their presence indicates severe disease and they are more often cited as an indication for surgical management than are fistulas (43). Because most abscesses are unlikely to respond to medical management, the presence of an abscess indicates the need for surgery (44). Crohn's abscesses that have been drained percutaneously are very likely to recur or to result in an enterocutaneous fistula, hence surgical resection is warranted even after successful drainage. Inflammatory masses indicate severe disease and often harbor an unrecognized abscess (45). Thus, inflammatory masses are considered an indication for surgical treatment.

Hemorrhage is an uncommon complication of CD. Massive gastrointestinal hemorrhage occurs more frequently in Crohn's colitis than small bowel CD. Hemorrhage from small bowel CD tends to be more indolent with episodes of chronic bleeding requiring intermittent transfusion (46).

Free perforation with peritonitis is a rare complication of CD and occurs in approx 1% of Crohn's patients. Free perforation is a clear indication for urgent operation (47).

Patients with CD are at increased risk for developing adenocarcinomas of the colon and small intestine. Preoperative diagnosis of carcinoma of the small bowel, however, is difficult as the symptoms, physical signs, and radiologic findings of small bowel cancer are similar to those of the underlying CD. The possibility of small intestinal carcinoma should be suspected in patients with long-standing disease, who develop a sudden change in symptoms, especially after a lengthy quiescent period. Small bowel cancer should also be considered when high-grade obstruction fails to resolve with conservative treatment. Defunctionalized segments of bowel seem to be at particular risk for malignancy. Therefore, bypass surgery should not be performed for small bowel CD and rectal stumps should be restored to their function or excised.

Preoperative Evaluation and Preparation

A complete preoperative assessment of the gastrointestinal tract should be undertaken prior to elective surgery for abdominal CD. The small bowel should be studied with contrast radiography. The colon and rectum are best evaluated with colonoscopy. Patients with suspected abscesses or inflammatory masses should undergo preoperative CT scanning of the abdomen and pelvis to determine the extent of the septic complication, the feasibility of percutaneous drainage and the relationship of the septic process with retroperitoneal structures.

Intestinal Resection

Resection of CD should be wide enough to encompass the limits of gross disease, but should not be extended to include an extended "margin" of normal bowel as wider resections offer no benefit in terms of lessening the risk of recurrence of disease (48). This is true even when the mucosal resection margins are positive for microscopic features of CD.

A wide variety of techniques for performing intestinal anastomoses have been applied for the treatment of CD. These include end-to-end, side-to-end, end-to-side, and side-to-side anastomoses. Regardless of the techniques employed, primary anastomosis can be performed in most CD patients with a high degree of safety (43). Patients with sepsis or profound malnutrition on the other hand are at high risk for anastomotic dehiscence, and hence, in these cases, a temporary intestinal stoma may be required.

Intestinal Strictureplasty

Intestinal strictureplasties involve a variety of techniques that allow for the release of intestinal strictures while preserving small bowel length (49). Strictureplasty can be applied for small bowel disease with single or multiple fibrotic strictures. Strictureplasty should be considered in cases where the alternative of resection would result in an extensive loss of bowel length. It should also be considered in patients with a history of multiple prior resections where preservation of length is a priority. Strictureplasty has also been applied to strictures of the duodenum where resection would carry high risk of morbidity. Although strictureplasty techniques are being utilized with increasing frequency, they are not appropriate for all surgical cases of CD. For instance, strictureplasty is, contraindicated in the face of generalized peritonitis and in patients with profound malnutrition. Strictureplasty is not appropriate for segments involved with fistulizing disease or where abscesses are involved. Additionally, long high-grade strictures that result from extremely thickened and rigid intestinal wall are often not amenable to strictureplasty and, therefore, require resection.

The two most common strictureplasty methods, the Heineke-Mikulicz and the Finney are named after the pyloroplasty methods from which they are derived. The Heineke-Mikulicz strictureplasty technique is appropriate for short segment strictures of less than 7 cm in length *(50)*. With this technique, a longitudinal incision is made along the antimesenteric border of the stricture. The longitudinal enterotomy is then closed in a transverse fashion to increase the width of the bowel at the point of the stricture. (Fig. 13). Once the enterotomy is made, the mucosal surface of the stricture is closely examined and areas of the stricture that are suspicious for adenocarcinoma are biopsied to rule out the possibility of an occult cancer.

The Finney strictureplasty can be utilized for longer strictures up to 15 cm in length *(51)*. With this technique, the affected bowel is folded onto itself in a U-shape and the two limbs are anastomosed together (Fig. 14).

For very long segments involving multiple areas of stenosis the side-to-side isoperistaltic strictureplasty can be employed *(52)*. With this technique, the diseased bowel loop is divided at its midpoint between bowel clamps and the mesentery is incised. The proximal intestinal loop is moved over the distal loop in a side-to-side fashion, and a long anastomosis between the two limbs is created (Fig. 15). The side to side isoperistaltic strictureplasty has been performed in diseased segments up to 75 cm in length *(53)*.

Unlike resection, after strictureplasty grossly diseased tissue remains *in situ*. This has given rise to concerns regarding the risk of early postoperative morbidity and recurrent symptomatic disease. The data, however, indicate that in appropriately selected patients perioperative morbidity after strictureplasty seems to be similar to resection *(50,54,55)*. The most common postoperative complication directly related to strictureplasty is hemorrhage from the suture line, occurring in up to nine percent of the cases. Gastrointestinal hemorrhage following strictureplasty is typically minor and can usually be managed conservatively with blood transfusions alone. Only in rare instances is reoperation required to control hemorrhage following strictureplasty. Septic complications such as dehiscence, intraabdominal abscess, and fistula formation occur in only two to three percent of strictureplasty cases *(50,56)*. The observed recurrence rates after strictureplasty seem to compare well to published recurrence rates after resection, and rapid recurrence of symptoms following strictureplasty has not proven to be a problem *(56–58)*.

As noted above, Crohn's disease patients are at increased risk for small bowel adenocarcinoma especially in segments of long standing disease. It has been suggested that persistent diseased intestine and continued long-term inflammation at the strictureplasty site may increase this risk for adenocarcinoma. Although there have been iso-

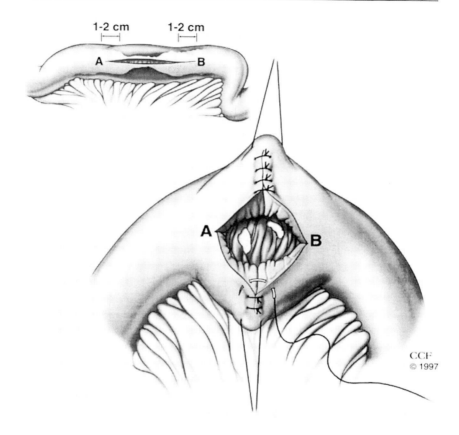

Fig. 13. Heineke-Mikulicz Strictureplasty adds to the bowel circumference at a focal stricture by closing a longitudinal incision in a transverse orientation. (Reprinted by permission from Milsom JW. Strictureplasty and Mechanical Dilation in Strictured Crohn's Disease. Operative Strategies in Inflammatory Bowel Disease, Springer-Verlag, 1999.)

lated reports of adenocarcinomas developing in the proximity or at the site of strictureplasty, the precise risk for neoplastic degeneration is not currently known, but remains a concern *(59)*.

Management of Complicated Crohn's Disease

ENTERIC FISTULAS

Fistulas are present in over one-third of CD cases, but only rarely do they represent the primary indication for operative intervention. Most patients with fistulizing disease come to surgery with coexisting stric-

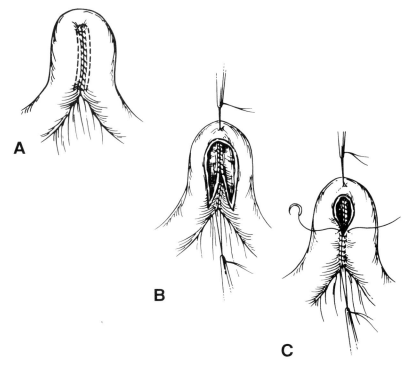

Fig. 14. Finney Strictureplasty can be used for strictures up to 15cm in length. (Reprinted by permission from Hurst RD and Michelassi F. Strictureplasty for Crohn's Disease: Techniques and Long-Term Results. World Journal of Surgery, Springer-Verlag, 1998.)

ture or abscess formation. Although fistulas are not often the primary reason for recommending surgery their coexistence with other complications of CD often pose challenging problems to the surgeon *(60)*.

Enteroenteric fistulas are a common manifestation of CD. Many enteroenteric fistulas, especially ileoileal or ileocecal fistulas, are completely contained within the diseased segments of the intestine and are thus managed by simple en bloc resection. In cases involving distant fistulization where en bloc resection would lead to extensive sacrifice of uninvolved intestine, an attempt to separate the normal appearing loops adherent to the diseased segment should be made.

Because of the proximity of the terminal ileum and the sigmoid colon ileosigmoid fistulas often develop with perforating CD of the terminal ileum. Typically the active CD is limited to the terminal ileum with the sigmoid colon only secondarily involved by the ileal inflammatory

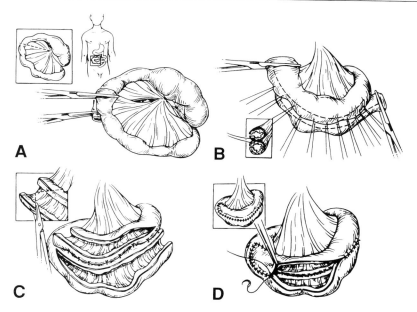

Fig. 15. Side-to-side isoperistaltic strictureplasty for extensive lengthily stricturing disease. (Reprinted by permission from Michelassi F. Side-to-Side Isoperistaltic Stricturoplasty for Multiple Crohn's Strictures. Williams & Wilkins, Diseases of the Colon & Rectum, 1996.)

adhesion and fistulization. Most ileosigmoid fistulas are asymptomatic. Large diameter fistulas particularly those originating proximal to a high-grade stricture can result in a functional bypass of the colon and give rise to significant diarrhea. Two-thirds of ileosigmoid fistulas are not recognized prior to operation *(61)*. For this reason, the surgeon must always be prepared for the possibility of encountering an ileosigmoid fistula in all cases of small bowel CD. Most ileosigmoid fistulas can be managed by dividing the fistulous adhesion, resecting the small bowel disease and then performing a simple closure of the colonic defect *(61,62)*. Sigmoid resection, however, is necessary when the sigmoid is primarily involved with active CD; when the sigmoid is extensively involved in an inflammatory ileal adhesion and is thus thickened and rigid; when debridement of the edges of the fistula results in a large sigmoid defect; or when the fistulous opening involves the mesenteric side of the colon and primary closure is therefore difficult.

Ileovesical fistulas are encountered in approx 5% of patients with CD *(43)*. Ileosigmoid and ileovesical fistulas often occur together with 60% of patients with an ileovesical fistula also having an ileosigmoid fistula

(62). Thus, the presence of an ileovesical fistula is often an indicator of complex fistulizing disease. Controversy exists regarding the timing of surgery for enterovesical fistulas. Some surgeons consider the simple presence of enteric fistulization to the urinary tract as an absolute indication for surgical treatment while others have argued that patients with enterovesical fistulas can be managed safely with conservative management for extended periods of time *(63)*. As with other Crohn's fistulas, the surgical treatment is based on resection of the diseased segment of intestine with extirpation of the fistulous tract. With ileovesical fistulas, the connection to the bladder is most commonly located at the dome and, therefore, the necessary debridement and primary closure can be affected without endangering the trigone.

Enterocutaneous fistulas occur in approx 4 % of patients with CD *(44)*. The presence of an enterocutaneous fistula does not necessarily dictate the need for surgical intervention. If the patient's underlying disease is under satisfactory control and the enterocutaneous fistula has minimal output then a period of conservative management may be appropriate. Yet with aggressive nonoperative management Crohn's related enterocutaneous fistulas are difficult to heal and surgical resection is often ultimately required.

INTESTINAL OBSTRUCTION

Small bowel stricturing disease can range from chronic low-grade obstruction with symptoms of crampy abdominal pain, bloating, food avoidance, and weight loss, to high-grade partial or even complete small bowel obstruction with vomiting, obstipation, and dehydration. CD resulting in intestinal obstruction does not require the same urgency that is advocated for the management of small bowel obstruction due to adhesions or herniation. Patients with high-grade partial or complete small bowel obstruction as a result of CD can be treated initially with nasogastric decompression, intravenous hydration, and steroid therapy. This allows for decompression of acutely distended and edematous bowel, and in most cases, results in resolution of the complete obstruction allowing for appropriate bowel preparation and overall safer conditions for surgery. If, however, there is concern that the obstruction is not Crohn's related, but may be because of adhesions or herniation, or if there is a question of intestinal injury, then conservative management should be abandoned and the abdomen explored. Patients with complete obstruction who respond well to initial therapy of nasogastric decompression and intravenous steroids remain at high risk for persistent or recurrent symptoms of obstruction and are best managed with surgery once adequate decompression is achieved.

INTRAABDOMINAL ABSCESS

Intra-abdominal abscesses that form from CD tend to be chronic with an indolent clinical course of modest fever, abdominal pain, and leukocytosis. These abscesses only rarely present with overwhelming systemic sepsis. In up to one-third of Crohn's abscesses there are no clinical signs of localized infection and the abscesses are discovered only at intraoperative exploration. A tender palpable abdominal mass is highly suspicious for an intraabdominal abscess as greater than 50% of inflammatory masses harbor an abscess collection. When an abscess is suspected or a mass palpated, preoperative CT scans should be obtained. CT scanning provides information regarding the size and location of the abscess, the feasibility of percutaneous drainage, and the relationship of the septic process with retroperitoneal structures such as the ureters, duodenum, and the inferior vena cava.

Many Crohn's abscesses are small collections that are nearly completely contained within the area of diseased intestine and associated mesentery. In these cases, resection of the affected segment of intestine results in extirpation of the abscess cavity such that placement of drains is not necessary and primary anastomosis can be performed without risk.

Whereas small abscesses can be readily managed at the time of surgical exploration larger abscesses are best managed with preoperative CT guided percutaneous drainage (64). Preoperative drainage of larger abscesses facilitates subsequent surgical intervention and may also allow for resection and primary anastomosis where the degree of sepsis and inflammation would otherwise dictate the need for a temporary ileostomy (65).

CD of the Duodenum

Because of the unique anatomical position of the duodenum, CD involving this segment of the gastrointestinal tract requires special consideration. Symptomatic CD of the duodenum is a rare entity and the need for surgical intervention is uncommon (66). Unlike jejunal or ileal resections, resection of the duodenum is an extreme undertaking. Fortunately, as a result of the peculiarities of duodenal CD, resection of the duodenum are almost never necessary.

The duodenum can either be primarily involved with CD or secondarily involved by inflammatory adhesions or fistulas originating from disease elsewhere in the gastrointestinal tract. Primary CD of the duodenum typically manifests with an inflammatory pattern resulting in ulceration and edema. This inflammation may give rise to stricture formation but almost never develops fistulas, sinuses, abscesses, or free perforation. For this reason, nonresectional techniques such as strictureplasty and bypass procedures are applicable in most cases of duodenal Crohn's disease. The optimal surgical strategies for managing duodenal Crohn's strictures are dependent upon the pattern of disease. Most duodenal Crohn's strictures are focal and can be managed with a Heineke-Mikulicz strictureplasty *(67)*. If the duodenal stricture is lengthy or the tissues are too rigid and unyielding then strictureplasty is not suitable and an intestinal bypass procedure should be performed. A simple side-to-side retrocolic gastrojejunostomy can be performed for obstructing disease of the duodenum. This procedure is effective at relieving the symptoms of duodenal obstruction but has the drawback in that the procedure is inherently ulcerogenic and a parietal cell vagotomy is often performed with the gastrojejunostomy.

Crohn's fistulas involving the duodenum, when they occur, are almost always the result of perforating disease originating elsewhere from small bowel or colon *(68)*. This most commonly occurs in recurrent CD at the site of a previous ileocolonic anastomosis that has become adherent to the duodenum. The surgical management of duodenal-enteric fistulas entails resection of the primary disease with repair of the duodenal defect. Most duodenal fistulas are located away from the juncture of the duodenal wall and the head of the pancreas, and thus can be managed by simple debridement and primary closure without difficulty. Larger fistulas or fistulas associated with more significant inflammatory adhesion may require more extensive debridement resulting in sizable duodenal defects which require closure with a Roux-en-Y duodeno-jejunostomy or with a jejunal serosal patch *(69)*. Duodenal resections are almost never necessary and should be held as the surgical option of last resort.

CD of the Colon

Surgical management of CD of the large intestine is contingent upon a variety of factors including the distribution and pattern of disease, the extent of rectal involvement and the adequacy of fecal continence. Surgical procedures commonly required include segmental colectomy or ileocolectomy with primary anastomosis, total abdominal colectomy with ileoproctostomy, and total proctocolectomy with permanent end ileostomy. Because of the recurrent nature of CD restorative procedures such as ileal pouch-anal anastomosis or continent ileostomies are not appropriate for patients with an established diagnosis of CD.

ILEOCOLITIS

Ileocecal or ileocolonic disease is managed similarly to disease limited to the terminal ileum. Resection to grossly normal margins with primary anastomosis is often the best surgical option. The long-term clinical course of terminal ileal disease with limited involvement of the proximal colon is similar to the clinical course seen with CD involving only terminal ileum. Recurrent disease tends to occur at the anastomosis and preanastomotic ileum. The risk for recurrent disease affecting the distal colon or rectum is low and, hence, the long-term risk for requiring a permanent stoma is low.

Extensive Crohn's Colitis with Rectal Sparing

CD that predominates in the colon often involves long segments of the colon. Surgical management of extensive Crohn's colitis requires total colectomy. Commonly, however, the rectum is spared from the disease and an ileorectal anastomosis can be performed and a permanent stoma avoided or at least delayed. Unfortunately, beacuse of recurrent disease in the rectum may of these patients ultimately require proctectomy with permanent ileostomy *(70)*. Yet, even with a high risk of recurrence, avoidance of a permanent stoma for several years can be achieved in large majority of patients whose rectum is uninvolved with disease *(71)*.

Segmental Crohn's Colitis

Crohn's colitis that involves a short length of focal disease with normal colon both proximal and distal is a relatively uncommon pattern of disease. Limited resection of the diseased portion of the colon with colo-colonic anastomosis has been advocated for short segment Crohn's colitis *(72,73)*. However, segmental colectomy is controversial because of the high risk of recurrence which at times, occurs rapidly in the preanastomotic colon. Clinical experience suggest the rate of recurrent disease can be lowered by resection of the entire proximal colon with subsequent anastomosis of the terminal ileum to the normal colon distal to the area of disease. Yet this approach results in extensive loss of normal colonic mucosa if used for disease limited to the distal left colon or sigmoid. Such an extensive loss of normal colon may result in frequent watery stools or even incontinence. Thus, a reasonable approach for the surgical management of segmental CD of the colon is to perform segmental resections with colo-colonic anastomosis for disease isolated to the distal descending or sigmoid colon and resections to normal ileum with ileo-colonic anastomosis for segmental colitis of the more proximal colon. This approach does not sacrifice the significant absorptive capacity of the proximal colon in patients with limited left sided disease, and avoids the risk of rapid recurrence in the proximal colon in patients with more extensive proximal disease.

RECTAL CROHN'S DISEASE

Crohn's limited to the rectum is an unusual pattern of disease. The surgical management of Crohn's proctitis mandates proctectomy. The extent of the proximal resection however is controversial. Performing an abdominal perineal resection with an end-sigmoid colostomy has been associated in some reports with a high risk for stomal complications when compared to total proctocolectomy with the Brooke ileostomy (74). Additionally, experience suggests that the residual colon may be at high risk for recurrent disease. For these reasons total proctocolectomy with ileostomy is often recommended for CD limited to the rectum and distal colon. This is particularly true for patients who have no history of small bowel CD. Total proctocolectomy, however, may not be appropriate for Crohn's proctitis patients who have undergone prior small bowel resection. These patients with foreshortened small intestine may be at risk for a high output ileostomy and therefore may benefit from attempts at preserving the colonic absorptive capacity. Hence, these patients may be better treated with proctectomy and end-colostomy. In general, however, permanent end-colostomy is generally avoided when treating rectal CD.

Perianal Crohn's Disease

Approximately one-third of CD patients will suffer from perianal manifestation. Perianal CD includes, abscesses, fistulas, fissures, anal stenosis, and hypertrophic skin tags (75). As a general rule, treatment of Crohn's-related perianal disease should be conservative as repeated operations with recurring disease can lead to significant injury to the anal sphincters with a risk of incontinence.

Surgical procedures commonly employed include incision and drainage of abscesses, simple fistulotomy, incision, and opening of fistulas tracts, application of "draining" and "cutting" setons, and rectal mucosal advancement flaps.

Surgical incision and drainage is mandated for perianal abscesses as attempts at treating purulent collections with medical therapy are invariably unsuccessful. Uncomplicated low-lying fistulas-in-ano are best treated initially with metranidazole or ciprofloxicin (76,77). These agents are moderately effective at promoting healing of Crohn's-related perianal fistulas and are associated with a very low risk for complication. If the response to antibiotic therapy is inadequate then simple fistulotomy should be performed for uncomplicated low-lying fistulas. More complex perianal fistulas, however, carry a higher risk for postsurgical complications and, thus, attempts at more aggressive medical treatment with anti-TNF antibody or 6-mp are warranted prior to recommending surgery.

Surgical options for treatment of complicated perianal fistulas include extensive opening of fistula tracts with use of setons. When managing these difficult cases, careful judgement is required as surgical fistulotomy or the application of cutting setons can result in incontinence with high-lying Crohn's fistulas. To avoid the risk of incontinence in these patients, rectal mucosal advancement flap procedures are often the best option for high-lying, supra-sphincteric, and complex fistulas *(78)* (Fig. 16).

Creation of a temporary stoma to divert the fecal stream is employed only in selected cases of complicated perianal disease. Fecal diversion is occasionally appropriate to help in the healing of difficult rectovaginal fistulas. For severe cases of perianal disease that do not respond to aggressive medical or local surgical treatment, fecal diversion often results in significant improvement. Unfortunately, in these cases disease actively typically recurs rapidly after reestablishment of the fecal stream.

Long-Term Morbidity and Recurrence of Disease

Because of the recurrent nature of CD, repeated operations are often required. Serial, massive, or injudicious resections of the small bowel for patients suffering from CD may result in permanent impairment of intestinal absorption. Resection of one-half to two-thirds of the small bowel represents the upper limit of safety. When resections exceed this, particularly in the absence of the colon, absorption is markedly altered and poses significant management problems. Fortunately, only in rare instances does a true short gut syndrome occur. In many such cases, the short gut syndrome can be managed with dietary manipulations and dependency on long-term hyperalimantation occurs in less than 1% of CD cases.

Loss of ileal function can result in bile salt malabsorption and diarrhea. This so-called "bile salt diarrhea" is often successfully treated with oral cholestyramine, which binds unabsorbed bile acids to prevent their effect upon the colon. Most patients who undergo resection of the terminal ileum do not suffer from significant malabsorption of vitamin B12. However, patients who have undergone lengthy or repeated resections of the terminal ileum should be monitored for possible B12 deficiency.

The most common long-term complication following surgery for CD is the risk of recurrent disease. Reported crude and cumulative recurrence rates vary greatly. Endoscopic evidence for recurrence has been reported to vary from 28% to 73% at 1 yr and from 77 to 85% at 3 yr after ileal resection *(79)*. In most instances, endoscopically detected recur-

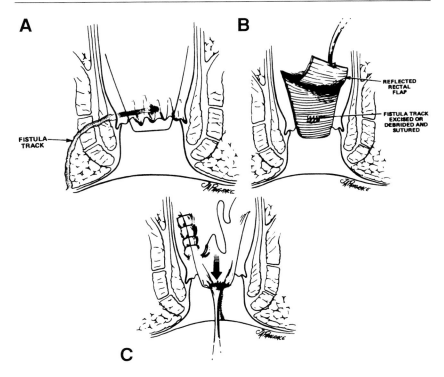

Figure 16. Rectal mucosal advancement flap designed to close the internal opening of a fistula-in-ano. (Reprinted by permission from Strong S and Fazio VW. The Surgical Management of Crohn's Disease. W.B. Saunders, Inflammatory Bowel Disease, 5th ed., 2000.)

rence is minor and asymptomatic and therefore not of great clinical significance. The recurrence of symptomatic CD is approx 60% at 5 yr and recurrences increase with time such that at 20 yr symptomatic recurrences occur in between 75 and 95% of cases *(80)*. Hence, the long-term risk for recurrence of Crohn's symptoms is very high. Reports vary, but the need for reoperation to treat recurrent disease is about 20% at 5 yr, 33% at 10 yr, and 50% at 20 yr *(42,81,82)*.

Recurrent CD is most likely to occur in proximity to the location of the previously resected intestinal segment, typically at the anastomosis and pre-anastomotic bowel. This is particularly true for terminal ileal disease. Additionally, the length of small bowel involved with recurrent disease parallels the length of disease originally resected *(83)*. Short segment disease tends to recur over a short segment of the pre-anastomotic bowel and lengthy disease typically is followed by lengthy recurrence. Also, to a lesser degree of concordance, stenotic disease tends to recur as stenotic disease and perforating disease tends to recur with perforating disease.

Many putative risk factors for recurrence have been studied. The cumulative literature, however, has validated few as true risk factors for postsurgical recurrence of disease. There is a growing body of evidence that indicates smoking can increase the risk of recurrence *(84–86)*. Additionally, there is some evidence to indicate that the use of NSAIDs may also promote recurrent disease *(87)*. All Crohn's patients should be strongly advised to refrain from smoking cigarettes or taking NSAIDs. Patients should also be considered for postoperative maintenance therapy with either control-release 5-ASA (Pentasa) or 6-Mercaptopurine *(88–90)*.

REFERENCES

1. Block GE. Surgical management of ulcerative colitis. Curr Concepts Gastroenterol 1979;4:6–20.
2. Michelassi F, Fichera A. Indications for surgery in inflammatory bowel disease: the surgeon's perspective. In: Kirsner JB, ed. Inflammatory Bowel Disease. W. B. Saunders, Philadelphia, PA, 2000, pp. 616–625.
3. Hurst RD, Finco C, Rubin M, Michelassi F. Prospective analysis of perioperative morbidity in one hundred consecutive colectomies for ulcerative colitis. Surgery 1995;118:748–755.
4. Hawley PR. Emergency surgery for ulcerative colitis. World J Surg 1988;12:169–173.
5. Block G. Emergency colectomy for inflammatory bowel disease. Surgery 1982; 91:249–53.
6. Colwell JC. Enterostomal care in inflammatory bowel disease. In: Kirsner JB, ed. Inflammatory Bowel Disease. W. B. Saunders, Baltimore, MD. 2000:710–717.
7. Oliveria L, Wexner SD, Daniel N, et al. Mechanical bowel preparation for elective colorectal surgery. Dis Colon Rectum 1977;40:585–591.
8. Kaiser AB. Antibiotic prophylaxis in surgery. N Engl J Med 1996;315:1129–1138.
9. Bauer JJ, Gelernt IM, Salky B, Kreel I. Sexual dysfunction following proctocolecotmy for benign disease of the colon and rectum. Ann Surg 1983;197:363–367.
10. Melville DM, Ritchie JK, Nicholls RJ, Hawley PR. Surgery for ulcerative colitis in the era of the pouch: the St Mark's Hospital experience. Gut 1994;35:1076–1080.
11. Brooke BN. The management of an ileostomy. Lancet 1952:102–104.
12. Lyttle JA, Parks AG. Intrasphincteric incision of the rectum. Br J Surg 1977; 413:64–67.
13. Leong AP, Londono-Schimmer EE, Phillips RK. Life-table analysis of stomal complications following ileostomy. Br J Surg 1994;81:727–729.
14. Marcello PW, Roberts PL, Schoetz DJ, Coller JA, Murry JJ, Veidenheimer MC. Obstruction after ileal pouch-anal anastomosis: a preventable complication? Dis Colon Rectum 1993;36:1105–1111.
15. Hurst RD. Complications of surgical treatment of ulcerative colitis and crohn's disease. In: Kirsner JB, ed. Inflammatory Bowel Disease. W. B. Saunders, Philadelphia, PA, 2000, pp. 718–735.
16. Kock NG. Intra-abdominal "reservoir" in patients with permanent ileostomy. Arch Surg 1969;99:223–231.

17. Barnett WO. Current experiences with continent intestinal reservoir. Surg Gynecol Obstet 1989;168:1–5.
18. Fogel SL. Continent Ileostomy (Kock Pouch). In: Bayless TM, Hanauer SB, eds. Advanced Therapy of Inflammatory Bowel Disease. B C Decker, Hamilton, 2001, pp. 191–195.
19. Kohler LW, Pemberton JH, Zinsmeister AR, Kelly KA. Quality of life after proctocolectomy; A comparison of Brooke ileostomy, Kock pouch, and ileal pouch-anal anastomosis. Gastroenterology 1991;101:679–684.
20. Cohen Z, McLeod RS, Stephen W, Stern HS, O'Connor B, Reznick R. Continuing evolution of the pelvic pouch procedure. Ann Surg 1992;216:506–511.
21. Seow-Choen, Tsunoda A, Nicholls RJ. Prospective randomized trial comparing anal function after handsewn ileo-anal anastomosis with mucosectomy versus stapled ileo-anal anastomosis without mucosectomy in restorative proctocolectomy. Br J Surg 1991;78:430–434.
22. Luukkonen P, Jarvinen H. Stapled vs hand-sutured ileoanal anastomosis in restorative proctocolectomy. A prospective randomized study. Arch Surg 1993;128:437–440.
23. O'Riordain MG, Fazio VW, Lavery IC, et al. Incidence and natural history of dysplasia of the anal transitional zone after ileal pouch-anal anastomosis: results of a five-year to ten-year follow up. Dis Colon Rectum 2000;43:1660–1665.
24. Fazio VW, Ziv Y, Church JM, et al. Ileal pouch-anal anastomosis: complications and function in 1005 patients. Ann Surg 1995;222:120–127.
25. Michelassi F, Hurst R. Restorative proctocolectomy with J-pouch ileoanal anastomosis. Arch Surg 2000;135:347–353.
26. Parks AG, Nicholls RJ. Proctocolectomy without ileostomy for ulcerative colitis. Br Med J 1978;2:85–88.
27. Parks AG, Nicholls RJ, Belliveau P. Proctocolectomy with ileal reservoir and anal anastomosis. Br J Surg 1980;67:533–538.
28. Harms BA, Hamilton JW, Yamamoto DT, Starling JR. Quadruple-loop (W) ileal pouch reconstruction after proctocolectomy: analysis and functional results. Surgery 1987;102:561–567.
29. Keighley MRB, Yoshioka K, Kmiot W. Prospective randomized trial to compare the stapled double lumen pouch and the sutured quadruple pouch for restorative proctocolectomy. Br J Surg 1988;75:1008–1011.
30. Smith L, Griend WG, Medwell SJ. The superior mesenteric artery: the critical factor in the pouch pull-through procedure. Dis Colon Rectum 1984;27:741–744.
31. Tjandra JJ, Fazio VW, Milsom JW, et al. Omission of temporary diversion in restorative proctocolectomy-is it safe? Dis Colon Rectum 1993;36:1007–1013.
32. Galandiuk S, Wolff B, Dozois RR, et al. Ileal pouch-anal anastomosis without ileostomy. Dis Colon Rectum 1991;34:870–873.
33. Everett WG, Pollard SG. Restorative proctocolectomy without temporary ileostomy. Br J Surg 1990;77:621–622.
34. Santos MC, Thompson JS. Late complications of the ileal pouch-anal anastomosis. Am J Gastroenterol 1993;88:3–10.
35. Sandborn WJ. Pouchitis following ileal pouch-anal anastomosis: Definition, pathogenesis, and treatment. Gastroenterology 1994;107:1756–1860.
36. Hurst RD, Chung TP, Rubin M, Michelassi F. Prospective study of the incidence, timing, and treatment of pouchitis in 104 consecutive patients after restorative proctocolectomy. Arch Surg 1996; In Press.
37. Becker JM, Raymond JL. Ileal pouch-anal anastomosis: A single surgeon's experience with 100 consecutive cases. Ann Surg 1986;204:375–383.

38. Keighley MRB, Grobler S, Bain I. An audit of restorative proctocolectomy. Gut 1993;34:680–684.
39. McIntyre PB, Pemberton JH, Wolff BG, Beart RW, Dozois RR. Comparing functional results one year and ten years after ileal pouch-anal anastomosis for chronic ulcerative colitis. Dis Colon Rectum 1994;37:303–307.
40. O'Connel PR, Pemberton JH, Brown ML, Kelly KA. Determinates of stool frequency after ileal pouch-anal anastomosis. Am J Surg 1987;153:157–164.
41. Pemberton JH, Kelly KA, Beart RW, Dozois RR, Wolff BG, Ilstrup DM. Ileal pouch-anal anastomosis for chronic ulcerative colitis: long-term results. Ann Surg 1987;206:504–513.
42. Michelassi F, Balestracci T, Chappell R, Block GE. Primary and recurrent Crohn's disease: Experience with 1379 patients. Ann Surg 1991;214:230–236.
43. Hurst RD, Molinari M, Chung TP, Rubin M, Michelassi F. Prospective study of the features, indications and surgical treatment in 513 consecutive patients affected by Crohn's disease. Surgery 1997;122:661–668.
44. Michelassi F, Stella M, Balestracci T, et al. Incidence, diagnosis and treatment of enteric and colorectal fistulas in patients with Crohn's disease. Ann Surg 1993; 218:660.
45. Michelassi F. Incidence, diagnosis and treatment of abdominal abscesses in Crohn's disease. Res Surg 1996;8.
46. Sparberg M, Kirsner JB. Recurrent hemorrhage in regional enteritis Report of 3 cases. Am J Dig Dis 1966;2:652–657.
47. Greenstein J, Mann D, Heimann T, et al. Spontaneous free perforation and perforated abscess in 30 patients with Crohn's disease. Ann Surg 1987;205:72–75.
48. Fazio VW, Marchetti F, Church J, et al. Effect of resection margins on the recurrence of Crohn's disease in the small bowel: a randomized controlled trial. Ann Surg 1996;224:563–573.
49. Milsom JW. Strictureplasty and mechanical dilation in strictured Crohn's disease. In: Michelassi F, Milsom JW, eds. Operative Strategies in Inflammatory Bowel Disease. New York: Springer-Verlag. 1999:259–267.
50. Fazio VW, Galandiuk S, Jagelman DG, Lavery IC. Strictureplasty in Crohn's disease. Ann Surg 1989;210:621–625.
51. Sharif H, Alexander-Williams J. The role of strictureplasty in Crohn's disease. Int Surg 1992;77:15–18.
52. Michelassi F. Sideto-side Isoperistaltic stricturoplasty for multiple Crohn's strictures. Dis Colon Rectum 1996;39:345–349.
53. Michelassi F, Hurst RD, Melis M, et al. Side-to-side isoperistaltic strictureplasty in extensive Crohn's disease: a prospective longitudinal study. Ann Surg 2000.
54. Nivatvongs S. Strictureplasty for Crohn's disease of small intestine. Present status in Western countries. J Gastsroenterol 1995;30:139–142.
55. Alexander-Williams J, Haynes IG. Conservative operations for Crohn's disease of the small bowel. World J Surg 1985;9:945–951.
56. Hurst RD, Michelassi F. Strictureplasty for Crohn's disease: Techniques and long-term results. World J Surg 1998;22:359–363.
57. Fazio VW, Tjandra JJ, Lavery IC, Church JM, Milsom JW, Oakley JR. Long term follow-up of strictureplasty in Crohn's disease. Dis Colon Rectum 1993;36:355–361.
58. Spencer MP, Nelson H, Wolff BG, Dozois RR. Strictureplasty for obstructive Crohn's disease: The Mayo experience. Mayo Clin Proc 1994 69:33–36.
59. Fleshman JW. Invited Editorial. Dis Colon Rectum 1997;40:238–239.
60. Broe PH, Bayless TM, Cameron JL. Crohn's disease: are enteroenteral fistulas an indication for surgery? Surgery 1982;91:249.

61. Block GE, Schraut WH. The operative treatment of Crohn's enteritis complicated by ileosigmoid fistula. Ann Surg 1982;196:356–360.

62. Schraut WH, Chapman C, Abraham VS. Operative treatment of Crohn's ileocolitis complicated by ileosigmoid and ileovesical fistulae. Ann Surg 1988;207:48–51.

63. Glass RE, Ritchie JK, Lennard-Jones JE, et al. Internal fistulas in Crohn's disease. Dis Colon Rectum 1985;28:557.

64. Doemeny JM, Burke DR, Meranze SG. Percutaneous drainage of abscesses in patients with Crohn's disease. Gastrointest Radiol 1988;13:237–241.

65. Bernini A, Spencer MP, Wong WD, et al. Computed Tomography-guided percutaneous abscess drainage in intestinal disease. Dis Colon Rectum 1997;40:1009–1013.

66. Schoetz DJ. Gastroduodenal Crohn's Disease. In: Michelassi F, Milsom JW, eds. Operative Strategies in Inflammatory Bowel Disease. Springer-Verlag, New York, 1999, pp. 389–393.

67. Poggioli G, Stocchi L, Laureti S, et al. Duodenal involvement of Crohn's disease. Dis Colon Rectum 1997;40:179–183.

68. Harold KL, Kelly KA. Duodenal Crohn Disease. Prob Gen Surg 1999;16:50–57.

69. Pichney L, Fantry G, Graham S. Gastrocolic and duodenocolic fistulas in Crohn's disease. J Clin Gastroenterol 1992;15:205–211.

70. Lefton HB, Farmer RG, Fazio V. Ileorectal anastomosis for Crohn's disease of the colon. Gastroenterology 1975;69:612–617.

71. Longo WE, Oakley JR, Lavery IC, al e. Outcome of ileorectal anastomosis for Crohn's colitis. Dis Colon Rectum 1992;35:1066–1071.

72. Sanfey H, Bayless TM, Cameron JL. Crohn's disease of the colon. Is there a role for limited resection? Ann J Surg 1984;147:38–42.

73. Allan A, Andrews MB, Hilton CJ, Keighley MRB, Allan RN, Alexander-Williams J. Segmental colonic resection is an appropriate operation for short skip lesions due to Crohn's disease of the colon. World J Surg 1989;13:611–616.

74. Post S, Herfarth C, Schumacher H, et al. Experience with ileostomy and colostomy in Crohn's disease. Br J Surg 1995; 82:1629–1633.

75. Homan WP, Tang CK, Thorbjarnarson B. Anal lesions complicating crohn's disease. Arch Surg 1976;111:1333–1336.

76. Turunen U, Farkkila M, Seppala K. Long-term treatment of perianal or fistulous Crohn's disease with ciprofloxacin. Scan J Gastroenterol Suppl 1989; 24:144.

77. Bernstein LH, Frank MS, Brandt LJ, et al. Healing of perineal Crohn's disease with metronidazole. Gastroenterology 1980;79:367–365.

78. Kodner IJ, Mazor A, Shemesh EI, et al. Endorectal advancement flap repair of rectovaginal and other complicated anorectal fistulas. Surgery 1993;114:682–690.

79. Rutgeerts P, Geboes K, Vantrappen G, Beyles J, Kerremans R, Hiele M. Predictability of the postoperative course of Crohn's disease. Gastroenterology 1990; 99:956–963.

80. Mekhjian HS, Switz DM, Watts HD, Deren JJ, Kanton RM, Beman FM. National cooperative Crohn's disease study: Factors determining recurrence of Crohn's disease after surgery. Gastroenterology 1979;77:907–913.

81. Post S, Herfath C, Bohm E, et al. The impact of disease pattern, surgical management, and individual surgeons on the risk for relaparotomy for recurrent Crohn's disease. Ann Surg 1996;223:253–260.

82. Greenstein AJ, Sachar DB, Pasternack BS, Janowitz HD. Reoperation and recurrence in Crohn's Colitis and ileocolitis: Crude and cumulative rates. N Engl J Med 1975;392:685–690.

83. D'Haens G, Baert F, Gasparaitis A, Hanauer S. Length and type of recurrent ileitis after ileal resection correlate with presurgical features in Crohn's disease. Inflamm Bowel Dis 1997;3:249–253.
84. Borley NR, Mortensen NJ, Jewell DP. Preventing postoperative recurrence of Crohn's disease. Br J Surg 1997;84:1493–1502.
85. Cottone M, Rosselli M, Orlando A, et al. Smoking habits and recurrence in crohn's disease. Gastroenterology 1994;106:643–648.
86. Cosnes J, Carbonnel F, Beaugerie L, Le Quintrec Y, Gendre JP. Effects of cigarette smoking on the long-term course of Crohn's disease. Gastroenterology 1996; 110:424–431.
87. Kaufman HJ, Taubin HL. Nonsteroidal anti-inflammatory drugs activate quiescent inflammatory bowel disease. Ann Int Med 1987;107:513–516.
88. Korelitz B, Hanauer S, Rutgeerts P, Present D, Peppercorn M. Post-operative prophylaxis with 6-MP, 5-ASS or placebo in Crohn's disease: A 2 year multicenter trial. Gastroenterology 1998;114:A1011.
89. Lochs H, Mayer M, Fleig WE, Mortensen PB, Bauer P, et al. Prophylaxis of postoperative relapse in Crohn's ideas with mesalamine (Pentasa) in comparison to placebo (abstract). Gastroenterology 1997;112:A1027.
90. McLeod RS, Wolff BG, Steinhart AH, et al. Prophylactic mesalamine treatment decreases postoperative recurrence of crohn's disease. Gastroenterology 1995; 109:404–413.

10 Ostomy Care

Janice C. Colwell, RN, MS, CWOCN

CONTENTS

INTRODUCTION

A fecal diversion is frequently recommended as part of the treatment plan of patients with inflammatory bowel disease (IBD). Fecal diversions consist of an incontinent stoma created from a portion of the small (ileostomy) or large (colostomy) intestine, which are managed with an odor-proof pouching system. The person with an ostomy must undergo significant adjustments in order to incorporate the stoma into their life. Living with a stoma means a person must master skin protection skills, learn how to utilize a pouching system, deal with clothing and intimacy issues, and learn to incorporate the ostomy into activities of daily living. The advanced practice nursing specialty, wound, ostomy and continence nursing, formally referred to as enterostomal therapy, was developed to assist individuals with ostomies in moving toward adjustment. The Enterostomal Therapy/Wound Ostomy and Continence (ET/WOC) Nurse provides the skills needed to ensure an appropriately placed

From: *Clinical Gastroenterology:*
Inflammatory Bowel Disease: Diagnosis and Therapeutics
Edited by: R. D. Cohen © Humana Press Inc., Totowa, NJ

stoma, assists the patient to master self-care, and facilitates the adjustment process, as well as manages stoma-related complications. The critical factors that can assure positive outcomes following ostomy surgery are stoma location, stoma creation, and support/education. It is the ET/WOC nurse, working along with medical and surgical team members, that can assist the patient to achieve the skills needed to learn to live with a stoma. This team approach will provide the patient with the support to make the necessary adjustments.

STOMA CREATION

All stomas should be matured at the time of surgery, everted to be approx 2–3 cm in length, and have a centrally located lumen *(1)*. A stoma that protrudes above the skin level will allow the effluent to be discharged directly into the pouching system, protecting the peristomal skin and preventing pouch leaks. Permanent end ileostomies are chiefly created for treatment of IBD. Other indications may include: colorectal cancer, familial polyposis, ischemia, trauma, and radiation proctitis. The number of permanent ileostomies has been decreasing, as a result of reconstructive surgery. The ileoanal anastomosis is a reconstructive surgical procedure offered primarily to patients with ulcerative colitis (UC) and familial polyposis. In this procedure, a proctocolectomy is performed, a pouch created with the last foot of terminal ileum, and attached to the anus. The patient undergoing this procedure generally will have a temporary diverting loop ileostomy for approx 3 mo to protect the anastomosis. Loop stomas do not protrude easily above the skin surface and may retract below skin level making management difficult even for the short duration that the patient has the stoma.

A colostomy is created in the treatment of IBD to either permanently or temporarily divert the fecal stream from the diseased rectum. The stoma is created from the descending or sigmoid colon and should meet the same requirements as an end ileostomy and protrude above the skin approx 2–3 cm. A transverse colostomy is not preferred, as the location of the stoma is above the belt line and the diameter of the transverse colon is approx 2", requiring a large pouching system. Should diversion be required above the descending colon, the creation of an ileostomy is recommended.

STOMA LOCATION

The optimal stoma location will help to minimize the incidence of technical complications. The selection of the stoma site preoperatively is a key factor in the ability of the patient to maintain a pouching system seal *(2)*. The ideal stoma site is located on a section of the abdomen that is free from creases and folds irregardless of the person's position, with approx 2–3" of flat surface surrounding the site and the area should be easy for the patient to visualize, ensuring the potential for self care. A poorly sited stoma can cause failure of the pouching system, resulting in leakage and peristomal skin problems. The ET/WOC nurse is generally responsible for choosing the site prior to surgery. The patient is examined in a sitting position, feet flat on the floor. The abdomen is assessed for dominant creases and folds that could prevent the pouch from adhering. The rectus muscle is located, as is the infraabdominal bulge. The risk for stoma herniation is thought to be decreased by placing the stoma through the rectus muscle. The infraabdominal bulge is identified because this frequently is an area that does not contain creases or bulges (even if weight gain or loss is anticipated) and most patients can readily see this area to facilitate stoma management. A stoma marking disk is held at the proposed site to determine if there is the presence of 2–3" of flat contours to provide an adhesive pouching surface. An additional criteria that is considered is stoma placement below the belt line, which would allow clothes to flatten and support the pouching system against the abdomen. Placing the stoma below the belt line in some men can be impossible because of the choice and style of clothing, for example, some men wear a belt low on the abdomen, generally into the low abdominal fold. Placement below the belt line in men who wear belts in the low abdominal fold becomes difficult as the stoma site will be located in a deep abdominal crease, preventing most pouching systems from sealing around the stoma. In these cases, the stoma is marked at or above the belt line and the patient must adjust clothing options. Once the proposed stoma site is located, the area is marked with a surgical marking pen and covered with a transparent dressing.

SUPPORT/EDUCATION

Preoperative Preparation

Prior to ostomy surgery, the patient and their family is provided with an overall description of what adjustments will be necessary to living with a stoma. There are a variety of educational tools that can be utilized along with discussion (Table 1). Patients should understand that the stoma will not have any sensation, that the output will pass without warning and that a pouching system will be worn at all times. They should be shown pictures of a stoma, or at least hear the description that the stoma tissue is similar to the mucosal lining of the mouth, as this will provide them with a point of reference. The pouching system should be

Table 1
Patient Resources

Organization	Description
United Ostomy Association 36 Executive Park, Suite 120 Irvine, CA 92714-6744 1-800-826-0826 www.uoa.org	The United Ostomy Association (UOA) is a volunteer-based health organization dedicated to assisting people who have had or will have intestinal or urinary diversions. The UOA provides local support and educational chapters and satellites throughout the United States. Publishes the Ostomy Quarterly Magazine, a source for people with ostomies to keep updated on product offerings. Offers preoperative and postoperative patient visiting and support, as well as publications covering ostomy issues. Participates in advocacy activities and national, state and regional conferences.
The International Ostomy Association c/o British Colostomy Association 15 Station Road, Reading, Berks. RG1 1LG England www.ostomyinternational.org	The International Ostomy Association provides an association for the benefit of ostomates, run by ostomates, to represent the viewpoint of ostomates on the international level. Some educational information offered.
World Ostomy Resource www.powerup.com.au	The World Ostomy Resource web site has one major function; to list links to all Ostomy sites in the world. An additional offering is support and promotion of ostomy-related projects such as research and books.
alt.support.ostomy	Newsgroup accessed via the internet with postings related to ostomy.
Crohn's & Colitis Foundation 800-932-2423, ext. 212	The Crohn's and Colitis Foundation's mission is to cure and prevent Crohn's disease and UC through research, and to improve the quality of life of children and adults affected by these digestive diseases through education and support. Provides educational resources and support.
Wound, Ostomy and Continence Nurses Society 4700 W. Lake Avenue Glenview, IL 60025 866-615-8560	An association of Enterostomal Therapy Nurses (ET), is a professional nursing society which supports its members by promoting educational, clinical, and research opportunities, to advance the practice and guide the delivery of expert health care to individuals with wounds, ostomies, and incontinence. The site includes a fact 1-800-224-WOCN sheet regarding the use of convexity and a search engine that allows users to search www.wocn.org for an ET nurse in any geographical area in the US.

204

Patient Educational Booklets: written information on living with an ileostomy and colostomy.

These companies provide ostomy related educational booklets available upon request. Both companies have educational information online via their web sites.

Staywell Krames
1100 Grundy Lane
San Bruno, CA 94066-3030
1-800-333-3032

Ostomy Product Manufacturers:
ConvaTec
P.O. Box 5254
Princeton, NJ 08543-5254
1-800-631-5244
www.convatec.com

Hollister Incorporated
2000 Hollister Drive
Libertyville, IL 60048
1-800-323-4060
www.hollister.com

205

described, and, if appropriate, an actual pouch should be available. The United Ostomy Association (UOA), a support group for people undergoing ostomy surgery can arrange a visit from a person whom has undergone ostomy surgery. Meeting with a person with an ostomy is an opportunity for the patient to talk about concerns, see someone who looks healthy, and is wearing clothes and they can note that the pouching system is not visible. It is usually at the preoperative educational session that the stoma site is marked in preparation for surgery. Self-ostomy care education will begin 1–2 d after surgery and will be ongoing.

Postoperative Stoma Education

The ostomy pouching system is applied in the operating room directly after the surgical procedure. Ostomy management instruction begins the first day after surgery. At this first session, the patient and, if appropriate, a family member watch as the postoperative pouch is changed. This gives the patient the opportunity to view the stoma and see what skills must be learned. The patient gives a return demonstration of how to open and close the clamp, as this is the first skill they will master. From this point on during the hospitalization, the patient participates in emptying the pouch. The next lesson, generally held on postoperative day 3, has the patient changing the pouch, handling both the stoma and the stoma pouching system. Length of stay after ostomy surgery is generally 5–7 d and there may only be the opportunity to have two lessons during this time. In order to be ready for discharge, the patient must be independently emptying the pouch; a home care nursing visit can be arranged if the patient has not progressed to independence in the pouching change.

OSTOMY MANAGEMENT PRINCIPLES

An ostomy pouching system should provide protection and maintenance of the peristomal skin from the effluent contain the output in an odorproof system, provide a reliable, consistent seal for at least 3 d, and allow the person using the system to participate in their lifestyle activities *(3)*. In order to achieve these goals, a pouching system is chosen with a strong resistant nonirritating skin barrier (to adhere the pouching system but maintain skin) and a pouch that is odorproof and can be concealed under clothing.

SKIN BARRIERS

The skin barrier is the portion of the ostomy pouching system that provides skin protection from the stomal output. Skin barriers are available in several types: solid sheets and washers, paste, powder, and liquid. The solid sheets and washers are available in two wear times: standard wear (approx 4 d) and extended wear (approx 7 d). All pouching systems utilize a solid skin barrier in the shape of a sheet or a washer integrated into the pouching system, either as a component that is part of the pouch or as a separate piece that will accept the ostomy pouch. The solid skin barrier is a thin flexible material manufactured of gelatin, pectin, and sodium carboxymethylcellulose, which will hold its shape when in contact with fecal output, but allow the user to move without detaching from the skin. A solid skin barrier is used to manage all fecal stomas and is placed directly around the base of the stoma to protect the peristomal skin from the fecal output. A precut skin barrier can be used with stomas that are round, a cut to fit skin barrier is preferred for a stoma that is not round, allowing the user to cut to fit. The back of the skin barrier is adhesive and secures the pouching system to the peristomal skin. Standard wear skin barriers are generally worn directly after surgery and changed every 3–4 d to allow stoma assessment and education. Extended wear barriers are worn after post operative edema has subsided or if the stoma output is high or the fecal consistency is highly liquid. A high output stoma will quickly "melt" the skin barrier allowing the effluent to be in contact with the peristomal skin and in extreme cases causing the pouch to detach from the skin.

Stoma barrier pastes are used to "caulk" the solid skin barrier. The skin barrier paste is placed on the cut edge of the solid skin barrier to prevent migration of the fecal output under the solid skin barrier and to fill uneven areas in the peristomal area. Skin barrier pastes contain alcohol which can irritate denuded skin and must be used with caution on impaired skin integrity.

Skin barrier powders are used to provide a drying effect on peristomal skin that is denuded. The powder is sprinkled on the affected skin, brushed into the area and the excess brushed off. The solid skin barrier is applied over the powdered area allowing the pouching system to adhere to the treated skin.

Liquid skin barriers are plasticized agents that place a protective coating on the peristomal area and are utilized to seal skin against stripping from aggressive adhesives and to seal denuded peristomal skin. Two types of liquid skin barriers are available, one with alcohol as a vehicle (which will cause burning if used on denuded skin) and "no sting" barrier wipes containing no alcohol. The most common form of liquid skin barriers are wipes, which are applied to the peristomal skin, allowed to dry (a shiny dry coating is observed) and then the pouching system is used.

Table 2
Ostomy Product Manufacturers

Coloplast	ConvaTec
1955 West Oak Circle	P.O. Box 5254
Marietta, GA 30062-2249	Princeton, NJ 08543-5254
1-800-533-0464	1-800-631-5244
www.coloplast.com	www.convatec.com
Hollister Incorporated	NuHope Laboratories, Inc.
2000 Hollister Drive	P.O. Box 331150
Libertyville, IL 60048	Pacoima, CA 91333
1-800-323-4060	1-800-899-5017
www.hollister.com	www.nu-hope.com

Pouches

All pouching systems must be made of odorproof material; there are very few commercially constructed pouches that are not odorproof. Although pouches are available in drainable or nondrainable styles, the preferred method of management is to use a drainable pouching system, that allows the user to drain the pouch contents without removing the pouch or the skin barrier. Pouches are available in either a one piece or a two piece system. A one piece system is composed of the pouch and the solid skin barrier as one unit. The two piece system consists of the pouch as one piece and the solid skin barrier as the other. The solid skin barrier with body side adhesive adheres to the skin and the top side of the skin barrier has a flange that accepts the pouch. The pouch can be changed as required without disturbing the skin barrier seal.

Pouching options include: clear or opaque film, short (9–10") or standard length (12"), and a variety of shapes dependent upon the manufacturer (Table 2). Some pouches have an absorbent material lining the back of the pouch that will absorb body moisture especially important in hot, humid climates.

The two piece system allows the wearer to change the pouch without changing the skin barrier and this may be an advantage for some people. The shorter pouch can be used as activity dictates and then "popped" off when no longer needed. This option is not available for the user of a one piece pouching system. *See* Table 3 for product listing and clinical tips.

Care Issues

The ostomy pouch must be emptied at the point where the pouch is approx one-third full. For most people with standard fecal diversions

Table 3
Ostomy Products

Product	Purpose	Clinical tips
Liquid Skin Barrier: Available in spray and wipe	Provides a film barrier on peristomal skin	Utilize single use wipes (get the product directly on the area). Most contain alcohol. If used on denuded skin use "nonsting" formulation.
Solid Skin Barrier: available in standard wear and extended wear wear washers	Protects peristomal skin from damaging effects of effluent	Cut to fit up up to stoma. High output stomas: utilize extended wear barrier.
Skin Barrier Paste: Avaiable in a tube and in paste strips	Acts as a "caulking" agent to prevent undermining of skin barrier seal when working with denuded skin	All tube paste contains alcohol and can harm denuded peristomal skin. Consider strip paste (does not contain alcohol).
Skin Barrier Powder: available in a bottle	Absorbs moisture on peristomal skin	Dust lightly on peristomal skin, a high buildup prevents pouching system adhesion.
One Piece Cut to Fit Pouching System	Skin barrier that can be custom cut to stoma size	Appropriate post operative. Used to fit irregular stomas.
Two Piece Pouching System	Skin barrier placed around the stoma and pouch snapped onto skin barrier	Allows user to change pouch (length and style) of pouch) and not skin barrier adhesive.
Convexity: rounded adhesive area	Provides pressure around a flush or retracted stoma to enhance seal, can provide a seal when a dominant peristomal crease or fold is present	Degrees of convexity available, used dependent on amount of stomal retraction, depth of peristomal creasing. The use of belt is suggested to enhance the convexity.
Pouch Deodorant	Neutralizes odor when emptying	Place in pouch upon application and after each emptying.
Pouch Cover	Absorbs moisture that can occur from plastic pouch and is often used to conceal pouch contents	If used to combat moisture buildup, patient side must be cotton. If moisture is a problem select a pouch with an integrated moisture pane.

this will varying between 4–6 times in 24 h. Emptying is dependent upon the amount of output, the consistency of the output and the size of the pouching system. There are a variety of pouching clamps, a clamp is placed at the bottom of the pouch to close the system. When emptying the pouch, the wearer holds the end of the pouch up, removes the clamp and allows the effluent to drain into the toilet. Most people find sitting upon the toilet the easiest way to empty the pouch as this minimizes splashing. If sitting on the toilet is not an option the patient drops toilet paper into the toilet to decrease splashing. Once the pouch contents have been emptied, the end and about 1 in of the inner pouch is wiped off and the closure reapplied. Emptying the pouch should be the only time that odor is noted, if this is unacceptable to the wearer, a liquid pouch deodorant can be inserted into the pouch when a fresh pouch is applied and after each emptying. The pouch deodorant will assist in neutralizing the odor prior to emptying. Rinsing of the pouch is not recommended as the water used in the rinsing process can loosen the skin barrier seal.

The outer portion of most pouching systems is water resistant allowing the wearer to shower, bathe, and swim wearing the system. For patients engaged in prolonged water sports a waterproof, occlusive tape is recommended.

Dietary discretion with an ostomy is dependent upon the nature of the disease that required the creation of a stoma, the location of the stoma and the patentcy of the stoma. As some stoma patients with inflammatory bowel disease may still have active disease, diets are based upon medical treatment of the disease. A patient with a temporary loop ileostomy for diversion after an ileal anal anastomosis pouch procedure will need to monitor foods that cause an increase in loose, watery stools and may need pharmaceutic intervention to prevent dehydration. A person with a snug stoma (at skin or fascial level) may require dietary discretion by avoiding roughage and totally indigestible foods. As a rule, for the first 6 wk following ostomy creation, a low-fiber diet is followed. After the postoperative edema has resolved, foods should be introduced slowly, noting the affect upon the consistency of the output and also noting if the patient complains of cramping at the stoma level as certain foods pass out of the stoma.

ISSUES OF DAILY LIVING

Concealing the pouching system is a major issue for people with an ostomy. As aforementioned, the stoma placement is attempted below the belt line. The importance of the belt line is noted when the patient dresses and pulls pants or skirts over the pouching system. If the pouching system can be placed below the belt line, the undergarments and the outer clothing can be used to conceal the pouch. Snug undergarments are key to flattening the pouching system and allowing the effluent to be equally distributed evenly through out the pouch. Outer garments can be form fitting if desired or can be loose, dependent upon the person's preference. Stomas that cannot be placed above the belt line will cause problems when the person dresses. Belts from pants or skirts can not cross over the pouch, as the belt will cut off the pouch, allowing effluent to sit at the level of the stoma and cause leakage. Clothing options for a person with a stoma placed above the belt line include suspenders, high waisted/high rise pants and the use of the tee shirt for men when swimming (otherwise the pouching system can be visualized when wearing swim trunks). Clothing considerations are greatly challenged when stoma placement is not ideal.

The creation of an ostomy causes the need for many adjustments, first and foremost the need to incorporate a new and changed body image. Stoma self-care must be mastered and along with this new mastery comes assurance that pouch leakage and odor will be controlled. Because a majority of people receive support from significant others and family these people must be included in the rehabilitation process *(4)*. The patient undergoing creation of a stoma should receive help in identifying resources for continued support and assistance. These resources should include professional follow-up and access to an ostomy support group, such as the United Ostomy Association.

Return to sexual function is frequently a concern for a person with a new ostomy. The person and their partner must recognize that the pouching system is secure and will not become dislodged or be harmed in anyway during sexual activity. Discussion about the return to intimacy should be included prior to discharge after ostomy creation. Some people with ostomies feel more comfortable if the pouch is covered or concealed with a pouch cover that resembles lingerie or clothing. Another alternative is the use of a mini pouch, a closed 2 in pouch that can be snapped onto the skin barrier and worn for short periods of time. The mini pouch remains flat against the wearer's abdomen, preventing the pouch for interfering while sexually active.

The economics of managing a stoma is an additional issue that requires attention from the patient. Pouching systems range from $3.00–10.00 per change and the average length of wear time is approx 5 d. Reimbursement for ostomy systems varies between health care programs. Medicare, or example, reimburses approx 80% of the used cost for a set number of pouches on a monthly basis. A person with an ostomy must determine the amount of assistance they will be entitled to before choosing a pouching system. The cost of the products can assist a person in making a cost-effective decision.

COMPLICATIONS

Peristomal Skin Breakdown

The most commonly presented stoma-related complication is breakdown of the peristomal skin. The reason for this complication is a poorly fitting ostomy pouching system. For approx 6 wk following surgery, the stoma size and shape will change as the postoperative edema resolves. The patient must be aware of the stoma size and decrease the diameter of the solid skin barrier to coincide with the shrinkage of the stoma. If this does not occur, the peristomal skin is exposed to the effluent and the epidermis becomes denuded. The solution to this problem is to resize the pouching system and utilize a skin barrier powder on the denuded skin to support healing *(5)*.

A second identified cause for peristomal skin breakdown and pouch leakage is use of an inappropriate pouching system for the person's stoma. A stoma should be evaluated in a sitting position to determine skin folds in the peristomal area as well as stoma or skin retraction. This assessment should include the observation of the stoma and the degree of protrusion. As aforementioned, a stoma should protrude 2–3 cm; if this amount of protrusion is not present in the sitting position, the stomal output may be expelled under the skin barrier, causing skin breakdown and pouch leakage. Immediately after surgery, the peristomal area may appear flat because of the presence of postoperative edema and the effects of corticosteroid administration causing a high distribution of abdominal fat. The pouching system should be reevaluated at frequent intervals. To level out a small dip around the stoma, skin barrier paste or a skin barrier washer can be used. To flatten out peristomal skin folds, to encourage protrusion of a less than ideal stoma or to manage a retracted stoma the use of a convex ostomy pouching system is recommended. A convex pouching system uses degrees of protrusion to apply pressure around the stoma to flatten out the skin and encourage drainage of the stomal output into the pouch. A belt can be attached to this system which will further enhance the seal.

Candidiasis

Peristomal candidiasis can occur under the solid skin barrier as well as under the outer water resistant tape. Factors that can predispose the person to an overgrowth of candida on the peristomal skin include: a dark moist area, use of systemic corticosteroids, and antibiotic therapy.

Treatment includes assessment of the pouching system to be assured that no moisture is in contact with the skin, and the application of an antifungal powder prior to pouch application. It is recommended that the pouching system be changed every 3 d to allow application of the antifungal powder. Cremes and ointments are contraindicated as they will interfere with the pouching seal.

Peristomal Herniation

The rate of peristomal hernia formation has been reported to be as high as 37% and is more likely to be found inpatients with colostomies, particularly loop colostomies (6). It is noted that to minimize the likelihood of hernia formation, the stoma should be brought out through the rectus muscle. The only definitive treatment of a peristomal hernia is surgical repair, however, recurrence rate is at least 50%. Local treatment consists of the use of a peristomal hernia support belt, a belt that fits around the stoma, allowing the stoma pouch to be accessed, while the belt applies firm pressure to the peristomal area.

Mucocutaneous Separation

Muco-cutaneous separation is a disconnection of the stoma and skin leaving a defect that is healed by secondary intention. This is seen in the immediate postoperative time frame. Causes are thought to include compromised healing, large skin opening, or excessive tension at the stoma/skin junction. Interventions include filling the defect with skin barrier powder and covering the area with a solid skin barrier.

Parastomal Pyoderma Gangrenosum

Parastomal pyoderma gangrenosum is an ulcerative, inflammatory cutaneous condition often associated with IBD patients. Skin lesions present in the peristomal area, generally present as pustules, break open and form full thickness ulcers with purple painful edges. Etiology is undetermined. Treatment is generally a combination of topical and systematic antiinflammatory, and absorptive dressings into the ulcers to provide a dry surface to apply the pouching system (7).

SUMMARY

The critical factors that can assure positive outcomes following ostomy surgery are stoma location, stoma creation, and support/education. The person living with a stoma requires preoperative consultation that will include the selection of a stoma site and the provision of information that should facilitate adjustment. The healthcare team must work together to ensure that the stoma is located in the best spot for the patient and that the stoma is created in a way which the patient can easily manage. Support and education must be ongoing and available to the person with an ostomy at the time of surgery, during the postoperative period, and for as long as the patient is working toward adjustment. The education of the patient in self-care activities, as well as the inclusion of the family in all aspects of rehabilitation remains key to facilitating the adjustment of a person with an ostomy. By conveying to a person with an ostomy a sense of acceptance and concern, along with the appropriate technical skills they require, the adjustment to and acceptance of the ostomy should be readily accomplished.

REFERENCES

1. Reasbeck PG, Smithers BM, Blackley P. Construction and management of ileostomies and colostomies. Digest Dis 1989;7:265–280.
2. Bass EM, DelPino A, Tan A. Does preoperative stoma marking and education by the enterostomal therapist affect outcome? Dis Colon Rectum 1997;40:440–442.
3. Erwin-Toth P, Doughty DB. Principles and procedures of stomal management. In: Ostomies and Cintinent Diversions: Nursing Management. Bryant R, and Hampton B, eds. Mosby-Year Book, St. Louis, MO, 1992.
4. Piwonka MA, Merino JM. A multidimensional modeling of predictors influencing the adjustment to colostomy. J Wound, Ostomy and Contin Nurs 1999;26:298–305.
5. Colwell JC. Enterostomal care in inflammatory bowel disease. In: Kirsner JB, ed. Inflammatory Bowel Disease. WB Saunders, Philadelphia, PA, 2000, pp.710–717.
6. Shellito PC. Complications of abdominal stoma surgery. Dis Colon Rectum 1998;14:1562–1572.
7. Sheldon, DG, Sawchuck L, Kozarch RA, Thirbly RC. Twenty cases of peristomal pyoderma gangrenosum. Arch Surg 2000;135:564–569.

11 Inflammatory Bowel Disease in Children and Adolescents

Ranjana Gokhale, MD
and Barbara S. Kirschner, MD

INTRODUCTION

The chronic inflammatory bowel diseases (IBD), Crohn's disease (CD) and ulcerative colitis (UC), are increasingly being recognized as a cause of chronic gastrointestinal disease in children and adolescents. About 20% of all patients with IBD develop symptoms during childhood *(1)* with about 5% being diagnosed before 10 yr of age *(2)*. Comprehensive studies from Scotland have reported a 4.4-fold increase in pediatric CD between 1968–1988. No such trend has been noted for UC *(3,4)*.

The variable age of onset, potential for growth failure because of disease activity and therapeutic interventions, and the special emotional needs of children are important considerations in the treatment of children with IBD.

From: *Clinical Gastroenterology:*
Inflammatory Bowel Disease: Diagnosis and Therapeutics
Edited by: R. D. Cohen © Humana Press Inc., Totowa, NJ

ETIOLOGY

The etiology of IBD remains unknown. Available evidence suggests that IBD results from immune-mediated bowel injury, triggered by environmental factors in a genetically predisposed individual. About 25% of affected children have a positive family history of IBD. A high concordance rate for CD has been noted among monozygotic as compared to dizygotic twins. The frequency of IBD in Ashkenazi jews is two to four times higher as compared to the general population. Boys and girls are equally affected in most studies. No differences have been noted between children with IBD and normal children regarding frequency of breast feeding, formula intolerance, prior gastrointestinal illness, or emotional stressors *(5)*. Many infectious and environmental agents have been postulated to cause IBD, although none have been proven. Recent clinical and experimental evidence suggests that chronic intestinal inflammation in IBD is a result of an abnormal heightened immune response to normal resident luminal bacterial components in a genetically predisposed individual *(6)*.

CLINICAL FEATURES OF CHILDREN WITH IBD

Ulcerative Colitis

The most consistent feature of UC is the presence of blood and mucus mixed with stool, accompanied with lower abdominal cramping, which is most intense during the passage of bowel movements. UC is usually diagnosed earlier after the onset of symptoms than CD as the presence of gross blood in the stools alerts the parents and physicians to a gastrointestinal problem. The location of abdominal pain depends on the extent of colonic involvement. Pain is in the left lower quadrant with distal disease and extends to the entire abdomen with pancolitis. Pediatric patients have a higher frequency of pancolonic involvement, likelihood of proximal extention of disease over time, and a higher risk of colectomy as compared to adult patients *(7)*. Abdominal distention, guarding, and rebound tenderness to palpation with decrease in bowel sounds requires close supervision because of the risk of developing toxic megacolon.

Crohn's Disease

In contrast to UC, the presentation in CD is subtle, often leading to a delay in diagnosis. Gastrointestinal symptoms depend upon the location, extent, and severity of involvement. In children, the most common location of disease is the ileocecal region (80%) with less frequent involvement of the terminal ileum alone, diffuse small bowel, and isolated colonic involvement. In patients with ileocolonic involvement, abdominal pain is usually postprandial and referred to the periumbilical area. Examination may localize tenderness to the right lower quadrant and an inflammatory mass may occasionally be felt. Gastroduodenal CD presents with early satiety, nausea, emesis, epigastric pain, or dysphagia. Because of postprandial pain and delay in gastric emptying, children with gastroduodenal CD often limit their caloric intake to diminish their discomfort. This may erroneously lead to a diagnosis of anorexia nervosa or other psychological disorders. Extensive small bowel disease causes diffuse abdominal pain, anorexia, diarrhea, and weight loss. Lactose malabsorption may occur either secondary to extensive small bowel involvement or primarily as a result of disaccharidase deficiency. Physical examination reveals diffuse abdominal tenderness. Clubbing of the distal phalanges is rare but seen most frequently in those children with extensive small bowel disease. Colonic CD may mimic UC, presenting with diarrhea with blood and mucus, associated with crampy lower abdominal pain often relieved by defecation. Perianal disease is common and occurs in 40% of children as anal tags, deep anal fissures, or fistulas (8). Increasing abdominal cramping, distention, and emesis accompanied with borborygmi are signs of progression of the inflammatory process to localized stenosis, partial, or complete obstruction.

EXTRAINTESTINAL FEATURES

Extraintestinal manifestations may precede or develop concurrently with intesinal symptoms and are common to both UC and CD. At least one extraintestinal manifestation is seen in about one third of children with IBD.

Fevers

Fevers are seen in 40% of patients with IBD at the time of presentation. Fevers are usually chronic, low-grade, and, hence, may frequently be unrecognized.

Weight Loss

Weight loss or a failure to maintain a normal growth velocity is the most common systemic feature of IBD, and is observed more frequently in children with CD than UC. In our patient population, 87% of children with CD and 68% of those with UC had weight loss at presentation.

Delayed Growth and Sexual Maturation

Delays in linear growth and sexual maturation may occasionally be the initial presentation of CD. Impaired growth can be demonstrated by a slowing of growth velocity (cm/yr) or a fall from previous height percentile of more than one channel (i.e., 50% to 10%). Previous measurements should be obtained for comparisons. Patients may also have concomittant delay in skeletal maturation, which is evaluated by radiologic determination of the nondominant hand. Delayed growth is more common in CD (60–88%) with the greatest frequency in prepubertal children, as compared to UC (6 –12%). Growth delay can also occur as a consequence of chronic corticosteroid use.

Chronic undernutrition is considered to be a major etiologic factor in growth delay. Undernutrition results from suboptimal enteral intake as a result of anorexia and abdominal discomfort as well as increased losses because of a protein losing enteropathy. Although malabsoprption of nutrients could also occur, it is rarely seen unless the patient has had extensive intestinal resection. Other contributing factors include low circulating levels of insulin-like growth factor (IGF-1) or somatomedin, which are seen in poorly nourished children and increase significantly following treatment *(10)* and elevated levels of circulating cytokines. Delayed sexual maturation or arrest of sexual maturation may occur concurrently with growth failure. Some females may also experience secondary amenorrhea caused by active disease or weight loss.

Arthralgia and Arthritis

Arthralgia and arthritis occur frequently in children with IBD and may occasionally precede intestinal manifestations of IBD. They usually coincide with disease activity and improve with medical treatment of underlying intestinal inflammation. Two forms of involvement are seen— a peripheral form and an axial form, including ankylosing spondylitis or sacroilitis. The peripheral form is usually pauciarticular affecting large joints, such as knees, ankles, hips, wrists, and elbows in decreasing order of frequency. Joint deformity is rare, although a destructive granulomatous synovitis has been described in CD. Ankylosing spondylitis is associated with HLA B27 in 50 to 80% of cases compared to over 90% in non-IBD-associated cases *(11)*. Progression is variable and does not appear to correlate with severity of bowel symptoms.

Mucocutaneous Lesions

Oral aphthoid ulcers occur in approx 20% of children with IBD. Ulcers usually cause minimal discomfort, although they may occasionally cause debilitating pain. They tend to parallel disease activity and treatment is directed toward underlying disease.

Cutaneous manifestations include erythema nodosum and pyoderma gangrenosum. Erythema nodosum is more common in CD and usually occurs in association with active intestinal inflammation; improvement coincides with treatment of the bowel disease. Pyoderma gangrenosum is an unusual manifestation usually seen in association with UC (<1%). It usually parallels active colonic disease, but on occasion may be refractory to systemic treatment and require intensive local therapy such as local corticosteroids, minocycline, dapsone, or clofazimine.

Ophthalmologic Complications

Ocular complications result from IBD itself or chronic corticosteroid therapy. Uveitis, iritis, and episcleritis are rare, occuring in <1% of pediatric patients. Episcleritis presents with scleral and conjunctival erythema with a burning sensation and photophobia. Local corticosteroid drops are usually effective. Iritis and uveitis present with eye pain, headache, and blurred vision or may be asymptomatic and detected by slit-lamp examination. Treatment consists of pupillary dilatation, covering the eye to decrease pain, and photophobia and local or systemic corticosteroid. Corticosteroids increase the frequency of posterior subcapsulsr cataracts and increased intraocular pressure. Individual corticosteroid susceptibility, rather than cumulative corticosteroid dose increases risk of these complications *(11)*. Ophthalmologic evaluation should be performed at six monthly intervals in children who are on long-term corticosteroids.

Hepatobiliary Disease

Hepatobiliary problems occur in about 4% of children with IBD. Primary sclerosing cholangitis (PSC), the most common, is usually seen in association with UC. PSC may be asymptomatic and is detected because of elevated alkaline phosphatase and γ-glutamyltransferase during routine blood screening. Children may occasionally present with pruritis and PSC prior to the development of intestinal symptoms from IBD. The course of PSC appears to be unrelated to underlying bowel disease and may progress after a colectomy. PSC is diagnosed either by liver biopsy or an endoscopic retrograde cholangiopancreatogram (ERCP) showing characteristic bile duct changes. Peripheral antineutrophilic cytoplasmic antibodies (pANCA) are positive in most patients with PSC and may be a marker for genetic susceptibility for this disease.

Autoimmune hepatitis in association with IBD is also well documented. Other infectious etiologies including occult viral infections should be excluded. Diagnosis is made following a liver biopsy and treatment includes corticosteroid and immunosuppressive medications.

Cholelithiasis is reported to be more common in CD with involvement of the terminal ileum or following resections. Other conditions including granulomatous cholecystitis and acalculous cholecystitis have also been described.

Renal Disease

Nephrolithiasis occurs in 1 to 2% of the pediatric population with IBD, predominantly as uric acid calculi in UC and oxalate calculi in CD. Hypercalciuria from prolonged bed rest or corticosteroid therapy appear to be risk factors. Secondary amyloidosis is extremely rare, but has been reported in CD. Obstructive complications may occur in CD as a result of ureteral compression by inflammatory mass or enterovesicular fistula.

Bone

Osteopenia or reduced bone mass can occur both at onset of IBD and as a complication of prolonged corticosteroid use. Osteopenia is an important potential complication of pediatric IBD as more than 90% of peak bone mass is attained during childhood and adolesence. Failure to attain peak bone mass increases future fracture potential. In the authors series of 99 children with IBD, low bone mineral density (BMD) was seen in 33% of children with CD and about half of those patients had severely reduced BMD (z score > 2 SD below mean). In contrast, approx 10% of patients with UC had low BMD at the lumbar spine *(13)*. Pubertal and postpubertal girls with CD were more likely to have low bone mass than pubertal children. Corticosteroid use was a predictor of low BMD, but other contributuing factors remain to be determined.

Aseptic or avascular necrosis is rare in the pediatric population and, although associated with corticosteroid use, the pathogenesis is unclear. Persistent joint pains, especially involving hip and knees, should prompt consideration of this complication. Chronic recurrent multifocal osteomyelitis (CRMO) has also been identified in six children with IBD. In all patients, onset of bony lesions preceded bowel symptoms by as much as 5 yr and responded to immunosuppressive therapy *(14)*.

DIAGNOSIS OF IBD IN CHILDREN

The diagnosis of IBD is based on clinical presentation, hematologic screening tests, radiologic examination, endoscopic appearance, and histologic findings (Table 1).

However, prior to testing, exclusion of enteric pathogens is of paramount importance in establishing the diagnosis of IBD. Pathogens that may mimic IBD include *Salmonella, Shigella, Campylobacter, Aeromonas, Plesiomonas, Yersinia, Eschericha coli 0157:H7, Clostridium difficile, Giardia Lamblia, Histoplasma,* and *Entamoeba Histolytica.* The role of an acute enteric infection in triggering the development of IBD is an area of active investigation. It is sometimes difficult to distinguish between acute infection and new-onset IBD, but children with IBD either fail to resolve symptoms or may have recurrent symptoms

Table 1
Establishing a Diagnosis of IBD in Children

History	Poor weight gain/weight loss
	Gastrointestinal symptoms
	Extraintestinal manifestations
	Family history of IBD
Physical Examination	Anthropometrics (height, weight)
	Pubertal (Tanner) staging
	Abdominal tenderness
	Perianal lesions
Screening Tests	
Complete Blood Counts	Microcytic anemia
	Leucocytosis with band forms
	Thrombocytosis
Acute Phase Reactants	Elevated sedimentation rate, serum
	orosomucoid, C-reactive protein
Chemistries	Low serum iron level, hypoalbuminemia,
	Elevated liver enzymes
Special Serologic Tests	pANCA, ASCA
Stool Examinations	exclude bacterial pathogens, C. difficile, ova
	and parasites, occult blood, fecal leucocytes
Endoscopic Evaluation	Esophagogastroduodenoscopy with biopsy
	Colonoscopy with biopsy
Radiologic Evaluation	Bone age X-ray (as indicated)
	Upper GI with small bowel follow-through
	Barium enema, enteroclysis (rarely used)

within days or weeks. Once enteric infections are excluded, work up can proceed as follows.

Hematologic Tests

Screening tests for IBD should include a complete blood count, inflammatory markers, and a metabolic profile that includes liver enzymes. Abnormal tests that are suggestive of IBD include elevated white blood count with increased band forms, microcytic anemia, and thrombocytosis. Acute-phase reactants like sedimentation rate, C-reactive protein, and serum orosomucoid are elevated in approx 90% of CD pediatric patients, but less frequently in UC. Hypoalbuminemia and a low-serum iron level may be seen. Elevated liver enzymes should prompt an evaluation for associated liver disease. Newer serologic tests include pANCA and antisaccharomyces cerevisiae antibodies (ASCA). These tests are used to support a diagnosis of IBD or as an aid in distinguishing UC from CD. P-ANCA is detected in 66–83% of children with UC and

14–19% of children with CD. Studies of ASCA in children show 44–54% sensitivity and 89–97% specificity *(15,16).*

Endoscopic Evaluation

Once a diagnosis of IBD is entertained, endoscopic examination with biopsies is indicated to establish the diagnosis. In most cases, histology can definatively differentiate between UC and CD, but in some instances of colitis, features may be atypical of either CD or UC and these children are categorized as having indeterminate colitis. Endoscopies in children are done under adequate conscious sedation using midazolam and demerol or fentanyl, or using deeper sedation with propofol administered by an anaesthesiologist. The latter approach is easier for children and adolescents and shortens procedure time. Bowel preparation is achieved by clear liquids for 1–2 d followed by Fleet's phosphosoda, 30–45 mL in 2 doses. We have found better compliance and adequate bowel preparation using phosphosoda, rather than magnesium citrate or polyethylene glycol solutions. On rare occasions, bowel preparation may be administered via nasogastric tube in an uncooperative child.

Radiologic Studies

Radiologic evaluations are usually reserved for patients with CD to assess involvement of small bowel loops and terminal ileum via a small bowel follow through X-ray. Although enteroclysis may provide superior images of the small intestine, the requirement for a nasoduodenal tube placement reduces the acceptance in children. Barium enemas are not used to diagnose UC, and should not be used in children with moderate or severe colitis to avoid inducing toxic megacolon. They may be beneficial in delineating stenotic segments, fistulas, or sinus tracts in CD.

TREATMENT OF IBD IN CHILDREN

Our goals in managing children with IBD include alleviation of gastrointestinal and extraintestinal manifestations, improving nutritional status to optimize growth and sexual maturation and attending to the emotional needs of children.

Emotional Needs

Most children with IBD have not experienced serious health problems prior to the onset of IBD. Therefore, they may be fearful of routine diagnostic and invasive procedures that are being performed on them, requiring sensitivity on the part of the physician. Discomfort from the disease process itself, delayed growth, and sexual maturation, as well as the cosmetic side effects from medications may affect the child's self-esteem and reinforce feelings of being different from their peers. Parents, as well as teachers who are important in the daily functioning of the child, need to be educated about the illness and we have found the brochures published by the CCFA to be very helpful in that regard. Children should be provided with special bathroom privileges and allowed to restrict gymnasium activities as needed, depending on their disease symptoms.

MEDICAL MANAGEMENT
Ulcerative Colitis: Mild Disease

Children with mild disease generally respond to oral sulfasalazine (SASP) alone or in combination with topical medications (Table 2). Oral SASP is started at 25–40 mg/kg/d in divided doses after meals and the dose can be gradually increased to 50–75 mg/kg/d. Folic acid supplementation should be given to patients on SASP. Side effects to SASP, mainly to the sulfa component, include headaches, gastrointestinal distress, especially nausea, and hypersensitivity reactions (skin eruptions, hemolytic anemia). Newer 5 aminosalicylic acid (5-ASA) meds: mesalamine, olsalazine, and balsalazide are useful in patients unable to tolerate SASP. Side effects seen with mesalamine are similar to SASP, although less common. Topical preparations: mesalamine and steroid enemas, mesalamine suppositories, and corticosteroid foam are very useful, but compliance in the pediatric population is somewhat limited. Most children respond to above measures, but about 27% require corticosteroids within the first year.

Moderate to Severe Disease

Children with systemic symptoms—including significant abdominal cramping, frequent bloody diarrhea, abdominal tenderness on palpation, anemia, and hypoalbuminemia, need to be hospitalized for close clinical observation and intravenous (iv) medications, fluids, and nutrition. Intravenous steroids (methylprednisone or hydrocortisone) are initiated at doses of 1–2 mg/kg/d (equivalent of prednisone) in divided doses to a maximum of 40–60 mg/d. Supportive care includes nothing or clear liquids by mouth and IV fluids or hyperalimentation. Oral SASP/5-ASA medications are held when oral intake is limited to avoid gastrointestinal distress. Antispasmodic agents should not be used because they predispose to the development of toxic megacolon. Blood counts and chemistries are closely monitored. Intravenous steroids are continued until abdominal cramping and hematochezia subside. Most children

Table 2
Medication Dosages in Pediatric IBD

Agent	Dosage
Corticosteroids	1.0–2.0 mg/kg/d prednisone equivalent iv or PO in divided doses (max 60 mg)
Budesonide	3–9 mg/d
Sulfasalazine	Starting dose 25–50 mg/kg/d Maximum 75 mg/kg/d (or 4 gms)
Aminosalicylates (oral)	30–60 mg/kg/d Mesalamine: max 4.8/g/d Olsalazine: max 2.0 g/d Balsalazide: max 6.75 g/d
Aminosalicylates (rectal)	Enemas: 4 g qhs Suppositories: 500 mg qd-bid
Metronidazole	10–20 mg/kg/d
Azathioprine	Starting dose 1–2 mg/kg/d Consider checking 6-MP metabolite levels
6-Mercaptopurine	Starting dose 1–1.5 mg/kg/d Consider checking 6-MP metabolite levels
Methotrexate	15 mg/m2/wk (max 25 mg)
Cyclosporine	4–8 mg/kg/d IV or PO Follow trough blood levels (200–250 mcg/ml)
Tacrolimus	0.15 mg/kg/d Follow trough blood levels, BUN, creatinine
Infliximab	5 mg/kg iv infusion

respond by 12 d and can then be given prednisone at equivalent doses for 4–6 wk as outpatients. Dietary restrictions include avoidance of high fiber, high residue, and spicy foods to prevent discomfort. Once clinical improvement occurs, prednisone is tapered by 2.5 mg to 5 mg every 1–2 wk as tolerated. Use of alternate-day prednisone is favored by many pediatric gastroenterologists so as to allow normal growth. Newer corticosteroid preparations, such as budesonide, which undergoes rapid first-pass metabolism in liver, have been recently approved for use in the United States.

IMMUNOSUPPRESSIVE THERAPY IN CHILDREN
Azathioprine and 6-Mercaptopurine

These drugs are being used with increasing frequency in children because of their steroid-sparing effects. Azathioprine (AZT) and 6-mercaptopurine (6MP) suppress disease activity in approx 70% of steroid-dependent or refractory children *(17)*. The long time required for beneficial effects preclude the use of these agents in acute episodes of severe colitis.

Methotrexate (MTX)

MTX has been reported to be beneficial in adult patients with UC and CD, especially in patients with CD. However, its use in pediatric UC patients has been limited.

Cyclosporine (CSA) and Tacrolimus (FK-506)

CSA has been used in children with acute steroid refractory UC, when surgery seems inevitable. Clinical improvement occurs in 7–10 d in 60–70% of children who enter remission. However, most children tend to relapse or have steroid-dependent disease, ultimately leading to colectomy. This effect has been reduced by the concomitant administration of AZA or 6-MP *(18)*. FK-506 use has recently been described in 16 children with colitis (10-UC, 4-CD, 2-indeterminate colitis) with improvement in 11 of 15 children within 14 d *(19)*. Four patients who initially responded ultimately required a colectomy. However, long-term safety of both these medications regarding toxicity and risk of lymphoproliferative disease remain to be seen.

CROHN'S DISEASE

Medical Management

The medical treatment approach for a child with CD needs to be individualized based on the severity of symptoms, degree and site of intestinal involvement, extraintestinal manifestations, and nutritional status.

CORTICOSTEROIDS

Corticosteroids are effective in decreasing disease activity in most patients. Dosing is similar to that described in UC. Once clinical remission is achieved, it is unproven whether low-dose alternate-day coricosteroid use should be continued or tapered. Children often have a recurrence of their symptoms when the dose is lowered below a threshold level. Under these circumstances, low-dose corticosteroids (≤5 mg/d), either daily or on alternate days, reduces disease activity and does not cause growth suppression.

Sulfasalazine and Mesalamine

SASP is useful for colonic and ileocolonic disease. Some of the newer preparations of 5-aminosalicylic acid (5-ASA) are useful for disease affecting the small bowel. However, 5-ASA preparations are not commercially available as a liquid formulation and, hence, cannot be administered to a young child. SASP can be prepared as a liquid and is useful in children with colonic CD. The dosing of these medications is similar to that described for UC. The long-term efficacy of SASP/5-ASA medications in maintaining remission of CD is unclear in contrast to UC.

ANTIBIOTICS: METRONIDAZOLE AND CIPROFLOXACIL

Perianal disease is seen in about 40% of children in CD *(8)*. Clinical experience has shown that metronidazole has been useful in the treatment of perianal disease both in adults and children. Rarely, children may develop sensory neuropathy, which resolves completely or improves after discontinuation of the drug. Ciprofloxacin has been used in adults with perianal disease, but its long-term use in children had been limited because of concerns of impaired cartilage growth. However a recent analysis of children with cystic fibrosis on long-term ciprofloxacin, did not demonstrate any radiologic evidence of cartilage damage or reduced linear growth.

Immunosuppressive Therapy

6-MERCAPTOPURINE AND AZATHIOPRINE

AZT and 6-MP are being increasingly used in children with CD. Indications include steroid dependency, extensive small bowel disease, history of previous resections, gastroduodenal disease, and perianal disease especially with refractory fistulae. In a recent study of 95 children with CD, AZT/6-MP was well tolerated in 82% of patients and led to a steroid reduction in 87% of patients *(17)*. Discontinuation of AZT or 6-MP was required in 18% of patients as a result of hypersensitivity reactions (pancreatitis, high fever) or infectious complications. Other side effects such as elevated aminotransferases and gastrointestinal intolerance respond to dose reduction.

METHOTREXATE

MTX has been used to maintain long-term remission in adult patients with CD. We recently described efficacy of subcutaneous use in 24 children with IBD. Improvement in clinical symptoms was seen in 70% of patients with CD resulting in a lowering of the corticosteroid dose *(20)*. Compliance with weekly injections is variable in this age group.

CYCLOSPORINE AND TACROLIMUS

Cyclosporine may be beneficial in children with refractory perianal disease. There is limited experience with tacrolimus in the treatment of CD in children.

Biologic Therapies

Increased production of inflammatory cytokines, especially tumor necrosis factor α (TNF-α) has been described in CD. TNF is found to be increased in amount both in histologically normal and in inflamed mucosa in CD. Infusions of anti-TNF antibody (infliximab) have been used successfully in adults and children with refractory CD, although optimal dosing and dosing regimens in children need to be clarified using prospective multicenter trials *(21)*. Open-label experiences with infliximab dosed at 5 mg/kg have been encouraging, and the drug's use has steadily increased among pediatric gastroenterologists. Thalidomide (an inhibitor of TNF-α production by monocytes) use is also not well described in pediatrics.

NUTRITIONAL INTERVENTION

Nutritional deficiencies caused by suboptimal caloric intakes, malabsorption or increased losses are common in children. Owing to potential effect on growth, pediatric gastroenterologists use nutritional intervention to control disease activity, provide restitution of deficiencies, and provide adequate calories to reverse growth failure. Caloric needs for newly diagnosed children are higher than normal children as most patients have lost weight at presentation. If the child is unable to drink elemental or semi-elemental formulas because of the taste, continuous nasogastric infusion at night has been useful. Up to one-third of children are unable or unwilling to pass a NG tube daily, and may require placement of a gastrostomy tube. Mineral deficiencies are also commonly seen in children with CD. Iron-deficiency anemia is the most common and is accompanied with microcytic anemia, low-serum iron levels, and low-serum ferritin. Zinc deficiency may contribute to growth failure and delayed sexual maturation. A low-serum alkaline phosphatase may be a clue to zinc deficiency. Mineral losses of calcium, magnesium, and phosphorus may also occur. All patients with IBD in our clinics are given a daily complete multivitamin with calcium supplementation, if their milk intake is suboptimal. Restriction of dairy products, which provide an excellent source of protein, calcium, and calories, should not be restricted unless the child is lactose intolerant. Even then, commercially available lactase products should be tried to improve tolerance of these foods *(22)*.

Indications for Referral to a Subspecialist

Children presenting with complaints of chronic recurrent abdominal pain in association with weight loss or failure to maintain a normal growth velocity, persistent diarrhea, or diarrhea with blood and mucus and extraintestinal manifestations should be referred to a subspecialist for further evaluation. Also children with a family history of IBD and persistent or recurrent gastrointestinal symptoms should be referred.

REFERENCES

1. Rogers BMG, Clark LM, Kirsner JB. The epidemiologic and demographic characteristics of inflammatory bowel disease: an analysis of a computerized file of 1400 patients. J Chronic Dis 1971;24:743–73.
2. Michener WM, Whelan G, Greenstreet RL, Farmer RG. Comparison of clinical features of Crohn's disease and ulcerative colitis with onset in childhood or adolescence. Cleveland Clinic Quarterly 1982;49:13–16.
3. Barton JR, Gillon S, Ferguson A. Incidence of inflammatory bowel disease in Scottish children between 1968 and 1983; marginal fall in ulcerative colitis, 3-fold rise in Crohn's disease. Gut 1989;30:618–622.
4. Ferguson A, Ghosh S, Choudari CP. Analysis of disease distribution, activity and complications in the patient with inflammatory bowel disease. Scand J Gastroenterol 1994;203:15–19.
5. Gilat T, Langman MJS. Childhood factors in the pathogenesis of inflammatory bowel disease: an international cooperative study. Scan J Gastroenterol 1987;22:1009–24.
6. Sartor RB. Current concepts of the etiology and pathogenesis of ulcerative colitis and Crohn's disease. Gastroenterol Clin North Am 1995;24(3):475–507.
7. Mir-Madjlessi SH, Michener WM, Farmer RG. Course and prognosis of idiopathic ulcerative proctosigmoiditis in young patients. J Pediatr Gastroenterol Nutr 1986;5:570–576.
8. Markowitz J, Daum F, Aiges H, Kahn E, Silverberg M, Fisher SE. Perianal disease in children and adolescents with Crohn's disease. Gastroenterology 1984;86:829–33.
9. Hyams JS. Extraintestinal manifestations of inflammatory bowel disease in children. J Pediatr Gastroenterol Nutr 1994;19:7–21.
10. Kirschner BS, Sutton MS. Somatomedin-C levels in growth-impaired children and adolescents with chronic inflammatory bowel disease. Gastroenterology 1986;91:830–836.
11. Mallas EG, Mackintosh P, Asquith P, Cooke WT. Histocompatibility antigens in inflammatory bowel disease. Their clinical significance and their association with arthropathy with special reference to HLA-B27(W27). Gut 1976;17:906–910.
12. Tripathi RC, Kirschner BS, Kipp M, Tripathi BJ, Slotwiner D, Borisuth NSC, et al. Corticosteroid treatment for inflammatory bowel disease in pediatric patients increases intraocular pressure. Gastroenterology 1992;102:1957–1961.
13. Gokhale R, Favus MJ, Karrison T, Sutton MS, Rich B, Kirschner BS. Bone mineral density assessment in children with inflammatory bowel disease. Gastroenterology 1998;114:902–11.
14. Bousvaros A, Marcon M, Treem W, Peters P, Issenman R, Couper R, et al. Chronic recurrent multifocal osteomyelitis associated with chronic inflammatory bowel disease in children. Dig Dis Sci 1999;44:2500–2507.
15. Olives JP, Breton A, Hugot JP, Oksman F, Johannet C, Ghisolfi J, et al. Antineutrophil cytoplamic antibodies in children with inflammatory bowel disease. J Pediatr Gastroenterol Nutr 1997;25:142–148.

16. Ruemmele FM, Targan SR, Levy G, Dubinsky M, Braun J, Seidman EG. Diagnostic accuracy of serological assays in pediatric inflammatory bowel disease. Gastroenterology 1998;115:822–829.

17. Kirschner BS. Safety of Azathioprine and 6-Mercaptopurine in pediatric patients with inflammatory bowel disease. Gastroenterology 1998;115:813–821.

18. Ramakrishna J, Langhans N, Calenda K, Grand RJ, Verhave M. Combined use of cyclosporine and azathioprine and 6-mercaptopurine in pediatric inflammatory bowel disease. J Pediatr Gastroenterol Nutr 1996;22:296–302.

19. Bousvaros A, Kirschner BS, Werlin S, Parker-Hartigan L, Daum F, Freeman K, et al. Oral Tacrolimus treatment of severe colitis in children: long term followup. J Pediatr 2000;137(6):794–799.

20. Gokhale R, Andrew H, Kirschner BK. Safety and efficacy of long term methotrexate in pediatric patients with inflammatory bowel disease. J Pediatr Gastroenterol Nutr 2000;31:A64.

21. Hyams JS, Markowitz J, Wyllie R. Use of infliximab in the treatment of Crohn's disease in children and adolescents. J Pediatr 2000:137:192–196.

22. Kirschner BS, DeFavaro MV, Jensen W. Lactose malabsorption in children and adolescents with inflammatory bowel disease. Gastroenterology 1981;81:829–832.

12 Nutritional/Metabolic Issues in the Management of Inflammatory Bowel Disease

Jeanette Newton Keith, MD
and Michael Sitrin, MD

Contents

INTRODUCTION

Nutritional management of the inflammatory bowel diseases (IBD), Crohn's disease (CD) and ulcerative colitis (UC), is an evolving field that changes with advances in the medical and surgical care of these disorders. As clinicians, it is essential to separately consider the various roles of nutritional treatments, and to understand their specific indications. In the literature, studies have attempted to address the following clinical issues: 1) the role of nutritional support in the induction of a remission in the setting of a newly identified disease or an acute exacerbation; 2) the role of nutrition in the maintenance of long-term remission; 3) nutrition support for the treatment of IBD complications; and 4) management of nutritional deficits and metabolic complications secondary to IBD.

Although in many situations the nutritional treatment of CD and UC is similar, in some situations, there are distinctly different responses to

From: *Clinical Gastroenterology:*
Inflammatory Bowel Disease: Diagnosis and Therapeutics
Edited by: R. D. Cohen © Humana Press Inc., Totowa, NJ

nutritional therapies. The primary focus of this chapter, therefore, will be an update regarding the indications for nutrition support in the management of IBD, as well as addressing the clinical limitations of the various nutritional interventions.

NUTRITIONAL SUPPORT AS PRIMARY THERAPY OF IBD

The Role of Enteral Nutrition Support as Primary Therapy for Crohn's Disease

Elemental diets, which are low-fat formulas containing dextrose polymers and free L-amino acids, were first introduced as part of NASA's space program in 1965. Key characteristics of this type of formula included its absorption in the proximal duodenum to mid-jejunum, low fecal debris production, limited fat content, and the ability to produce positive nitrogen balance (1). Elemental diets were subsequently used as preoperative nutrition to control catabolism in patients awaiting surgical intervention for many disease states including CD (2). In this setting, patients with CD were noted to have a greater than expected improvement in disease activity scores and sometimes went into remission, thereby, avoiding surgery, and suggesting a primary therapeutic role for enteral nutrition (3). Open trials reported favorable outcomes with the exclusive use of elemental diets as the primary therapeutic intervention in CD (4,5).

O'Morain et al. conducted the first prospective randomized controlled trial in 1984. The purpose was to assess the efficacy of elemental diets as a primary therapeutic modality in CD (6). In this study, the use of an elemental diet (Vivonex®) was compared with conventional steroid therapy to assess its ability to induce remission of an acute exacerbation. The elemental diet successfully induced remission in 82% of patients, compared with an 80% remission rate in those patients who received steroid therapy. Other groups showed similar beneficial effects of an elemental diet when used in combination with nonabsorbable antibiotics. The combination therapy was equal to prednisolone therapy when parameters such as CD Activity Index (CDAI), ESR, and fecal granulocyte excretion were compared (7).

In two subsequent multicenter trials, 21 of 51 patients (41%) receiving a protein hydrolysate-containing defined liquid diet orally in the European Cooperative CD Study III, and 29 of 55 patients (53%) receiving an oligopeptide diet via nasogastric or nasoduodenal tube in Study IV entered into clinical remission, respectively. The median time to clinical remission for the enterally fed group was 30.7 d in Study IV. Of note, 29 of the 51 patients receiving an oral liquid diet in study III dropped out of the study, mainly because of unpalatability of the formula. In comparison, 32 of 44 patients in Study III (73%) and 41 of 52 patients in Study IV (78%) receiving conventional steroid therapy entered into clinical remission in a median time of 8.2 d. Therefore, it was concluded that enteral nutrition, as primary therapy, was inferior to conventional steroid therapy. No influence of initial disease activity severity or disease location on the response to formula diet could be shown in these two studies *(8,9)*.

To further understand the seemingly conflicting results, Okada et al. *(10)* performed a nonrandomized controlled trial lasting 6 wk on 20 patients with CD who had never received specific therapy. The first group of 10 patients was placed on an elemental diet and the second group of 10 patients was prescribed prednisolone, while continuing their habitual diet. Clinical and radiographic disease activity assessments, in addition to markers of inflammation and nutritional status were measured for a total of 6 wk in the elemental diet group and for a total of 10 wk in the steroid-treated group. At the end of the first treatment period, the enterally fed group showed greater improvement in all parameters, including radiographic evidence of disease, than did the steroid-treated group. In light of the clinical response in the enterally fed group, the steroid-treated patients subsequently received an elemental diet for 4 wk in addition to the corticosteroids, with improvement in radiographic evidence of disease as well as further reduction of the markers of inflammation. It is important to note that patients with stenosis had difficulty with the enteral feeding. One of two patients with stenosis who received an elemental diet required surgical intervention. It was concluded that the elemental diet, in the absence of stenotic disease, was superior to steroid treatment as primary therapy. Second, it was suggested that enteral nutrition might have a role as adjunctive therapy based on the clinical improvement of the steroid-treated group following the addition of an enteral diet to their treatment.

Potential explanations for outcome differences in the various trials included small sample sizes in the original study by O'Morain, and the use of different liquid diets in the subsequent studies *(11)*. Others suggested that disease location might play a role in the variable clinical outcomes *(12)*. There are reports that enteral feeding is most effective in disease limited to the small bowel, whereas Crohn's colitis is less responsive to nutritional therapy *(13)*.

Multiple studies attempted to determine if there was a type of feeding or specific nutrient component responsible for inducing disease remission. Royall et al. *(14)* compared the efficacy of an elemental diet (Vivonex®) vs a formula with normal fat content containing peptides

(Peptamen®) in 40 patients with moderate to severe CD. There was a substantial increase in the total body nitrogen in the group receiving the amino acid-based formula that was not seen in the group receiving the peptide-based feeding. In addition, there was a reduction in the proinflammatory precursor, linoleic acid, in the group receiving the elemental diet. In spite of these subtle changes, there was no difference in remission rates or reduction in the CDAI between groups. The relapse rate for both groups was equivalent at 12 mo. It was noted that a gain in total body nitrogen was required for sustained disease remission.

A review of additional studies by Griffiths et al. assessing the efficacy of liquid formula diets as primary therapy found no advantage of elemental diets over semielemental or polymeric formulas *(11)*.

In all, three meta-analyses have been performed to assess the efficacy of enteral nutrition vs conventional steroid therapy *(15,6)*. The average response rate to steroids was 80% as compared to 60% for the enterally fed groups. One major limitation to all of the studies was the lack of a placebo control group. However, when one considers the placebo control response rate of 20% to 40% in the control groups from earlier drug therapy trials, it is highly suggestive that there are therapeutic benefits from enteral feedings *(17)*. The meta-analyses found no differences between elemental and more complex formulas.

The exact mechanism(s) by which enteral nutrition induces a remission in CD remains an enigma. It has been postulated that one of the potential benefits of the formula diets is that they are less antigenic compared to the normal diet. The removal of intraluminal antigens is postulated to reduce inflammation *(7)*. This theory was challenged by Greenberg et al. *(18)* who conducted a randomized control trial in 51 patients with active CD unresponsive to other medical management. Patients were randomized to one of three regimens: 1) total parenteral nutrition (TPN) and nil per os (npo) ($n = 17$); 2) defined formula administered through a nasogastric tube ($n = 21$); or 3) partial parenteral nutrition and a low residue diet as tolerated ($n = 15$). Clinical remission occurred in 71% of patients receiving TPN, 58% in the enterally fed group, and 60% in the group receiving partial nutritional support, which were not significantly different. When the 1-yr relapse rate was reviewed, there was no statistical differences between the three groups, suggesting that avoidance of normal food was not a factor in disease remission, nor did it influence clinical outcome at 1 yr.

Others have postulated that altered gut flora, provision of essential luminal nutrients, bowel rest, improvement in nutritional parameters, or reduction in gastrointestinal protein loss by enteral formulas account for the clinical and radiographic improvement in the disease *(19)*. Recent preliminary data suggests that the amount and type of fat in the formula may be important determinants of the therapeutic response *(20)*.

In summary, enteral nutrition remains as a viable therapeutic modality for the primary treatment of CD in patients who refuse steroid therapy, and in those circumstances in which steroid-related side-effects need to be avoided, such as children with growth failure. Future studies evaluating the efficacy of enteral nutrition in the patient who is steroid-resistant or -dependent are needed to further clarify the role of enteral nutrition as primary therapy in CD.

The Role of Parenteral Nutrition Support as Primary Therapy in Crohn's Disease

Total parenteral nutrition (TPN) has been used mainly as adjunctive therapy in patients with exacerbations of CD that were unresponsive to corticosteroid therapy, or in patients whose disease could only be controlled by high-dose steroids. Most of the studies have been uncontrolled, and because of the initiation or modification of medical treatments during the study period, the specific role of TPN has been difficult to define. Some studies, however, have found excellent responses to TPN in patients continued on the some dose of steroids and in patients treated with TPN alone. Overall, response rates of 40–90% have been reported in steroid-resistant or -dependent patients *(21–24)*. Some studies found that Crohn's colitis was less responsive to TPN than ileocolitis or small bowel disease. For example, one study reported that 73% of patient's with small bowel CD, vs 57% of patients with colonic CD avoided surgery when TPN was used as adjunctive therapy *(25)*. These findings were supported by other studies *(26)*, but additional series have not found an effect of disease location on response rate. TPN improved the nutritional status of virtually all patients.

The duration of the disease remission achieved with TPN has been evaluated by several investigators. Kushner et al. found that prolonged bowel rest and home parenteral nutrition was an effective therapeutic modality in severe, active CD unresponsive to conventional medical management. For patients with nonfistulous disease, there was partial healing of mucosal lesions and a reduction in corticosteroid requirements in most patients, but almost all relapsed within 2 yr *(27)*. Similar results were noted when Lerebours et al. studied the use of TPN in 20 steroid-dependent and -resistant patients with nonfistulous disease. Although initial disease remissions were often achieved, the risk of long-term recurrence was not affected by TPN use *(28)*. Muller et al. found that 25 of 30 patients with CD achieved remission after 12 wk of TPN as sole therapy, but the relapse rate was 60% at 2 yr and 85% at 4 yr *(29)*.

Several studies have compared TPN and enteral nutrition support in patients with CD. Greenberg et al. *(18)* compared TPN, enteral nutrition, and partial parenteral nutrition plus a low residue diet. In all three groups, the remission rates were similar. Wright, Adler, and Jones also found no difference in the number of remissions or time until remission between enteral and parenteral nutrition support *(30,31)*. Based on these findings and the generally favorable responses to enteral nutrition, tube feedings should the preferred modality of nutritional support for the majority of patients with CD. TPN should be reserved for those with very short bowel, high-grade obstruction, certain types of fistulas, and those who do not tolerate tube feedings.

The Role of Nutrition Support
as Primary Therapy for Ulcerative Colitis

In contrast to the generally favorable responses to nutrition support in CD, UC generally responds poorly to nutritional interventions. Initial uncontrolled studies with very small patient numbers suggested a potential role for TPN as primary therapy *(32,33)*. Subsequent controlled trials, however, found that ulcerative colitis patients receiving TPN fared no better than those receiving conventional medical therapy alone, and over half of the patients in the trials required colectomy during that hospitalization *(34,35)*, The different response of Crohn's colitis and ulcerative colitis to TPN was highlighted in the study by Sitzman et al. *(36)*. In a retrospective review, they compared the clinical course of 16 patients with Crohn's colitis compared to 22 patients with UC. The patients were placed on TPN, corticosteroids, antibiotics (primarily metronidazole), sulfasalazine, and/or azathioprine. Of the 22 patients with UC, 16 required colectomy during the initial hospitalization, one subsequently had surgery, and one died refusing on operation. Of the 16 Crohn's colitis patients, only one required surgery during the initial hospitalization. Two additional patients treated with TPN for Crohn's colitis required surgical intervention at 2 and 4 yr postintervention. The remaining 13 patients remained in remission on medical therapy.

Gonzalex-Huix et al. found that enteral nutrition support was as effective as TPN as adjunctive therapy with steroids in acute UC *(37)*. As an added benefit, patients receiving enteral support had fewer complications, including postoperative infections.

In conclusion, nutritional support appears to have minimal benefit as treatment for acute UC. In those severely malnourished patients undergoing medical therapy with steroids, cyclosporine, or other drug treatments, nutritional support may be useful to avoid further nutritional depletion, and enteral nutrition should generally be employed rather than TPN.

The Role of Specific Nutrients as Primary Therapy

Glutamine, fish oils, and short chain fatty acids have been studied to determine if these specific nutrients have beneficial therapeutic effects in patients with IBD.

Glutamine is the primary substrate for enterocytes and is key to the maintenance of normal small intestinal metabolism, structure, and function *(38)*. Although it is not an essential amino acid in healthy individuals, it has been shown to be a conditionally essential amino acid during periods of severe stress and catabolism. In this setting, glutamine demands exceed production capacity leading to a deficiency state *(39)*. Studies in animal models of enterocolitis suggested that glutamine-enriched enteral diets may lead to an improved intestinal morphology, preserved barrier function, reduced bacterial translocation, diminished disease activity, and improved nitrogen balance *(40,41)*. In a recent clinical trial, however, when a glutamine-enriched polymeric diet was used in the treatment of CD, there was no benefit over the standard glutamine-poor diet *(42)*. In a small pilot study, 6 of 10 patients with ileal-anal anastomosis and pouchitis treated with a 21-d course of glutamine suppositories had symptomatic resolution of symptoms vs only 3 of 9 patients treated with butyrate suppositories *(43)*.

Short-chain fatty acids (SCFA) are the preferred fuel of colonocytes, providing most of the metabolic energy for these cells. SCFA are derived from the fermentation products of unabsorbed carbohydrates and proteins, with the predominant ions in fecal water being butyrate, acetate, and propionate. In both experimental animals and humans, diversion of the fecal stream and deprivation of the colon of SCFA is associated with colitis. SCFA enemas have been reported to decrease inflammation in diversion colitis by some investigators, but others have not been able to duplicate these results. Differences in the duration of treatment, the concentration of the SCFA solution and the reason for the diversion may explain the variability in outcome *(44)*. SCFA enemas have diminished inflammation in patients with distal ulcerative colitis in some, but not all studies *(45–48)*.

Fish oils have been used to treat animals with experimentally induced inflammatory states and humans with inflammatory diseases such as rheumatoid arthritis and psoriasis *(49–51)*. Fish oils contain omega-3 fatty acids that competitively inhibit prostaglandin and leukotriene synthesis. Eicosapentanoic acid (EPA), which is an unsaturated fatty acid in the omega-3 family of fish oils, is metabolized through the cyclooxygenase pathway to prostaglandin and thromboxanes of the omega-3 series. It is metabolized by the 5-lipoxygenase pathway to leukotriene B_5 that is 30 times less potent than leukotriene B_4 as a neutrophil chemotactic agent. In addition, other beneficial antiinflammatory effects of fish oils include suppression of interleukin 1 (IL-1) and platelet activating factor, free radical scavenging, alterations of membrane fluidity, and inhibition of platelet aggregation *(52)*.

In IBD, there are increased levels of the arachidonic acid metabolites prostaglandin E_2 and leukotriene B4. Prostaglandin E_2, which is found predominantly in enterocytes and macrophages, increases vascular permeability, dilates blood vessels, and downregulates immune function. Inflammatory cells, including polymorphonuclear cells, macrophages and mast cells, on the other hand, form leukotriene B_4. B_4 is a potent chemotactic agent for neutrophils and is responsible for the recruitment of neutrophils into the inflamed tissue.

Stenson et al. conducted a randomized double-blind placebo-controlled crossover trial of fish oils vs placebo in UC. There was reduction in the levels of leukotriene B4 in the rectal dialysate, improvement in colonic histological scores, slight corticosteroid dose reduction, and clinical evidence of weight gain following a 4-mo treatment period with fish oil supplements. Those patients receiving placebo required a slight increase in their corticosteroid doses *(53)*. These findings were supported by the work done of Hawthorne et al. who reported a modest beneficial effect of fish oil supplementation in UC. There was increased leukotriene B_5 production and a 53% reduction in the production of leukotriene B_4. There was significant dose reduction of corticosteroids after 1 and 2 mo of treatment, as well as a trend toward a faster rate of remission with fish oil treatment. Unfortunately, there was no difference in the rate of relapse *(54)*. Alsan et al. also evaluated the role of fish oil supplementation in UC and found a 56% reduction in disease activity in the treatment group compared to a 4% reduction in the placebo group, in spite of no changes in histopathologic scores or mucosal leukotriene B_4 levels *(55)*. In conclusion, there may be a modest clinical benefit from fish oil supplementation in UC. Further work is needed to clarify the mechanism of action and to further define the optimal treatment regimen.

Role of Diet and Nutrients in the Maintenance of Remission in IBD

Many investigators have attempted to define dietary factors that contribute to the onset or exacerbation of IBD. Consumption of increased amounts of omega-6 fatty acids, refined sugar, animal protein, animal fat, dairy products, margarine, ultrafine dietary particles, and other foods have been linked to both ulcerative colitis and CD in epidemiological studies *(56–60)*. None of these observations, however, have been sufficiently reproducible to convincingly link any specific type of food with inflammatory bowel disease.

Exclusion diets have been suggested as a therapeutic strategy by some groups, but are difficult to use clinically, require highly motivated patients, and are subject to high dropout rates *(61,62)*. Patients treated with a low carbohydrate diet or an omega-3 fatty acid supplement have relapse rates no different from those receiving their habitual diet and dietary compliance with the low carbohydrate diet was poor *(63)*.

The ability of fish oil supplements to maintain remission of CD has been evaluated with inconsistent results. A study by Lorenz-Meyer et al. showed no benefit of fish oil over placebo in the maintenance of CD remissions *(63)*. A subsequent study by Belluzzi et al., however, demonstrated a reduction in disease relapses in patients with CD receiving an enteric-coated fish oil preparation. This preparation was much better absorbed than previously used products, and was associated with fewer adverse reactions *(64)*.

As aforementioned, treatment with enteral nutrition support appears to induce remission of CD in many patients. With resumption of normal dietary intake, however, the disease typically relapses fairly quickly, with most studies reporting a 60–70% relapse rate within 12 mo *(65)*. Several recent studies have demonstrated that enteral nutrition support prolongs disease remission in children with CD *(66–68)*. In a retrospective analysis of children with CD successfully treated with tube feedings, a questionnaire was used to assess long-term outcome. Of the 28 patients who continued intermittent nocturnal tube feedings 4 to 5 d per wk along with a normal diet during the day, only five relapsed at 6 mo and 12 at 12 mo. In contrast, 15 of the 19 patients who stopped nocturnal enteral feedings relapsed by 6 mo *(66)*.

NUTRITION THERAPY OF IBD COMPLICATIONS

Preoperative Nutrition Support

Poor wound healing, infections of various types, anastomotic leaks, prolonged ileus, decubitus pressure sores, and increased mortality are well-known postoperative complications of malnutrition *(67)*. Parenteral and enteral nutrition support have been shown to be effective therapeutic modalities for correction of nutritional deficiencies in patients undergoing surgery, but the use of nutrition support to prevent postoperative complications remains a controversial topic. Controlled clinical trials of perioperative nutrition support specifically in patients with IBD are lacking, and most of our information comes from studies on general surgical patients.

In a retrospective study, Mullen et al. examined whether preoperative TPN improved the clinical outcome in a heterogeneous surgical population. They compared patients who received at least 7 d of pre-operative TPN with those who received no TPN prior to surgery. In the subset of patients at the highest risk of developing nutrition-related complications based on the Prognostic Nutritional Index, a validated objective nutrition assessment tool, preoperative TPN resulted in a 2.5-fold reduction in complications, a seven-fold reduction in major sepsis, and a five-fold reduction in mortality *(68)*. Rombeau et al. retrospectively reviewed the efficacy of preoperative TPN for patients undergoing surgery for IBD. Their results showed an overall reduction in total and septic complications in patients who had received at least 5 d of preoperative TPN. Patients with evidence of malnutrition (serum albumin <3.4 g/dL and a transferrin level of <150 mg/dL) had an increased incidence of post-operative complications. Those patients who were not malnourished (transferrin >150 mg/dL) did not have a postoperative complication, even when less than 5 d of TPN was provided *(69)*.

These findings were supported by a prospective randomized control trial of preoperative TPN is patients in Veterans Administration hospitals undergoing elective abdominal or chest surgery. Patients receiving TPN for 7 to 14 d prior to surgery and 3 d afterward were compared to those who received no TPN. Patients with mild malnutrition receiving TPN had more infections than the controls, and did not have a significant reduction in other complications. In contrast, patients with clinical evidence of severe malnutrition treated with preoperative TPN had a reduction in noninfectious complications, such as wound dehiscence, prolonged ileus, and so on, with no increase in postoperative infections *(70)*.

These and other studies point out the importance of a careful nutritional assessment in evaluating patients for preoperative TPN. Those with significant malnutrition will likely benefit from preoperative TPN, whereas those with good or borderline nutritional status may experience net harm from this treatment. Based on the studies described earlier, it has been estimated that preoperative nutrition support of malnourished patients reduces the risk of postoperative complications by 10% *(71)*. One case-control study has reported that preoperative TPN of CD patients was associated with a reduction in the length of bowel resection *(72)*.

The appropriate duration of TPN prior to surgery has also been debated. Christie and Hill examined 19 patients with active IBD undergoing elective surgery treated with preoperative TPN. Serial measurements of total body protein, plasma proteins, respiratory muscle function, and skeletal muscle function were performed prior to and after surgery. The patients in this study had a baseline deficit of 35% of total body protein stores, associated with a 20–40% impairment of physiologic functions compared to controls. By day 4 of TPN, there was significant improvement in the physiologic measurements, at a time when there was no detectable change in total body protein. Subsequently, physiologic function continued to improve, but at a much slower rate. Very gradual recovery of total body protein stores and further gain in muscle function occurred during convalescence from surgery *(73)*. Based on these and other observations, a 7–14 d period of preoperative TPN is recommended for malnourished patients. Longer periods of repletion have not been proven beneficial.

Controlled clinical trials have not evaluated the effect of preoperative enteral nutrition support on postoperative complications. Tube feedings can provide excellent bowel preparation for surgery, and as aforementioned are generally well tolerated in patients with IBD. Home enteral support has been used for nutritional repletion of children prior to surgery *(74)*. Further research is needed to see whether enteral nutrition support avoids the infectious complications associated with TPN, thereby providing greater net benefit.

Nutrition Support for Intestinal Fistula Management

Patients with CD and enteric fistulas are commonly (55–90%) malnourished. Malnutrition occurs because of poor food intake, small bowel bacterial overgrowth causing malabsorption, infection, and increased energy requirements, and loss of enteric secretions rich in protein and other nutrients. Sepsis is the most common complication that occurs with enterocutaneous and enteroenteric fistulas *(75)*.

Studies assessing the efficacy of TPN and bowel rest as primary therapy for fistulas in patients with CD have reported very different rates of fistula closure. The variability in outcome is likely related to the different types of fistulas seen in these patients. Fistulas that occur in the postoperative setting secondary to anastomotic leaks or drainage tubes, in the absence to active IBD and other co-morbidities such as malnutrition or distal bowel obstruction, and that have a tract <2 cm in length with a defect <1 cm^2 are associated with high closure rates. Unfavorable features that predict low rates of spontaneous closure are fistulas arising from active CD or cancer, a long tract with epithelialization, anastomotic disruption, repair of an enterotomy or multiple prior surgeries, distal bowel obstruction, and comorbidities such as malnutrition and sepsis. In some cases, there is spontaneous closure with TPN and bowel rest, but the fistulas recur with resumption of a normal diet. The long-term closure rate of fistulas caused by active CD with TPN is less than 30%, and surgery is usually required. Even when permanent fistula closure cannot be achieved, nutritional support may be useful to replete the patient prior to surgery *(76)*.

Studies assessing the benefits of enteral nutrition support as therapy for fistulas are limited to case reports and small series. In general, tube feedings are well tolerated, achieve nutritional repletion, and are associated with spontaneous closure rates similar to those seen with TPN *(77,78)*. Patients with colocutaneous fistulas, ileal fistulas with low output, or proximal fistulas where the feeding tube can be placed beyond the origin of the fistula are the best candidates for enteral feedings. TPN is preferred for those with high output fistulas, proximal fistulas that cannot be bypassed with a feeding tube, and in the setting of ileus or distal obstruction.

Many clinicians prefer to use elemental diets in patients with CD and fistulas because these formulas are rapidly and completely absorbed, induce minimal secretion of digestive enzymes, cause little fecal output, and often change the character of the fistula effluent so it is less corrosive on the skin. There is some concern, however, that prolonged use of elemental feedings may cause distal small bowel and colonic atrophy.

Nutritional and Growth Failure

Growth failure is seen in as many as 20–30% of pediatric CD patients and to a lesser extent in ulcerative colitis *(79)*. The major causes of growth failure include active IBD, inadequate energy intake, and prolonged treatment with daily corticosteroids *(80)*. The goals of therapy must be to achieve adequate nutritional intake while at the same time inducing a disease remission and reduction in steroid requirements. Growth can be restored in some children by aggressive dietary management and oral nutritional supplements in addition to their medical therapy *(81)*. Many, however, will have difficulty sustaining the use of oral supplements because of taste fatigue. Because of the excellent response to enteral nutrition support, the desirability of avoiding steroid-related side effects such as acne, Cushingnoid features, and osteoporosis, and the finding in some studies that growth is better with enteral feedings when compared to steroid therapy, some pediatricians feel that enteral nutrition support is the preferred treatment modality for IBD exacerbations *(82)*. Older children and adolescents can be taught to self-intubate nightly with a small bore feeding tube and administer their tube feedings during sleep, thereby minimizing interference with usual daily activities and socialization. Younger children may benefit from endoscopic gastrostomy tube placement for long-term tube feeding. Placement of a feeding gastrostomy tube has not been associated with fistula formation *(83)*. Home TPN for the treatment of children with IBD and growth failure should be reserved for those with short bowel, certain fistulas, obstruction, or extensive disease than cannot be managed with enteral nutrition.

Home TPN

Patients with CD and gut failure secondary to extensive resection and/or active disease are now supported by home total parenteral nutrition. Overall, the rehabilitation of patients with CD on home TPN is excellent, and mortality is low *(84)*. Home TPN is associated with improved quality of life, reduced steroid requirements, and nutritional repletion. Despite these benefits, home TPN is also associated with significant morbidity because of catheter-related sepsis, catheter occlusion, venous thrombosis, dehydration, and electrolyte derangements. Home TPN also fails to prevent relapses of disease, and there is no decrease in surgical procedures *(85)*. Metabolic bone disease and liver dysfunction, which can progress to cirrhosis and liver failure, are severe complications of home TPN. Every effort, therefore, should be made to preserve bowel function and maintain oral or enteral nutritional intake whenever possible.

TREATMENT OF NUTRITIONAL DEFICITS

Mechanisms of Malnutrition in IBD

Malnutrition can occur in inflammatory bowel disease for a variety of reasons (Table 1). The most common cause is decreased oral intake secondary to reduced appetite, avoidance of eating because of meal-induced symptoms, and restrictive diets prescribed in an attempt to manage gastrointestinal complaints *(86)*.

Increased caloric need in the setting of fever and infections may also be a contributing factor in the development of malnutrition in IBD. In general, however, in the absence of infectious complications, most patients will have normal resting metabolic rates, as predicted by the Harris-Benedict equation. Those patients with the most severe weight loss may have a higher-than-predicted metabolic rate, perhaps reflecting altered body composition or metabolism. Some authors have found an aberration in lipid oxidation in CD, with increased utilization of fat compared with controls and increased diet-induced thermogenesis *(87)*. The average total daily caloric need for outpatients with quiescent IBD is approx 1.7 times the basal energy requirement *(88,89)*.

Pharmacologic therapies used in the management of both CD and UC also have nutritional consequences. For example, corticosteroids affect vitamin D and calcium metabolism, contributing to osteoporosis *(91–94)*. Sulfasalazine can cause folate malabsorption and in severe cases, megaloblastic anemia *(95)*.

Table 1
Causes of Malnutrition in IBD[1]

Cause	
Inadequate intake	Reduced appetite, restrictive diet
Malabsorption	Loss of luminal surface, nutrient, and drug interactions
Maldigestion	Bacterial overgrowth, bile acid deficiency
Drugs	Sulfasalazine, corticosteroids, cholestyramine, colestipol, cyclosporine, azathioprine
Increased GI losses	Mineral, protein, fat, electrolyte, trace element or blood losses
Increased energy expenditure	Infection, inflammation, increased cell turnover

[1]Adapted from: Zurita VF, Rawls DE, Dyck WP. Nutritional support in inflammatory bowel disease. Dig Dis 1995;13:93.

Prevalence of Nutritional Deficiencies

Because of the many abnormalities in nutrient intake, absorption, and metabolism seen in IBD, there is a high prevalence of protein-calorie malnutrition and vitamin and mineral deficiencies as outlined in Table 2. Weight loss at the time of presentation has been reported in 65–75% of patients with CD and 18–62% of patients with UC. Growth failure and delayed puberty in pediatric patients typically reflect inadequate energy intake. Hypoalbuminemia and edema are commonly observed, secondary to both inadequate protein intake and absorption and to protein-losing enteropathy, which is characteristic for active inflammatory bowel disease and can be measured by monitoring fecal excretion of alpha-1 antitrypsin (96).

Deficiencies of all classes of micronutrients have been reported in patients with IBD. Patients with CD and ileal disease or resection are at greatest risk for vitamin deficiencies. Vitamin B_{12} malabsorption has been reported with as little as 35 cm of ileal resection or disease (97). Deficits of vitamins A and D are seen about 25% of patients with CD and steatorrhea because of ileal dysfunction (14). Folate deficiency is commonly seen as a result of inadequate intake and malabsorption secondary to intestinal disease and/or sulfasalazine use (95).

Mineral deficiencies are also commonly observed. Iron deficiency anemia is a frequently complication secondary to chronic blood loss and poor intake and absorption (98). Zinc deficiency is closely correlated with disease activity, and fecal zinc losses typically reflect the severity of diarrhea (99,100). Inadequate intake and malabsorption also contribute to zinc deficiency. The most common signs and symptoms associ-

Table 2
Incidence of Nutritional Deficiencies in IBD[1]

	CD%	UC%
Vitamin D	75	35
Weight Loss	65–75	18–62
Folic Acid	54–67	30–40
Vitamin B$_{12}$	48	5
Iron	39	81
Selenium	35–41	NR
Growth Failure	31	10
Delayed Puberty	30	20
Hypoalbuminemia	25–80	25–50
Anemia	25–85	66
Magnesium	14–33	ND
Calcium	13	ND
Vitamin C	12	NR
Vitamin A	11	NR
Zinc	10–50	NR
Vitamin K	10–25	NR
Potassium	5–20	ND
Copper	ND	ND

NR = Not reported: ND = reported, but no data to accurately estimate incidence.
[1]Adapted from: Zurita VF, Rawls DE, Dyck WP. Nutritional support in inflammatory bowel disease. Dig Dis 1995; 13:94.

ated with zinc deficiency include growth retardation in children, loss of taste (dysguesia), skin lesions that range from acne to seborrheic in nature, alopecia, night blindness, apathy, and poor wound healing *(101)*. Magnesium deficiency is commonly observed in CD patients with extensive distal bowel resections *(102)*. Magnesium is an essential cofactor involved in more than 250 enzymatic processes that are part of key metabolic pathways. Of note, magnesium deficiency can be associated with impaired parathyroid hormone metabolism and correction of the magnesium deficiency often normalizes the serum calcium level *(103)*. Therefore, magnesium status should be monitored on a regular basis, especially in the setting of chronic diarrhea or extensive disease. One limitation in monitoring magnesium status is the poor correlation between total body magnesium stores and serum levels, as 98% of magnesium is intracellular. Signs and symptoms of magnesium deficiency include hyperreflexia, muscle cramps, prolongation of the QTc interval on ECG, hypotension, tremor, depression, and apathy. In severe cases, heart rhythm disturbances, and cardiac arrest can occur *(104,105)*. For the clinician, a high index of suspicion is key to the diagnosis of magnesium deficiency. Calcium deficiency is an important factor in the osteoporosis that often complicates IBD. Calcium intake is often poor because of anorexia and lactose intolerance. Steatorrhea, loss of absorptive surface, vitamin D deficiency, and corticosteroid treatment are important causes of calcium malabsorption in patients with IBD. Careful monitoring of calcium status including bone density studies should be performed, particularly in post-menopausal women, the elderly, and others at risk for osteoporosis *(91–94)*. Selenium deficiency also occurs in patients when >200 cm of small bowel is resected *(106)*.

Management of Nutritional Deficiencies

Because of the high prevalence of nutritional deficiencies in IBD, these patients should be periodically screened for the presence of clinical and subclinical nutritional deficits. Monitoring of the overall nutrition status can best be done using the Subjective Global Assessment (SGA). This assessment tool, described in Table 3, incorporates key historical information and specific physical examination findings in order to stratify patients according to the degree of malnutrition. Although clinically useful, the SGA is somewhat limited by the lack of a neurologic examination that is essential for detection of some vitamin and mineral deficiencies, such as vitamin B_{12}. In combination with a serum albumin level, however, the SGA is an effective tool for identifying malnutrition in the clinical setting *(107)*. Histories and physical examinations of patients with IBD should carefully seek signs and symptoms of vitamin and mineral deficiencies. In addition, laboratory assessments of micronutrients, mainly serum levels, should be obtained in at-risk patients in order to detect subclinical nutritional depletion, and to initiate dietary treatment or supplementation before the onset of clinical deficiency.

The dietary treatment of patients with IBD must be individualized and appropriate for their degree of impairment of gastrointestinal function. Many physicians impose unnecessary restrictions that are detrimental to adequate nutritional intake. Restriction of dietary fiber is often recommended, but Heaton et al. showed that treatment of CD with an unrefined-carbohydrate, fiber-rich diet is well tolerated and associated with the need for fewer surgeries than a typical low-fiber diet *(108)*. Dietary fiber is a heterogeneous mixture of substances with different physiologic effects. Insoluble fibers such as bran tend to decrease gastrointestinal transit time and increase bowel frequency. In contrast, soluble fiber that includes pectins and guars, increase transit time and

Table 3
Features of Subjective Global Assessment (SGA)

Select appropriate category with a checkmark, or enter numerical value where indicated by A "#".
A. History
   1. Weight change and height
      Overall loss in past 6 mo: Amt. + #___kg; % loss = #___; height = #___cm
      Change in past 2 wk:___increase;___no change;___decrease
   2. Dietary intake change (relative to normal)
      ___No change
      ___Change:___duration = #___weeks
      Type:___suboptimal solid diet;___full liquid diet;___hypocaloric liquids;___starvation
      Supplement: (circle) nil, vitamin, minerals, #___frequency/wk
   3. Gastroinestinal symptoms (that persisted for >2 wk)
      ___None;___nausea;___vomiting;___diarrhea;___anorexia
   4. Functional capacity
      ___No dysfunction (e.g., full capacity)
      ___Dysfunction: duration #___wk
         Type: ___working suboptimally;___ambulatory;___bedridden
   5. Disease and its relation to nutritional requirements
      Primary diagnosis (specify):_____
      Metabolic demand (stress):___no stress;___low stress;___moderate stress;___high stress
B. Physical (for each trait specify: 0 = normal; 1+ = mild; 2+ = moderate; 3+ = severe)
   #___Loss of subcutaneous fat (triceps, chest)   #___Ascites
   #___Muscle wasting (quadriceps, deltoids, temporalis)   #___Mucosal lesions
   #___Ankle edema   #___Cutaneous lesions
   #___Sacral edema   #___Hair change
C. SGA rating (select one)
   ___Well nourished
   ___Moderately (or suspected of being) malnourished
   ___Severely malnourished

Reproduced with permission from Shils, Olson, and Shike, Modern Nutrition in Health and Disease, 1999, Lippincott, Williams, & Wilkins, Philadelphia, PA.

retain water, may be beneficial in the treatment of patients with loose stools or diarrhea *(17)*. Fiber consumption, should, therefore, be individualized according to the patient's symptoms, and needs restriction only in those patients with stenosis and obstruction.

Lactose malabsorption is related to ethnicity as opposed to disease-state or location in children with IBD *(81)*. In adults with CD, Pironi et al. found a slight increase in the prevalence of lactose malabsorption by hydrogen breath test, but only 8% of the adults experienced clinical symptoms with the ingestion of 250 mL of milk *(109)*. In UC, the incidence of lactose intolerance was 44% vs 36% in controls when challenged with a 50-gram dose of lactose. In contrast, only 28% of patients were intolerant when given a 12.5-g dose. Therefore, patients with IBD can typically tolerate moderate amounts of lactose in their diets, and severe restriction is rarely warranted *(110)*. Dairy foods are a rich source of calcium, vitamin D, protein, and other nutrients and should not be routinely eliminated from the diets of patients with IBD. In those patients who are severely lactose intolerant, smaller doses of lactose-containing foods can be given more frequently. Lactase enzyme supplements, consumption of lactose-free or reduced-lactose milk products, and calcium and vitamin D supplements can be measured to ensure adequate intake.

The restriction of dietary fat may be beneficial for patients who have evidence of fat malabsorption and steatorrhea. Steatorrhea induces fluid and electrolyte secretion by the colon, contributing to diarrhea. High fecal fat excretion also increases fecal losses of divalent cations and fat-soluble vitamins. Steatorrhea also increases colonic absorption of dietary oxalate, contributing to hyperoxaluria and kidney stones. Increased fecal fat bind calcium in the intestinal lumen, which normally precipitates oxalate and prevents absorption, and also increases colonic permeability for oxalate. A low-fat diet with 50–70 gm/d is recommended for CD patients with steatorrhea because of ileal resection or disease and an intact colon *(17)*. For patients with steatorrhea and an ileostomy or jejunostomy, a less-severe fat restriction is needed, as dietary fat does not affect ostomy output and these patients do not develop enteric hyperoxaluria *(111)*. Dietary fat needs to be limited only to the extent necessary to prevent fat-soluble vitamin and mineral depletion. Excessive restriction of fat can lead to inadequate energy intake and weight loss.

Many physicians recommend that all patients with inflammatory bowel disease receive a therapeutic multivitamin and mineral supplement that provides one to five times the recommended dietary allowance of various micronutrients. It should be noted that most multivitamins do not contain adequate magnesium or calcium, and specific supplementation may be needed. Additional vitamin and mineral therapy is based on demonstrated deficiency, usually documented by low serum levels, and the dose is adjusted to achieve a normal serum nutrient concentration. In those with CD and ileal dysfunction, vitamin B_{12} replacement can be achieved by intramuscular injection of 100 µg per mo or 1000 µg every 2–3 mo. Alternatively, large doses of oral B_{12} or a B_{12} nasal spray can be used *(112)*. Repletion of magnesium deficiency is often difficult with oral supplementation, because magnesium preparations are cathartics and may worsen the patient's diarrhea. Parenteral magnesium supplements may be required.

SUMMARY

Careful nutritional evaluation should be a part of the medical care of all patients with IBD. Nutritional therapies can effectively be used in the management of various clinical problems, but the goals of therapy need to be clearly defined, and the treatment based on a detailed understanding of pathophysiology and the patient's disease status. Properly applied, nutritional treatment can play an important role in the reduction of morbidity from these chronic diseases.

REFERENCES

1. Winitz M, Graff J, Gallagher N., Narkin A, Seedman D. Evaluation of chemical diets as nutrition for man-in-space. Nature 1965;205:742–743.
2. Stephens RV, Randall HT. Use of a concentrated, balanced, liquid elemental diet for nutritional management of catabolic states. Ann Surg 1969;170:642–667.
3. Voitk AJ, Echave V, Feller JH, Brown RA, Gurd FN. Experience with elemental diet in the treatment of inflammatory bowel disease: is this primary therapy? Arch Surg 1973;107:329–333.
4. O'Morain C, Segal AW, Levi AJ. Elemental diet in the treatment of acute Crohn's disease. Br J Med 1980;781:1173–1175.
5. Axelsson C, Jarnum S. Assessment of the therapeutic value of an elemental diet in chronic inflammatory bowel disease. Scand J Gastroenterol 1977;12:89–95.
6. Saverymuttu S, Hodgson HJF, Chadwick VS. Controlled trial comparing prednisolone with an elemental diet plus non-absorbable antibiotics in active Crohn's disease. Gut 1985;26:994–998.
7. Malchow H, Steinhardt HJ, Lorenz-Meyer H, Strohm WD, Rasmussen S, Sommer H, et al. Feasibility and effectiveness of a defined-formula diet regimen in treating active Crohn's disease: European Cooperative Crohn's Disease Study III. Scand J Gastroenterol 1990;25:235–244.
8. Lochs H;Steinhardt HJ, Klaus-Wentz B, Zeitz M, Vogelsang H, Sommer H, et al. Comparison of enteral nutrition and drug treatment in active Crohn's Disease: results of the European Cooperative Crohn's Disease Study IV. Gastroenterology 1991;101:881–888.
9. Okada M, Yao T, Yamamoto T, Takenaka K, Imamura K, Maeda K, et al. Controlled trial comparing an elemental diet with prednisolone in the treatment of active Crohn's disease. Hepato-gastroenterol 1990;37:72–80.
10. Griffiths AM, Ohlsson A, Sherman PM, Sutherland LR. Meta-analysis of enteral nutrition as a primary treatment of active Crohn's disease. Gastroenterology 1995;108:1056–1067.
11. King TS, Woolner JT, Hunter JO. Review article:the dietary management of Crohn's disease. Aliment Pharmacol Ther 1996;11:17–31.
12. O'Morain CA. Does nutritional therapy in inflammatory bowel disease have a primary or an adjunctive role? Scand J Gastroenterol 1990;25:29–34.
13. Royall D, Jeejeebhoy KN, Baker JP, Allard JP, Habal FM, Cunnane SC, et al. Comparison of amino acid {v} peptide based enteral diets in active Crohn's disease:clinical and nutritional outcome. Gut 1994;35:783–787.
14. Fernandez-Banares F, Cabre E, Esteve-Comas M, Gussull, MA. How effective is enteral nutrition in inducing clinical remission in active Crohn's disease? A meta-analysis of the randomized clinical trials. JPEN 1985;19:356–364.

15. Messori A, Trallori G, D'Albasio G, Milla M, Vannozi G, Pacini F. Defined-formula diets versus steroids in the treatment of active Crohn's disease. A meta-analysis. Scand J Gastroenterol 1996;31:267–272.

16. Sitrin MD. Nutrition and inflammatory bowel disease. In:Kirsner JB, ed. Inflammatory Bowel Disease. 5th Edition. W.B. Saunders, Philadelphia, PA, 2000, pp. 598–607.

17. Greenburg GR, Fleming CR, Jeejeebhoy KN, Rosenberg IH, Sales D, Tremaine WJ. Controlled trial of bowel rest and nutritional support in the management of Crohn's disease. Gut 1988;29:1309–1315.

18. Ruemmele FM, Roy CC, Levy E, Seidman EG. Nutrition as primary therapy in pediatric Crohn's disease:fact or fantasy? J Ped 2000;136:285–291.

19. Gassull MA, Fernandez-Benares F, Cabre E, Papo M, Giaffer MH, Sanchez-Lombrana JL, Quer J, Malchow H, Gonzalez Huix F. European Group on Enteral Nutrition in Crohn's Disease. Fat composition is the differential factor to explain the primary therapeutic effect of enteral nutrition in Crohn's disease:results of A double-blind, randomized, multi-center European trial. Gastroenterology 2000;118:A740.

20. Fischer JE, Foster GS, Abel RM, Abbott WM, Ryan JA. Hyperalimentation as primary therapy for inflammatory bowel disease. Arch Surg 1973;125:165–175.

21. Vogel CM, Corwin TR, Baue AS. Intravenous hyperalimentation:in the treatment of inflammatory diseases of the bowel. Arch Surg 1974;108:460–467.

22. Driscoll RH, Rosenberg IH. Total parenteral nutrition in inflammatory bowel disease. Med Clin North Am 1978;62:185–201.

23. Ostro MJ, Greenberg GR, Jeejeebhoy KN. Total parenteral nutrition and complete bowel rest in the management of Crohn's disease. JPEN 1985;9:280.

24. Reilly J, Ryan JA, Strole W, Fischer JE. Hyperalimentation in inflammatory bowel disease. Amer J Surg 1976;131:192–200.

25. Elson CO, Layden TJ, Nemchausky BA, Rosenberg JL, Rosenberg IH. An evaluation of total parenteral nutrition in the management of inflammatory bowel disease. Dig Dis Sci 1980;25:42–48.

26. Kushner RF, Shapir J, Sitrin MD. Endoscopic, radiographic, and clinical response to prolonged bowel rest and home parenteral nutrition in Crohn's disease. JPEN 1986;10:568–573.

27. Lerebours E, Messing B, Chevalier B, Bories C, Colin, R, Bernier JJ. An evaluation of total parenteral nutrition in the management of steroid-dependent and steroid-resistant patients with Crohn's disease. JPEN 1986;10:274–278.

28. Muller JK, Keller HW, Erasoni H, Pichlmaier H. Total parenteral nutrition as sole therapy in Crohn's disease: a prospective study. Br J Surg 1983;70:40–43.

29. Wright RA, Adler EC. Peripheral parenteral nutrition is no better than enteral nutrition in acute exacerbation of Crohn's disease: a prospective trial. J Clin Gastroenterol 1990;12:396–399.

30. Jones VA, Workman E, Freeman AH, Dickinson RJ, Wilson AJ, Hunter JO. Crohn's disease: maintenance of remission by diet. Lancet 1985;2:177–180.

31. Dean RE, Campos MM, Barrett B. Hyperalimentation in the management of chronic inflammatory intestinal disease. Dis Colon Rectum 1976;19:601–604.

32. Fazio VW, Alexander-William J, Oberhelman HA, Goligher JC, Brotman M. Inflammatory disease of the bowel. Dis Colon Rectum 1976;19:574–578.

33. McIntyre PB, Powell-Tuck J, Wood SR, Lennard-Jones JE, Lerebours E, Hecketsweiler P, et al. Controlled trial of bowel rest in the treatment of severe acute colitis. Gut 1986;27:481–485.

34. Dickinson RJ, Ashton MG, Axon ATR, Smith RC, Yeung CK, Hill GL. Controlled trial of intravenous hyperalimentation and total bowel rest as an adjunct to the routine therapy of acute colitis. Gastroenterology 1980;79:1199–1204.

35. Sitzmann JV, Converse RL, Bayless TM. Favorable response to parenteral nutrition and medical therapy in Crohn's colitis. Gastroenterology 1990;99:1647–1652.
36. Gonzalez-Huix F, Fernandez-Banares F, Esteve-Comas M, Abad-Lacruz A, Cabre E, Acero D, et al. Enteral versus parenteral nutrition as adjunct therapy in acute ulcerative colitis. Amer J Gastroenterol 1993;88:227–232.
37. Souba WW, Herskowitz K, Salloum RM, Chen MK, Austgen TR. Gut glutamine metabolism. JPEN 1990;14:45S–50S.
38. Hall JC, Heel K, McCauley R. Glutamine. Br J Surg 1996;83:305–312.
39. Rombeau JL. A review of the effects of glutamine-enriched diets on experimentally induced enterocolitis. JPEN 1990;14:100S–105S.
40. Fujita T, Sakurai K. Efficacy of glutamine-enriched enteral nutrition in an experimental model of mucosal ulcerative colitis. Br J Surg 1995;82:749–751.
41. Akobeng AK, Miller V, Stanton J, Elbadri AM, Thomas AG. Double-blind randomized controlled trial of glutamine-enriched polymeric diet in the treatment of active Crohn's disease. J Ped Gastroenterol Nutr 2000;30:78–84.
42. Wischmeyer P, Pemberton JH, Phillips SF. Chronic pouchitis after ileal pouch-anal anastomosis: responses to butyrate and glutamine suppositories in a pilot study. Mayo Clin Proc 1993;68:978–981.
43. Guillemot F, Colombel JF, Neut C, Verplanck N, Lecomte M, Romond C, et al. Treatment of diversion colitis by short-chain fatty acids. Dis Colon Rectum 1991;34:861–864.
44. Patz J, Jacobsohn WZ, Gottschalk-Sabag S, Zeides S, Braverman DZ. Treatment of refractory distal ulcerative colitis with short chain fatty acid enemas. Am J Gastroenterol 1996;91:731–734.
45. Breuer RI, Buto SL, Christ ML, Bean J, Vernia P, Paoluzi P, et al. Rectal irrigation with short-chain fatty acids for distal ulcerative colitis: preliminary report. Dig Dis Sci 1991;36:185–187.
46. Breuer RI, Soergel KH, Lashner BA, Christ ML, Hanauer SB, Vanagunas A, et al. Short chain fatty acid rectal irrigation for left-sided ulcerative colitis: a randomized, placebo controlled trial. Gut 1997;40:485–491.
47. Treem WR, Ahsan N, Shoup M, Hyams JS. Fecal short-chain fatty acids in children with inflammatory bowel disease. J Pediatr Gastroenterol Nutr 1994;18:159–164.
48. Kremer JM, Jubiz W, Michalek A, Rynes RI, Bartholomew LE, Bigaquette J, et al. Fish-oil fatty acid supplementation in active rheumatoid arthritis: a double-blinded, controlled, crossover study. Ann Intern Med 1987;106:497–503.
49. Kremer JM, Lawrence DA, Jubiz W, DiGiacomo R, Rynes R, Bartholomew LE, et al. Dietary fish oil and olive oil supplementation in patients with rheumatoid arthritis: clinical and immunologic fffects. Arthritis Rheumatism 1990;33:810–820.
50. Bjørneboe A, Smith AK, Bjørneboe GA, Thune PO, Drevon CA. Effect of dietary supplementation with n-3 fatty acids on clinical manifestations of psoriasis. Br J Dermatology 1988;118:77–83.
51. Marotta F, Chui DH, Safran P, Rezakovic I, Zhong GG, Ideo G. Shark fin enriched diet prevents mucosal lipid abnormalities in experimental acute colitis. Digestion 1995;56:46–51.
52. Stenson WF, Cort D, Rodgers J, Burakoff R, DeSchryver-Keeskemeti K, Cramlich TL, et al. Dietary supplementation with fish oil in ulcerative colitis. Annals of Internal Medicine 1992;116:609–614.
53. Hawthorne AB, Daneshmend TK, Hawkey CJ, Belluzzi A, Everitt SJ, Holmes GKT, et al. Treatment of ulcerative colitis with fish oil supplementation:a prospective 12 month randomised controlled trial. Gut 1992;33:922–928.
54. Aslan A, Triadafilopoulos G. Fish oil fatty acid supplementation in active ulcerative colitis. A double-blind, placebo-controlled, crossover study. Amer J Gastroenterol 1992;87:432–437.

55. Geerling BJ, Dagnelie PC, Badart-Smook A, Russel MG, Stockbrugger RW, Brummer RJM. Diet as a risk factor for the development of ulcerative colitis. Amer J Gastroenterol 2000;95:1008–1013.

56. Shoda R, Matsueda K, Yamato S, Umeda N. Epidemiologic analysis of Crohn's disease in Japan:increased dietary intake of n-6 polyunsaturated fatty acids and animal protein relates to the increased incidence of Crohn's disease in Japan. Am J Clin Nutr 1996;63:741–745.

57. Russel MG, Engels LG, Muris JW, Limonard CB, Volovics A, Brummer RJM, et al. "Modern life" in the epidemiology of inflammatory bowel disease:a case-control study with special emphasis on nutritional factors. Eur J Gastroenterol Hepatol 1998;10:243–249.

58. The Epidemiology Group of the Research Committee of Inflammatory Bowel Disease in Japan. A case-control study of ulcerative colitis in relation to dietary and other factors in Japan. J Gastroenterology 1995;30:9–12.

59. Powell JJ, Harvey RSJ, Ashwood P, Wolstencroft R, Gershwin ME, Thompson RPH. Immune potentiation of ultrafine dietary particles in normal subjects and patients with inflammatory bowel disease. J Autoimmunity 2000;14:99–105.

60. Riordan AM, Hunter JO, Cowan RE, Crampton JR, Davidson AR, Dickinson RJ, et al. Treatment of active Crohn's disease by exclusion diet:East Anglian Multicentre Controlled Trial. Lancet 1993;342:1131–1134.

61. Green TJ, Issenman RM, Jacobson K. Patients' diets and preferences in a pediatric population with inflammatory bowel disease. Can J Gastroenterol 1998;12:544–549.

62. Lorenz-Meyer H, Bauer P, Nicolay C, Schulz B, Purrmann SJ, Fleig WE, et al. Study Group Members (German Crohn's Disease Study Group). Omega-3 fatty acids and low carbohydrate diet for maintenance of remission in Crohn's disease:A randomized controlled multicenter trial. Scand J Gastroenterol 1996;31:778–785.

63. Belluzzi A, Brignola C, Campieri M, Pera A, Boschi S, Miglioli M. Effect of an enteric-coated fish-oil preparation on relapses in Crohn's disease. NEJM 1996;334:1557–1560.

64. Rigaud D, Cosnes J, Le Quintrec Y, Rene E, Gendre JP, Mignon M. Controlled trial comparing two types of enteral nutrition in treatment of active Crohn's disease: elemental versus polymeric diet. Gut 1991;32:1492–1497.

65. Wilschanski M, Sherman P, Pencharz P, Davis L Corey M, Griffiths A. Supplementary enteral nutrition maintains remission in paediatric Crohn's disease. Gut 1996;38:543–548.

66. Heuschkel RB, Walker-Smith JA. Enteral nutrition in inflammatory bowel disease of childhood. JPEN 1999;23:S29–S32.

67. Seidman E, Leleiko N, Ament M, Berman W, Caplan D, Evans J, et al. Nutritional issues in pediatric inflammatory bowel disease. J Pediatr Gastro 1991;12:424–438.

68. Belli DC, Seidman E, Bouthillier L, Weber AM, Roy CC, Pletincx M, et al. Chronic intermittent elemental diet improves failure in children with Crohn's disease. Gastroenterology 1988;94:603–610.

69. Mullen JL, Gertner MH, Buzby GP, Goodhart GL, Rosato EF. Implications of malnutrition in the surgical patient. Arch Surg 1979;114:121–125.

70. Mullen JL, Buzby GP, Matthews DC, Smale BF, Rosato EF. Reduction of operative morbidity and mortality by combined preoperative and postoperative nutritional support. Ann Surg 1980;192:604–613.

71. Rombeau JL, Barot LR, Williamson CE, Mull JL. Preoperative total parenteral nutrition and surgical outcome in patients with inflammatory bowel disease. Amer J Surg 1982;143:139–142.

72. The Veterans Affairs Total Parenteral Nutrition Cooperative Study Group. Perioperative total parenteral nutrition in surgical patients. N Engl J Med 1991;325:525–532.

73. Klein S, Kinney J, Jeejeebhoy K, Alpers D, Hellerstein M, Murray M, et al. Nutrition support in clinical practice: review of published data and recommendations for future research directions. JPEN 1997;21:133–156.

74. Lashner BA, Evans AA, Hanauer SB. Preoperative total parenteral nutrition for bowel resection in Crohn's disease. Dig Dis Sci 1989;34:741–746.

75. Christie PM, Hill GL. Effect of Intravenous nutrition on nutrition and function in acute attacks of inflammatory bowel disease. Gastroenterology 1990;99:730–736.

76. Blair GK, Yaman M, Wesson DE. Preoperative home elemental enteral nutrition in complicated Crohn's disease. J Pediatr Surg 1986;21:769–771.

77. Fukuchi S, Seeburger J, Parquet G, Rolandelli R. Nutrition support of patient with enterocutaneous fistulas. Nut Clinl Prac 1998;13:59–56.

78. Bury KD, Stephens RV, Randall HT. Use of a chemically defined, liquid, elemental diet for nutritional management of fistulas of the alimentary tract. Am J Surg 1971;121:174–183.

79. Deital M. Elemental diet and enterocutaneous fistula. World J Surg 1983; 7:451–454.

80. Voitk AJ, Echave V, Brown RA, McArdle AH, Gurd FN. Elemental diet in the treatment of fistulas of the alimentary tract. Surg Gynecol Obstet 1973;137:68–72.

81. Rosenthal SR, Snyder JD, Hendricks, Walker WA. Growth failure and inflammatory bowel disease: approach to treatment of a complicated adolescent problem. Pediatrics 1983;72:481–490.

82. Kirschner BS, Voinchet O, Rosenberg IH. Growth retardation in inflammatory bowel disease. Gastroenterology 1978;75:504–511.

83. Kirschner BS, Klich JR, Kalman SS, DeFavaro MV, Rosenberg IH. Reversal of growth retardation in Crohn's disease with therapy emphasizing oral nutritional restitution. Gastroenterology 1981;80:10–15.

84. Walker-Smith JA. Management of growth failure in Crohn's disease. Arch Dis Childhood 1996;75:351–354.

85. Israel DM, Hassall E. Prolonged use of gastrostomy for enteral hyperalimentation in children with Crohn's disease. Amer. J Gastroenterol 1995;90:1084–1088.

86. Howard L, Hassan N. Home parenteral nutrition 25 years later. Gastroenterol Clin North Am 1998;27:481–512.

87. Galandiuk S, O'Neill M, McDonald P, Fazio VW, Steiger E. A century of home parenteral nutrition for Crohn's disease. Amer J Surg 1990;159:540–545.

88. Sitrin MD, Rosenberg IH, Chawla K, Meredith S, Sellin J, Rabb JM, et al. Nutritional and metabolic complications in a patient with Crohn's disease and ileal resection. Gastroenterology 1980;78:1069–1079.

89. Chan ATH, Fleming R, O'Fallon WM, Huizenga KA. Estimated versus measured basal energy requirements in patients with Crohn's disease. Gastroenterology 1986;91:75–78.

90. Barot LR, Rombeau JL, Steinberg JJ, Crosby LO, Feurer ID, Mullen JL. Energy expenditure in patients with inflammatory bowel disease. Arch Surg 1981;116: 460–462.

91. Mingrone G, Capristo E, Greco AV, Benedetti G, De Gaetan A, Tataranni PA, et al. Elevated diet-induced thermogenesis and lipid oxidation rate in Crohn's disease1-3. Am J Clin Nutr 1999;69:325–330.

92. Kushner RF, Schoeller DA. Resting and total energy expenditure in patients with inflammatory bowel disease. Am J Clin Nutr 1991;53:161–165.

93. Blodgett H, Burgin L, Iezzoni D. Effect of prolonged cortisone treatment on statural growth skeletal maturation and metabolic status of children. N Engl J Med 1956;254:636–641.

94. Luckert BP, Raisz LG. Glucocorticoid induced osteoporosis pathogenesis and management. Ann Int Med 1990;112:352–364.

95. Compston JE, Horton LWL. Oral 25-hydroxyvitamin D3 in treatment of osteomalacia associated with ileal resection and cholestyramine therapy. Gastroenterology 1978;74:900–902.

96. Issenman RM. Bone mineral metabolism in pediatric inflammatory bowel disease. Inflammatory Bowel Dis 1999;5:192–199.

97. Franklin JL, Rosenberg IH. Impaired folic acid absorption in inflammatory bowel disease:effects of salicyclazosufapyridine (Azulfidine). Gastroenterology 1973;64:517–525.

98. Florent C, L'Hirondel C. Desmazures C, Aymes C. Bernier JJ. Intestinal clearance of (1-antitrypsin: a sensitive method for the detection of protein-losing enteropathy. Gastroenterology 1981;81:777–780.

99. Behrend C, Jeppesen PB, Mertensen PB. Vitamin B 12 absorption after ileorectal anastomosis for Crohn's disease. Eur J Gastroenterol-Hepatol 1995;7:397.

100. Gasche C, Reinisch W, Lochs H, Parsaei B, Bakos S, Wyatt J, et al. Anemia in Crohn's disease: importance of inadequate erythroprotein production and iron deficiency. Dig Dis Sci 1994;39:1930–1934.

101. Schoelmerich J, Becher MS, Hoppe-Seyler P, Matern S, Haeussinger D, Loehle E, et al. Zinc and vitamin A deficiency in patients with Crohn's disease is correlated with activity but not with localization or extent of the disease. Hepatogastroenterol 1985;32:34–38.

102. Valberg LS, Flanagan PR, Kertesz A, Bondy DC. Zinc absorption in inflammatory bowel disease. Dig Dis Sci 1986;31:724–731.

103. Alpers DH, Klein S. Approach to the patient requiring nutritional supplementation. In:Textbook of Gastroenterology. Lippincott, Williams & Wilkens, Philadelphia, 1999, pp. 1081–1107.

104. Galland L. Magnesium and inflammatory bowel disease. Magnesium 1988; 7:78–83.

105. Leicht E, Schmidt-Gayk H, Langer HJ, Sneige N, Biro G. Hypomagnesaemia-induced hypocalcaemia:concentrations of parathyroid hormone, prolactin and 1,25-dihydroxyvitamin D during magnesium replenishment. Magnes Res 1992;5:33–36.

106. Abott LG, Rude RK. Clinical manifestations of magnesium deficiency. Miner Electrolyte Metab 1993;19:314–322.

107. Hessov I, Hasselblad C, Fasth S, Hulten L. Magnesium deficiency after Ileal resections for Crohn's disease. Scand J Gastroenterol 1983;18:643–649.

108. Rannem T, Ladefoged K, Hylander E, Hegnhøj, Jarnum S. Selenium status in patients with Crohn's disease. Am J Clin Nutr 1992;56:933–937.

109. Detsky AS, McLaughlin JR, Baker JP, Johnston N, Whittaker S, Mendelson RA, Jeejeebhoy KN. What is subjective global assessment of nutritional status? JPEN 1987;11:8–13.

110. Heaton KW, Thornton JR, Emmett PM. Treatment of Crohn's disease with an unrefined carbohydrate, fibre-rich diet. BMJ 1979;2:764–766.

111. Kirschner BS, DeFavaro MV, Jensen W. Lactose malabsorption in children and adolescents with inflammatory bowel disease. Gastroenterology 1981; 81:829–832.

112. Pironi L, Callegari C, Cornia GL, Lami F, Miglioli M, Barbara L. Lactose malabsorption in adult patients with Crohn's disease. Am J Gastroentol 1988;83: 1267–1271.

113. Bernstein CN, Ament M, Artinian L, Ridgeway J, Shanahan F. Milk tolerance in adults with ulcerative colitis. Am J Gastroenterol 1994;89:872–877.
114. Ovesen L, Chu R, Howard L. The influence of dietary fat on jejunostomy output in patients with severe short bowel syndrome. Am J Clin Nutr 1983;38:271–277.
115. Lambert D, Benhayoun S, Adjalla C, Gelot MA, Renkes P, Felden F, et al. Crohn's disease and vitamin B12 metabolism. Dig Dis Sci 1996;41:1417–1422.

13 Extraintestinal Manifestations of Inflamamtory Bowel Disease

Elena Ricart, MD
and William J. Sandborn, MD

CONTENTS

INTRODUCTION

Ulcerative colitis (UC) and Crohn's disease (CD) are associated with a wide variety of extraintestinal manifestations (EIM) that often make their management difficult and are significant causes of morbidity and mortality (Fig. 1). An EIM can occur before, concomitant with, or after

From: *Clinical Gastroenterology:*
Inflammatory Bowel Disease: Diagnosis and Therapeutics
Edited by: R. D. Cohen © Humana Press Inc., Totowa, NJ

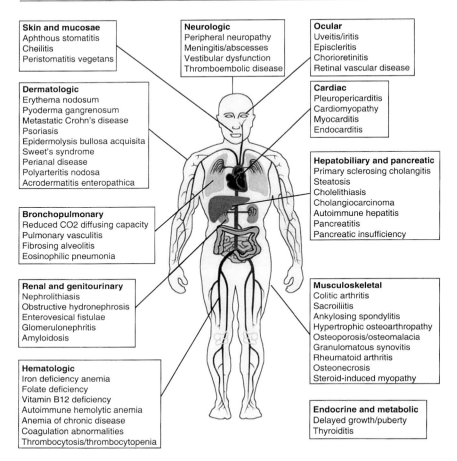

Skin and mucosae
Aphthous stomatitis
Cheilitis
Peristomatitis vegetans

Dermatologic
Erythema nodosum
Pyoderma gangrenosum
Metastatic Crohn's disease
Psoriasis
Epidermolysis bullosa acquisita
Sweet's syndrome
Perianal disease
Polyarteritis nodosa
Acrodermatitis enteropathica

Bronchopulmonary
Reduced CO_2 diffusing capacity
Pulmonary vasculitis
Fibrosing alveolitis
Eosinophilic pneumonia

Renal and genitourinary
Nephrolithiasis
Obstructive hydronephrosis
Enterovesical fistulae
Glomerulonephritis
Amyloidosis

Hematologic
Iron deficiency anemia
Folate deficiency
Vitamin B12 deficiency
Autoimmune hemolytic anemia
Anemia of chronic disease
Coagulation abnormalities
Thrombocytosis/thrombocytopenia

Neurologic
Peripheral neuropathy
Meningitis/abscesses
Vestibular dysfunction
Thromboembolic disease

Ocular
Uveitis/iritis
Episcleritis
Chorioretinitis
Retinal vascular disease

Cardiac
Pleuropericarditis
Cardiomyopathy
Myocarditis
Endocarditis

Hepatobiliary and pancreatic
Primary sclerosing cholangitis
Steatosis
Cholelithiasis
Cholangiocarcinoma
Autoimmune hepatitis
Pancreatitis
Pancreatic insufficiency

Musculoskeletal
Colitic arthritis
Sacroiliitis
Ankylosing spondylitis
Hypertrophic osteoarthropathy
Osteoporosis/osteomalacia
Granulomatous synovitis
Rheumatoid arthritis
Osteonecrosis
Steroid-induced myopathy

Endocrine and metabolic
Delayed growth/puberty
Thyroiditis

Fig. 1. Extraintestinal Manifestations of Inflammatory Bowel Disease

the diagnosis of the specific type of inflammatory bowel disease (IBD), and in some cases may even follow surgical removal of the diseased bowel. Large case studies have demonstrated that between 25% and 35% of patients with either type of IBD will have at least one EIM *(1,2)*. Multiple EIMs may occur in the same patient with the triad of joint-eye-skin involvement being the most common.

There have been several attempts to classify the EIMs of IBD (Table 1). Greenstein classified them into three groups according to the location of intestinal inflammation: colon related (joint, eye, skin, and oral manifestations); small bowel related (malabsorption, nephrolithiasis, cholelithiasis); and nonspecific manifestations (osteoporosis, liver disease, amyloidosis) *(1)*. An alternative classification based on the

Table 1
Classification of EIM of IBD

1. According to the location of intestinal inflammation[a]
   a. Colon-related manifestations: joint, eye, skin, and oral manifestations
   b. Small bowel related manifestations: malabsorption, cholelithiasis, genitourinary manifestations
   c. Nonspecific manifestations: osteoporosis, liver disease, amyloidosis
2. According to the inflammatory bowel activity[b]
   a. Bowel disease activity related: colitic arthritis, episcleritis, erythema nodosum
   b. Bowel disease activity unrelated: ankylosing spondylitis, pyoderma gangrenosum, primary sclerosing cholangitis
   c. Direct result of diseased bowel: fistulas, ureteral obstruction, nutritional deficiencies

[a]Greenstein AJ, Janowitz HD, Sachar DB. The extraintestinal complications of Crohn's disease and ulcerative colitis: a study of 700 patients. Medicine 1976;55:401–411.
[b]Monsen U, Sorstad J, Hellers G, Johansson C. Extracolonic diagnosis in ulcerative colitis: an epidemiological study. Am J Gastroenterol 1990;85:711–716.

inflammatory bowel activity divided EIMs into three categories: those related to the intestinal disease activity that usually respond to treatment of the underlying bowel disease (colitic arthritis, episcleritis, erythema nodosum); those whose course appears to be independent of the underlying bowel disease activity (ankylosing spondylitis, pyoderma gangrenosum, primary sclerosing cholangitis); and those that are a direct result of the presence of diseased bowel (fistulas, ureteral obstruction, nutritional deficiencies) (3).

This chapter provides an overview of the clinical aspects of the more common extraintestinal manifestations associated with UC and CD.

PATHOGENESIS

Little is known about the basis for the different organ distribution and the characteristic combinations of EIMs in IBD patients. While some extracolonic manifestations have clear etiologic factors (e.g., cholelithiasis, fistulous communications, or side effects of drugs used to treat IBD), the pathophysiology of the main groups of EIM is not clearly understood, and both autoimmunity and genetic susceptibility seem to play an important role. Several observations support the importance of autoimmunity in the pathogenesis of the EIM in IBD: relationship between EIM and the extent of colonic involvement, association of IBD with a number of autoimmune diseases (e.g., psoriasis, rheumatoid arthritis, thyroid diseases), increased incidence of autoimmune disorders in patients with UC compared to the general population, clinical response of EIM to immunosuppressive therapy, and humoral and cellular abnormalities in patients with IBD (activation of complement, presence of antineutrophilic cytoplasmic antibodies (ANCAs) in patients with UC and primary sclerosing cholangitis, and autoantibodies against pancreas, skin, and intestinal extracts) *(4–7)*. The importance of genetic susceptibility is supported by the observation that the incidence of EIM is higher in familial IBD *(8)*. Whatever genetic or environmental factors initiate IBD, the presence of altered mucosal permeability, reduced oral tolerance, cytokine imbalances, and influx of protein sequences allow constant stimulation of an abnormally regulated inflammatory reaction. Increased permeability of endothelial cells allows the combination of bacteria, their antigens and metabolic products, proinflammatory cytokines, and activated lymphocytes and neutrophils to get into the general circulation. Distant organs, such as the eyes or the peripheral joints, lose their normal immunologic tolerance and develop an inflammatory response that corresponds to an extraintestinal manifestation *(9)*.

MUSCULOSKELETAL MANIFESTATIONS

Peripheral arthritis, axial arthropathy, and ankylosing spondylitis are the three more important patterns of musculoskeletal manifestations in patients with IBD.

Peripheral colitic arthritis is the most common EIM in IBD and occurs in about 20% of patients. A recent clinical classification describes two types of peripheral arthropathy that are immunogenetically distinct entities: type 1 (pauciarticular) is related to HLA-B27 and is an acute, self-limiting arthropathy lasting a median of 5 wk, affects less than five joints, correlates with relapses of IBD, and is strongly associated with both erythema nodosum and uveitis; type 2 (polyarticular) is a symmetrical seronegative polyarthropathy not associated with HLA-B27, that runs a course independent of IBD, affects more than five joints, tends to cause persistent symptoms with a median duration of 3 yr, and is associated with uveitis but not with other extraintestinal manifestations *(10,11)* (Table 2). Both forms are migratory, and nondeforming arthritis that mostly affect the large joints of the lower extremities. The knees are most commonly affected followed by the hips, ankles, wrists, and elbows, and less often the hands and shoulders. The involved joints are swollen, erythematous, warm, and painful. The risk for peripheral arthritis increases with the amount of involved colon, although episodes of acute arthritis have been reported in patients with disease limited to the rectum, or after a colectomy with ileoanal anastomosis *(12)*. Treat-

Table 2
Classification of Peripheral Arthropathy in Inflammatory Bowel Disease

Type 1 (pauciarticular)
- Less than five joints
- Acute, self-limiting attacks (<10 wk)
- Associated with relapses of IBD
- Strongly associated with extraintestinal manifestations of IBD

Type 2 (polyarticular)
- Five or more joints
- Symptoms usually persist for months to years
- Runs a course independent of IBD
- Associated with uveitis, but not with other extraintestinal manifestations

Adapted from Orchard TR, Wordsworth BP, Jewell DP. Peripheral arthropathies in inflammatory bowel disease: their articular distribution and natural history. Gut 1998;42:387–39.

ment of peripheral arthropathy associated with IBD should be directed toward decreasing gut inflammation; and total proctocolectomy usually resolves it. If joint symptoms persist, additional therapies may include nonsteroidal antiinflammatory agents (NSAIDs), intraarticular corti-costeroid injections, and physical therapy. NSAIDs should be used with caution because exacerbation of IBD with NSAID has been reported *(13)*.

Axial arthropathy occurs in 3–5% of IBD patients. It frequently presents before identification of IBD and does not parallel bowel disease activity. It involves sacroiliac joints (more frequently), spine, hips, and shoulders. Asymptomatic sacroiliitis is a common radiographic finding, but this entity may also be a cause of low back pain. Most of the patients with sacroiliitis are HLA-B27 negative and do not progress to ankylosing spondylitis *(14)*.

Ankylosing spondylitis (AS) affects 3–6% of patients with IBD, whereas 2%–18% of patients with AS have associated IBD *(15)*. It is related to HLA-B27 in 50–80% of patients compared to over 90% of those with non-IBD associated AS *(16)*. Typical symptoms of AS include insidious onset of back pain and morning stiffness. The pain typically exacerbates with rest and relieves with exercise. Progression of the disease is variable and does not run parallel to the severity of bowel symptoms. In early cases, radiographs may be normal or show only minimal sclerosis, whereas in advanced cases there are squaring of vertebral bodies, and marginal syndesmophytes leading to bony prolif-eration and ankylosis called "bamboo spine" (Figs. 2A,B). Treatment for AS with IBD is the same as for idiopathic AS, and includes NSAIDs and physiotherapy, with some reported benefits with other agents includ-

A

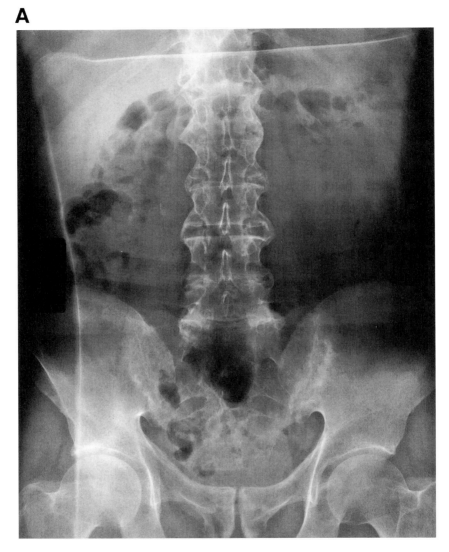

Fig. 2. (**A**) and (**B**) Ankylosing Spondylitis. Spine radiographs of a patient with long-standing ankylosing spondylitis showing squaring of vertebral bodies, marginal and symmetric syndesmophytes, and bilateral sacroiliitis.

ing sulfasalazine, methotrexate, and azathioprine. Proctocolectomy does not affect AS *(14)*. Recent reports suggest marked improvement with the anti-tumor necrosis factor agents etanercept and infliximab.

B

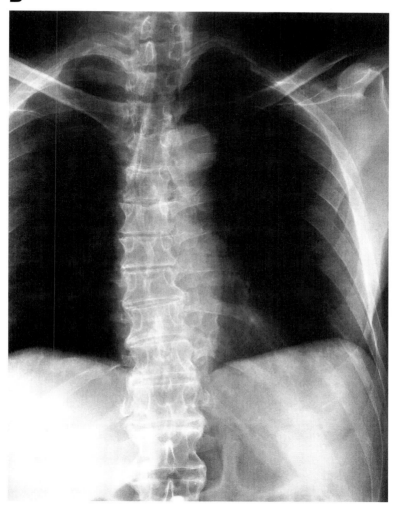

Fig. 2. *Continued*

Numerous other rheumatic conditions have been reported in patients with IBD *(15)*: osteomalacia and osteoporosis (secondary to vitamin D and calcium deficiency from impaired dietary intake, malabsorption, or corticosteroid use), hypertrophic osteoarthropathy, polymyositis, isolated atlantoaxial subluxation, and avascular necrosis of the hip secondary to corticosteroids use.

DERMATOLOGIC MANIFESTATIONS

More than 40 different dermatologic manifestations have been described in IBD *(17)*. The incidence of dermatologic manifestations varies from 9% to 19%, with a higher incidence when the large intestine is involved *(1,18)*. Conversely, an increased risk of pouchitis after total colectomy with ileal pouch anal anastomosis has been reported in patients with extraintestinal manifestations, particularly on the skin and the eyes *(19)*.

Erythema nodosum (EN) and pyoderma gangrenosum (PG) are the most common dermatologic conditions observed. EN appears in up to 9% of patients with UC and 15% of patients with CD *(17)*. It usually reflects increasing bowel activity, but not severity or extent of the bowel disease. EN presents as one or several hot, red, tender, and symmetrically distributed subcutaneous nodules, generally on the extensor surfaces of the lower legs but occurring also on the ankles, calves, thighs, and arms (Fig. 3). Approximately 75% of patients developing EN also present with peripheral arthritis. Most lesions usually respond to medical or surgical treatment of the bowel disease; however, recurrences are common and may be seen after colectomy *(20)*.

PG has been associated classically with UC with a reported incidence of 5% of patients with UC, although it can also occur in CD, particularly in Crohn's colitis. PG develops commonly during earlier stages of IBD, but does not show any relation to the clinical activity of the bowel disease. PG begins as pustules or fluctuant nodules that increase rapidly involving adjacent areas of healthy skin. Lesions then ulcerate showing violaceous edges delimited by a margin of erythema (Fig. 4). Lesions can be single or multiple and vary in size and location, although they occur more frequently on extensor surfaces of the lower limbs or other sites susceptible to trauma (surgical scars, and skin adjacent to ileostomy can often be the site for PG). Up to 50% of patients with PG have associated manifestations involving joints and/or eyes. Total colectomy, dapsone, cyclosporine A, and more recently thalidomide and infliximab have been found to be effective for the treatment of PG *(20–22)*.

Aphthous stomatitis appears in 20% of CD patients and in 5% of UC patients. Oral lesions occur spontaneously, with or without relation to the bowel disease activity and, in general, cause minimal discomfort, although some patients may complain of debilitating pain. Treatment regimens have included systemic or topical steroids, immunosuppressives, clofazimine, dapsone, and cyanoacrylate adhesive. Thalidomide, chloroquine, and infliximab can be tried for patients with refractory lesions *(22)*.

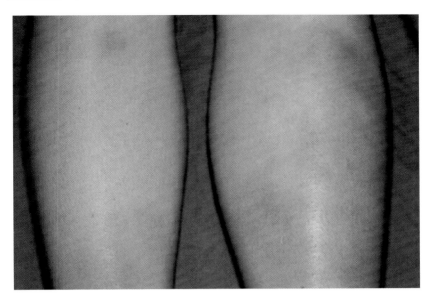

Fig. 3. Erythema Nodosum. The lesions of erythema nodosum are characterized as raised, red, tender subcutaneous nodules characteristically located on
the anterior tibial surfaces of the lower extremities. (Adapted with permission
from: Callen, Greer, Hood, Paller, Swinyier. Color Atlas of Dermatology.
W.B. Saunders, Philadelphia, PA, 1993.)

Metastatic Crohn's disease (MCD) is a rare cutaneous manifestation
defined as the presence of granulomatous dermatitis occurring distant
from, or non-contiguous with, the bowel lesions in CD. Clinical presentation may be diverse and includes genitalia ulcerations, papules and
nodules of trunk and extremities, ulcerating and nonulcerating plaques,
and hidradenitis or erysipelas-like facial eruption *(23)* (Figs. 5A,B).
Therapy for MCD includes corticosteroids, dapsone, sulfasalazine, azathioprine, 6-mercaptopurine, metronidazole, and in resistant cases,
hyperbaric oxygen *(17)*. Most recently, the chimeric monoclonal antibody anti-TNF α, infliximab, showed efficacy in two cases of therapy-
resistant perineal MCD *(24)*.

Other skin manifestations include vesiculopustular eruption and
pyoderma vegetans that occur mainly in UC; aphthous ulcers, necrotizing vesiculitis, and cutaneous polyarteritis nodosa which are more common in CD; and other autoimmune diseases such as psoriasis, vitiligo,
and epidermolysis bullosa acquisita. Other cutaneous changes are
caused by nutritional deficiencies. Acrodermatitis enteropathica, as a

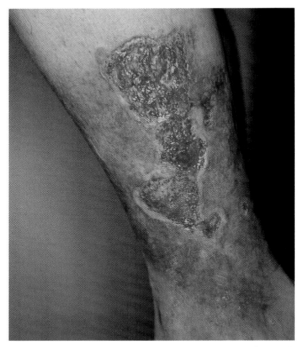

Fig. 4. Pyoderma gangrenosum in the anterior tibial surface, showing a deep ulceration with a necrotic center, an undermined border, and violaceous skin surrounding the lesion. (Adapted with permission from: Callen, Greer, Hood, Paller, Swinyier. Color Atlas of Dermatology. W.B. Saunders, Philadelphia, PA, 1993.)

result of zinc deficiency, is common in patients with draining fistulas and patients with long-term total parenteral nutrition *(25)*.

HEPATOBILIARY MANIFESTATIONS

Hepatobiliary complications are the most serious EIMs that occur in patients with IBD and include small duct and large duct primary sclerosing cholangitis (PSC), hepatitis (chronic active, viral, drug induced, granulomatous), cirrhosis, cholangiocarcinoma, steatosis, amyloidosis, hepatic abscess, and cholelithiasis.

The incidence of steatosis among patients with IBD has been reported as occurring in up to 80% of patients *(26)*. Fat deposition is of macrovesicular type, nonspecific, and usually reversible. The pathogenesis is likely to be multifactorial with malabsorption, protein loss, bacterial metabolites, drug injuries including corticosteroids and methotrexate,

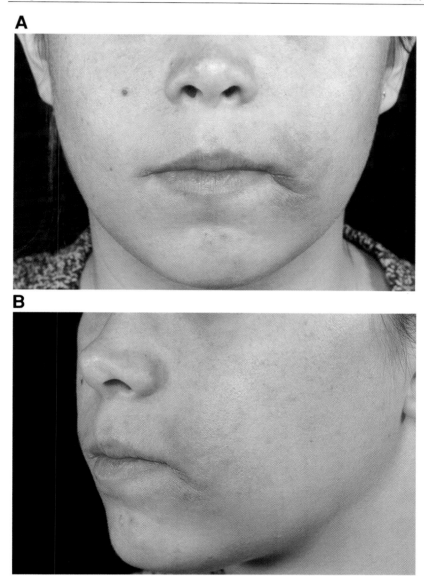

Fig. 5. **(A)** and **(B)** Metastatic Crohn's Disease. Patient with diffuse swelling on the left side of the mouth with superficial skin corrugations, diffuse erythema, and a textural change to the surface of the skin.

and in rare cases total parenteral nutrition associated cholestasis, as contributing factors. Patients tend to be asymptomatic unless they may have hepatomegaly, which may cause discomfort.

Cholelithiasis is a frequent complication in patients with IBD (30%). It usually occurs in patients with CD involving the terminal ileum or following ileal resection, and is secondary to bile salt malabsorption *(27)*.

Primary sclerosing cholangitis (PSC) is the most specific hepato-biliary complication of IBD and it has been reported in up to 4% of patients with IBD. In 70–90% of patients with PSC, especially young males, the disorder is associated with UC *(28)*. PSC is a chronic cholestatic syndrome characterized by fibrosing inflammation of the biliary system resulting in bile duct obliteration, biliary cirrhosis, and hepatic failure. Clinically, PSC presents most commonly with progressive fatigue, weight loss, pruritus, jaundice, and a cholestatic biochemical profile with marked elevations of the serum alkaline phosphatase. Visualization of irregularities, strictures, and dilatations in the biliary tree is essential to confirm the diagnosis (Fig. 6). Endoscopic retrograde cholangiopancreatography is the diagnostic method of choice. Although there is a strong association of UC with PSC, there is no relation to the onset, duration, extent, or activity of colitis, and indeed, the colitis is usually total but symptomatically mild and characterized by prolonged remissions *(29)*. Total colectomy does not alter the course of PSC, and liver disease may develop after years a total colectomy has been performed *(30)*. Patients with UC and PSC are at increased risk of developing pouchitis following ileoanal anastomosis *(31)*.

Although only 5% of UC patients have associated PSC, the majority of PSC patients will develop IBD. Therefore, patients with newly diagnosed PSC should undergo colonoscopy even if no symptoms of bowel disease are present; similarly, patients with IBD and increased concentrations of serum alkaline phosphatase should have an examination of the bile ducts.

Patients with PSC, with or without concomitant IBD, are at higher risk of developing cholangiocarcinoma (1–15% of patients) *(32)*. Malignancy should be suspected in patients with a rapid clinical deterioration and the presence of a dominant stricture or mass effect on imaging studies. The prognosis for cholangiocarcinoma is poor, with most patients dying within 1 yr of diagnosis. The occurrence of PSC also appears to be an additional risk factor for the development of dysplasia and carcinoma in patients with long-standing UC *(33)*. There is now general consensus that annual surveillance colonoscopy is indicated in these patients.

At present, there are no medical or endoscopic treatments with proven benefit for PSC. Immunosuppressive agents such as prednisone, azathioprine, methotrexate, and penicillamine have failed to demonstrate efficacy *(34–38)*. A study from the Mayo Clinic using ursodeoxycholic acid showed no clinical benefit in retarding disease progression but

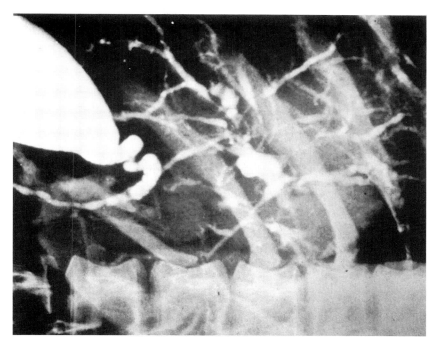

Fig. 6. Endoscopic retrograde cholangiopancreatography (ERCP) showing the typical irregularities, strictures, and dilatations in the biliary tree in a patient with primary sclerosing cholangitis.

demonstrated an improvement in cholestatic biochemistry markers *(39)*. Several authors have reported favorable results with endoscopic dilatation of symptomatic dominant strictures *(40)*. Additional studies comparing the efficacy and safety of various endoscopic treatment approaches are needed. Orthotopic liver transplantation is presently, the ultimate therapy for end-stage PSC and should be considered in patients with signs of decompensating liver cirrhosis, recurrent cholangitis, or intractable pruritus *(41)*.

OCULAR MANIFESTATIONS

A wide variety of ocular manifestations may be seen in patients with IBD including episcleritis, uveitis, marginal keratitis, conjunctivitis, scleritis, orbital inflammatory disease, optic neuritis, ischemic optic neuropathy, and retinal vasculitis. Some ocular problems may run a course independent of the activity of the underlying bowel disease (e.g., uveitis, scleritis) or may reflect bowel activity (e.g., episcleritis) *(42)*.

There is a clear association between eye lesions and other EIM especially those involving the joints.

Episcleritis is the most common ocular complication and develops in 5% of patients with active IBD. Clinically it appears as a painless hyperemia of the sclera and conjunctiva and does not affect the visual acuity. Episcleritis responds to antiinflammatory therapy, and local corticosteroids are usually effective.

Uveitis is a general term used to describe any inflammatory condition involving the uveal tract that is composed by the iris, ciliary body, and choroid, whereas the term iritis describes inflammation limited to the iris. Uveitis/iritis appear in 1–3% of patients and manifest with eye pain, blurred vision, photophobia, headache, iridospasm, and abnormal pupillary response to light. In patients positive for HLA-B27, uveitis is usually sudden in onset, anterior, and unilateral, whereas in patients negative for HLA-B27 uveitis is often insidious, posterior, and bilateral *(43)*. Diagnosis is confirmed by slit-lamp examination and treatment consists of pupillary dilatation, covering the eye to reduce pain and photophobia, and topical or systemic corticosteroids. Refractory cases of uveitis, usually in HLA-B27 positive patients, may require immunosuppressive therapy. Treatment is important to prevent iris atrophy and synechial formation. The incidence of asymptomatic uveitis in pediatric IBD patients (6%) may warrant periodic ocular screening in this age group *(44)*.

RENAL/UROLOGIC MANIFESTATIONS

Renal and urologic complications are not unusual in patients with IBD and have been reported in 4–23% of patients. The most common manifestations are kidney stones, enterovesical fistulas, and ureteral obstruction *(45)*.

Patients with IBD have a risk of nephrolithiasis that is 10–100 times greater than that for the general hospital patients, ranging from 1% to 25% *(46)*. Classically described risk factors for renal stone development include presence of ileostomy, extensive ileal disease, and extensive ileal resection. Other potential lithogenic factors include dehydration, diminished water absorption, urinary tract obstruction, abnormal urate excretion, alterations in oxalate absorption and excretion, steroids, and prolonged bedrest. Renal stones in IBD patients are mainly composed of calcium oxalate or uric acid. During an episode of nephrolithiasis, aggressive hydration, adequate analgesia, and occasionally lithotripsy may be required. Patients with an ileostomy should be encouraged to drink adequate fluids.

Bladder involvement by CD results from the direct extension of the inflammatory process from an adjacent segment of inflamed bowel. The majority of enterovesical fistulas involve the sigmoid colon or the terminal ileum. Clinically, patients have dysuria, urinary frequency and urgency, and suprapubic discomfort. Pneumaturia and fecaluria are considered pathognomonic. Computed tomography is the diagnostic test of choice *(47)*. Other diagnostic techniques include magnetic resonance imaging, cystoscopy, and cystography. Spontaneous resolution of enterovesical fistulas can occur but is uncommon. Surgical resection of the fistula and involved bowel is the definitive treatment *(48)*. If resection is not possible, a diverting colostomy may be performed. In addition, cyclosporine *(49)* and 6-mercaptopurine *(50)* have been successfully used.

Ureteral obstruction is not secondary to stones in 50–70% of patients with IBD *(51)*. In CD, it is usually caused by retroperitoneal inflammation, whereas in UC patients, obstruction is often secondary to surgical complications (e.g., suture in or near the ureter) or to colon cancer. Most of the nonstone-related ureteral obstructions associated with IBD improve with conservative therapy alone. If this does not occur, bowel surgery is recommended.

Glomerulonephritis, tubulointerstitial abnormalities, and amyloidosis have also been reported in the setting of IBD.

PANCREATIC MANIFESTATIONS

Pancreatitis may occur in patients with CD or UC. Many of these cases are either acute pancreatitis related to choledocholithiasis, or drug-induced pancreatitis from 5-ASA, sulfasalazine, corticosteroids, azathioprine or 6-mercaptopurine *(52)*. In addition, clinically significant and nondrug-related pancreatitis has been reported in two subgroups of inflammatory bowel disease patients. First, patients with duodenal CD may have reflux of duodenal contents into pancreatic ducts through an incompetent ampulla, or direct ampullary involvement with stenosis, resulting in pancreatitis. Second, pancreatitis may occur in patients with UC and primary sclerosing cholangitis or pericholangitis. Finally, cases of pancreatitis have been reported in IBD patients with none of the previous mentioned risk factors *(53)*. Whether these patients have idiopathic pancreatitis or can be considered as a rare EIM of IBD is unclear.

PULMONARY MANIFESTATIONS

Symptomatic bronchopulmonary manifestations have been described only rarely in patients with CD or UC. However, several recent studies have reported a significantly higher rate of findings compatible with interstitial lung disease in pulmonary function tests in asymptomatic IBD patients compared to controls *(54)*. Pulmonary manifestations in patients with IBD can be divided as sulfasalazine related or unrelated. Sulfasalazine-associated lung problems usually occur after 2 mo of therapy and include eosinophilic pneumonia, fibrosing alveolitis, and interstitial pneumonitis *(55)*. Nonsulfasalazine-related disorders include pulmonary vasculitis, chronic bronchitis and bronchiectasis, and interstitial pulmonary disease *(56)*. Whether or not there is truly a relationship or only a coincidental association between these entities and IBD is unknown.

CARDIAC MANIFESTATIONS

Myopericarditis and pleuropericarditis have been reported in patients with both UC and CD although the incidence is <1% in patients with IBD *(57)*. The clinical course can range from mild to pericardial tamponade requiring drainage. Treatment with corticosteroids is effective.

Aortic insufficiency and conduction defects are often associated with idiopathic ankylosing spondylitis and can be seen also in patients with IBD with or without ankylosing spondylitis *(58)*.

NEUROLOGIC MANIFESTATIONS

Association of IBD with neurologic involvement is rare and often controversial. Cerebrovascular thromboembolic disease can occur at any age and tend to correlate with bowel disease activity *(59)*. Direct extension of inflammatory masses or abscesses into neural structures has been reported in patients with CD and may lead to meningitis or epidural abscesses *(60)*. Peripheral neuropathy occurs relatively frequently with metronidazole therapy *(61)*. About 50% of patients will present with paresthesias after 6 mo or more of receiving metronidazole (mean dose 15–20mg/kg/d) and 80% develop a sensory peripheral neuropathy. Multiple sclerosis has also been associated with IBD. The two diseases coexist at three times the expected frequency, and familial aggregation occur at about nine times more often than would be expected by chance *(62)*. An idiopathic chronic inflammatory demyelinating polyneuropathy may also occur *(63)*.

HEMATOLOGIC MANIFESTATIONS

Anemia is seen in 50% of patients with IBD and is usually caused by iron deficiency. Other causes include folic acid deficiency, vitamin B_{12} deficiency, malnutrition, hemolysis (drug-induced, e.g., sulfasalazine or autoimmune), and bone marrow suppression (drug-induced, e.g., azathioprine). Anemia of chronic disease is also seen in patients with IBD and is characterized by a decrease in serum iron and iron binding capacity, decreased saturation of serum iron-binding capacity, normal or increased serum ferritin, increased bone marrow storage of iron, and decreased bone marrow sideroblasts *(64)*.

Patients with IBD may have abnormalities in the coagulation profile that predispose to thromboembolic complications. These include: thrombocytosis, increased plasma levels of fibrinogen, and factors V and VIII, decreased levels of antithrombin III, spontaneous platelet aggregation, impaired fibrinolytic capability, and mutation of factor V Leiden *(65)*. Venous thrombosis involving the lower extremities is the most commonly described, but thrombosis may also appear in brain, lung, and liver. Budd-Chiari syndrome and portal vein thrombosis have been described in the setting of UC. Deep vein thrombosis leading to pulmonary embolism is the third most frequent cause of death in patients with UC, following peritonitis and cancer. Thus, a high index of suspicion for venous thrombosis must be maintained in patients with IBD.

METABOLIC AND ENDOCRINE MANIFESTATIONS

Growth retardation accompanied by a delay in sexual maturation is more common in children with CD, but may be seen also in UC. About 50% of children have weight-for-age measurements less than 90% of expected, with absolute height deficits seen in 10–40% of children with IBD *(66)*. Nonspecific endocrine abnormalities have been documented in these IBD children. Chronic undernutrition is considered the primary etiologic factor in the pathogenesis of growth impairment and is considered to be secondary to diminished intake, malabsorption of nutrients, and protein loss enteropathy. A significant iatrogenic cause of growth failure is the chronic administration of high-dose daily corticosteroid therapy. Alternate-day treatment with corticosteroids may have less effect on growth retardation *(67)*. Thus, the suppression of gastrointestinal symptoms using high doses of corticosteroids with the concomitant compromise of growth is not considered a successful medical therapy in children. In these patients, surgical therapy should be considered *(68)*.

SUMMARY

About one-third of patients with IBD will develop one or more extraintestinal manifestations that can involve virtually all the organs of the body. EIMs may precede or follow the diagnosis of IBD and may occur with exacerbations of bowel symptoms or independently. Identified pathogenetic mechanisms include genetic susceptibility, and abnormally regulated autoimmune and inflammatory reactions. Systematic assessment, early recognition, and adequate therapy are essential aims in the management of patients with inflammatory bowel disease and extraintestinal manifestations to prevent severe complications and improve their quality of life.

ACKNOWLEDGMENT

We greatly acknowledge the support of Centocor, Inc. for their sponsorship of the color artwork in this chapter.

REFERENCES

1. Greenstein AJ, Janowitz HD, Sachar DB. The extraintestinal complications of Crohn's disease and ulcerative colitis: a study of 700 patients. Medicine 1976;55:401–411.
2. Rankin GB, Watts HD, Melynk CS, Kelley ML Jr. The National Cooperative Crohn's Disease Study: extraintestinal manifestations and perianal complications. Gastroenterology 1979;77:914–920.
3. Mayer L, Janowitz HD. Extraintestinal manifestations of inflammatory bowel disease. In: Kirsner JB, Shorter RG, eds. Inflammatory Bowel Disease. Lea & Febiger, Philadelphia, PA, 1988:299–317.
4. Monsen U, Sorstad J, Hellers G, Johansson C. Extracolonic diagnosis in ulcerative colitis: an epidemiological study. Am J Gastroenterol 1990;85:711–716.
5. Snook JA, de Silva HJ, Jewell DP. The association of autoimmune disorders with inflammatory bowel disease. Q J Med 1989;269:835–840.
6. Seibold F, Mork H, Tanza S, Muller A, Holzhuter C, Weber P, et al. Pancreatic autoantibodies in Crohn's disease. A family study. Gut 1997;40:481–484.
7. Seibold F, Brandwein S, Simpson S, Tehorst C, Elson CO. p-ANCA represents a cross-reactivity to enteric bacterial antigens. J Clin Immunol 1998;18:153–160.
8. Satsangi J, Grootscholten C, Holt H, Jewell DP. Clinical patterns of familial inflammatory bowel disease. Gut 1996;38:738–741.
9. Levine JB. Extraintestinal manifestations of inflammatory bowel disease. In: Kirsner JB, ed. Inflammatory Bowel Disease. 5th ed. WB Saunders, Philadelphia, PA, 2000, pp. 397–409.
10. Orchard TR, Wordsworth BP, Jewell DP. Peripheral arthropathies in inflammatory bowel disease: their articular distribution and natural history. Gut 1998; 42:387–391.
11. Orchard TR, Thiyagaraja S, Welsh KI, Wordsworth BP, Hill Gaston JS, Jewell DP. Clinical phenotype is related to HLA genotype in the peripheral arthropathies of inflammatory bowel disease. Gastroenterology 2000;118:274–278.
12. Andreyev H, Kamm M, Forbes A, Nicholls RJ. Joint symptoms after restorative proctocolectomy in ulcerative colitis and familial polyposis coli. J Clin Gastroenterol 1996;23:35–39.
13. Kaufmann HJ, Taubin HL. Non-steroidal antiinflammatory drugs activate quiescent IBD. Ann Intern Med 1987;107:513–516.
14. Katz JP, Lichtenstein GR. Rheumatologic manifestations of gastrointestinal diseases. Gastroenterology Clin North Am 1998;27:533–562.

15. Weiner SR, Clare J, Taggart NA. Rheumatic manifestations of IBD. Semin Arthritis Rheum 1991;20:353–366.
16. Mallas EG, Mackintosh P, Asquith P, Cooke WT. Histocompatibility antigens in inflammatory bowel disease. Their clinical significance and their association with arthropathy with special reference to HLA-B27. Gut 1976;17:906–910.
17. Apgar JT. Newer aspects of inflammatory bowel disease and its cutaneous manifestations: a selective review. Sem Derm 1991;10:138–147.
18. Gregory B, Ho VC. Cutaneous manifestations of gastrointestinal disorders. Part II. J Am Acad Dermatol 1992;26:371–383.
19. Lohmuller JL, Pemberton JH, Dozois RR, Ilstrup D, van-Heerden J. Pouchitis and extraintestinal manifestations of inflammatory bowel disease after ileal-pouch anal anastomosis. Ann Surg 1990;211:622–629.
20. Mir-Madjlessi SD, Taylor JS, Farmer RG. Clinical course and evolution of erythema nodosum and pyoderma gangrenosum in chronic ulcerative colitis: a study of 42 patients. Am J Gastroenterol 1985;80:615–620.
21. Carp JM, Onuma E, Das KM, Gottlieb AB. Intravenous cyclosporine therapy in the treatment of pyoderma gangrenosum secondary to Crohn's disease. Cutis 1997;60:135–138.
22. Tremaine WJ. Treatment of erythema nodosum, aphthous stomatitis, and pyoderma gangrenosum in patients with IBD. Inflam Bowel Dis 1998;4:68–69.
23. Sutphen JL, Cooper PH, Mackel SE, Nelson DL. Metastatic cutaneous Crohn's disease. Gastroenterology 1984;86:941–944.
24. Van Dullemen HM, Jong E, Slors F, Tytgat GNJ, van Deventer SJH. Treatment of therapy-resistant perineal metastatic Crohn's disease after proctocolectomy using anti-tumor necrosis factor chimeric monoclonal antibody, cA2. Dis Colon Rectum 1998;41:98–102.
25. Hendricks KM, Walker WA. Zinc deficiency in inflammatory bowel disease. Nutr Rev 1988;46:401–408.
26. Desmet VJ, Geboes K. Liver lesions in inflammatory bowel disease. J Path 1987;151:247–255.
27. Brink MA, Slors JF, Keulemans YC, Mok KS, DeWaart DR, Carey MC, et al. Enterohepatic cycling of bilirubin: a putative mechanism for pigment gallstone formation in ileal Crohn's disease. Gastroenterology 1999;116:1492–1494.
28. Olsson R, Danielsson A, Jarnerot G, Lindstrom E, Loof L, Rolny P, et al. Prevalence of primary sclerosing cholangitis in patients with ulcerative colitis. Gastroenterology 1991;100:1319–1323.
29. Lundqvist K, Broome U. Differences in colonic disease activity in patients with ulcerative colitis with and without primary sclerosing cholangitis: a case control study. Dis Colon Rectum 1997;40:451–456.
30. Cangemi JR, Wiesner RH, Beaver SJ, Ludwig J. The effect of proctocolectomy for chronic ulcerative colitis on the natural history of primary sclerosing cholangitis. Gastroenterology 1989;96:790–794.
31. Penna C, Dozois R, Tremaine W, Sandborn W, LaRusso N, Schleck C, et al. Pouchitis after ileal pouch-anal anastomosis for ulcerative colitis occurs with increased frequency in patients with associated primary sclerosing cholangitis. Gut 1996;38:234–239.
32. Nashan B, Schiltt HJ, Tusch G, Oldhafer KJ, Ringe B, Wagner S, et al. Biliary malignancies in primary sclerosing cholangitis. Hepatology 1996;23:1105–1111.
33. Kornfeld D, Ekbom A, Ihre T. Is there an excess risk for colorectal cancer in patients with ulcerative colitis and concomitant primary sclarosing cholangitis? A population based study. Gut 1997;41:522–525.

34. Lindor KD, Wiesner RH, Colwell LJ, Steiner B, Beaver S, LaRusso NF. The combination of prednisone and colchicine in patients with primary sclerosing cholangitis. Am J Gastroenterol 1991;86:57–61.
35. Wagner A. Azathioprine treatment in primary sclerosing cholangitis. Lancet 1971;ii:663–664.
36. Javett SL. Azathioprine in primary sclerosing cholangitis. Lancet 1971;ii:810–811.
37. Knox TA, Kaplan MM. A double-blind controlled trial of oral-pulse methotrexate therapy in the treatment of primary sclerosing cholangitis. Gastroenterology 1994;106:494–499.
38. LaRusso NF, Wiesner RH, Ludwig J, McCarty RL, Beaver SJ, Zinsmeister AR. Prospective trial of penicillamine in primary sclerosing cholangitis. Gastroenterology 1988;95:1036–1042.
39. Lindor KD. Ursodiol for primary sclerosing cholangitis. Mayo Primary Sclerosing Cholangitis-Ursodeoxycholic Acid Study Group. New Engl J Med 1997;336:691–695.
40. Lee JG, Schutz SM, England RE, Leung JW, Cotton PB. Endoscopic therapy of sclerosing cholangitis. Hepatology 1995;21:661–667.
41. Wiesner RH, Porayko MK, Dickson ER, Gores GJ, LaRusso NF, Hay JE, et al. Selection and timing of liver transplantation in primary biliary cirrhosis and primary sclerosing cholangitis. Hepatology 1992;16:1290–1299.
42. Salmon JF, Wright JP, Murray AND. Ocular inflammation in Crohn's disease. Ophthalmology 1991;98:480–484.
43. Lyons JL, Rosenbaum JT. Uveitis associated with inflammatory bowel disease compared with uveitis associated with spondyloarthropathy. Arch Ophthalmol 1997;115:61–64.
44. Hofley P, Roarty J, McGinnity G, Griffiths AM, Marcon M, Kraft S, et al. Asymptomatic uveitis in children with chronic inflammatory bowel diseases. J Pediatr Gastroenterol Nutr 1993;17:397–400.
45. Pardi DS, Tremaine WJ, Sandborn WJ, McCarthy JT. Renal and urologic complications of inflammatory bowel disease. Am J Gastroenterol 1998;93:504–514.
46. Shield DE, Lytton B, Weiss RM, Schiff M Jr. Urologic complications of inflammatory bowel disease. J Urol 1976;115:701–706.
47. Goldman SM, Fishman EK, Gatewood OM, Jones B, Siegelman SS. Computerized tomography in the diagnosis of enterovesical fistulas. AJR 1985;144:1229–1233.
48. McNamara MJ, Fazio W, Lavery IC, Weakley FL, Farmer RG. Surgical treatment of enterovesical fistulas in Crohn's disease. Dis Colon Rectum 1990:33:271–276.
49. Hanauer SB, Smith MD. Rapid closure of Crohn's disease fistulas with continuous intravenous cyclosporine. Am J Gastroenterol 1993;88:646–649.
50. Korelitz BI, Adler DJ, Mendelsohn RA, Sacknoff AL. Long-term experience with 6-mercaptopurine in the treatment of Crohn's disease. Am J Gastroenterol 1993;88:1198–1205.
51. Fleckenstein P, Knudson L, Petersen EB, Marcussen H, Jarnum S. Obstructive uropathy in inflammatory bowel disease. Scand J Gastroenterol 1977;12:519–523.
52. Lankish PG, Droge M, Gottesleben F. Drug induced acute pancreatitis: incidence and severity. Gut 1995;37:565–567.
53. Eisner TD, Goldman IS, McKinley MJ. Crohn's disease and the pancreas. Am J Gastroenterol 1993;88:583–586.
54. Kuzela L, Vavreck A, Prikazska M, Drugda B, Hronec J, Senkova A, et al. Pulmonary complications in patients with inflammatory bowel disease. Hepato-Gastroenterol 1999;46:1714–1719.
55. Moseley RH, Barwixh KW, Dobuler K, DeLuka VA. Sulfasalazine-induced pulmonary disease. Dig Dis Sci 1985;30:901–904.

56. Gionchetti P, Schiavina M, Campieri M, Fabiani A, Cornia BM, Belluzzi A, et al. Bronchopulmonary involvement in ulcerative colitis. J Clin Gastroenterol 1990;12:647–650.

57. Patwardhan RV, Heilpern J, Brewster AC, Darrah JJ. Pleuropericarditis: an extraintestinal complication of inflammatory bowel disease. Report of three cases and review of the literature. Arch Intern Med 1983;143:94–96.

58. Burdick S, Tresch DD, Komokowski RA. Cardiac valvular dysfunction associated with Crohn's disease in the absence of ankylosing spondylitis. Am Heart J 1989;118:174–176.

59. Markowitz RL, Ment LR, Gryboski JD. Cerebral thromboembolic disease in pediatric and adult inflammatory bowel disease: case report and review of the literature. J Pediatr Gastroentrol Nutr 1989;8:413–420.

60. Hefter H, Piontek M, Aulich A. Bacterial meningitis and dorsal spinal epidural abscess caused by Crohn's disease. Neurology 1991;41:606–608.

61. Duffy LF, Daum F, Fisher SE, Delman J, Vishnubhakat SM, Aiges HW, et al. Peripheral neuropathy in Crohn's disease patients treated with metronidazole. Gastroenterology 1985;88:681–684.

62. Sadovnick AD, Paty DW, Yannakoulias G. Concurrence of multiple sclerosis and inflammatory bowel disease. New Engl J Med 1989;321:762–763.

63. Chad DA, Smith TW, DeGirolami U, Hammer K. Perineuritis and ulcerative colitis. Neurology 1986;36:1377–1379.

64. Means RT Jr, Krantz SB. Progress in understanding the pathogenesis of anemia of chronic disease. Blood 1992;80:1639–1647.

65. Liebman HA, Kashani N, Sutherland D, McGehee W, Kam AL. The factor V Leiden mutation increases the risk of venous thrombosis in patients with inflammatory bowel disease. Gastroenterol 1998;115:830–834.

66. Motil KJ, Grand RJ, Davis-Kraft L, Ferlic LL, Smith EO. Growth failure in children with inflammatory bowel disease: a prospective study. Gastroenterology 1993;105:681–691.

67. Hyams JS, Carey DE. Corticosteroids and growth. J Pediatr 1988;113:249–254.

68. Hyams JS. Extraintestinal manifestations of inflammatory bowel disease in children. J Pediatr Gastroenterol Nutr 1994;19:7–21.

14 Cancer in Inflammatory Bowel Disease

William M. Bauer, MD
and Bret A. Lashner, MD

INTRODUCTION

Inflammatory bowel disease (IBD)—ulcerative colitis (UC) and Crohn's disease (CD), inclusive—predisposes one to an increased risk of gastrointestinal malignancies. Identifying those patients at greatest risk of malignancy for cancer surveillance will allow the clinician to make the largest impact in lowering the cancer-related mortality in IBD. The approach to cancer surveillance for patients with long-standing IBD, though, is controversial.

From: *Clinical Gastroenterology:*
Inflammatory Bowel Disease: Diagnosis and Therapeutics
Edited by: R. D. Cohen © Humana Press Inc., Totowa, NJ

279

COLORECTAL CANCER

Ulcerative Colitis

The increased risk of developing colorectal cancer (CRC) in patients with UC is well established *(1,2)*. The lifetime incidence of CRC in a patient with UC approaches 6% and the cancer-related mortality is approx 3%. Up to 1% of all cases of CRC seen in the general population may be associated with IBD *(3)*. Long duration of disease and the presence of extensive colonic disease are important risk factors for the development of CRC associated with IBD *(4–9)*.

The risk of developing CRC is low until 8 yr of disease, after which the risk rises exponentially with increasing disease duration to as high as 56 times the general population by the fourth decade of disease *(3,5,10)*. Younger age at onset of the underlying colitis also has been suggested as an independent risk factor for the development of CRC *(1,6,9)*. Of note, cancer in UC occurs at a younger age than in sporadic CRC *(11)*.

Colorectal cancers can extend over several colonic segments. The cancer may be endoscopically undetectable, or be annular and involve the bowel wall causing a stricture *(4)*. Cancers are sometimes multiple and can develop without giving usual clinical signs and symptoms of obstruction, weight loss, abdominal or rectal masses, or excessive bleeding. In one series, 30% of CRCs were found to be clinically silent *(11)*.

Surveillance Colonoscopy

Periodic colonoscopic surveillance with biopsies is currently recommended as the standard of care to monitor for the risk of cancer associated with UC *(12)* (Fig. 1). Surveillance programs for patients with UC can detect dysplasia, a benign but premalignant neoplastic lesion, and, with colectomy following the detection of dysplasia, can improve cancer-related mortality *(13,14)*. Unresolved issues related to surveillance include the sensitivity of the detection of dysplasia, the predictive value of dysplasia, the lead-time between dysplasia and cancer, and the emotional and financial impact of the surveillance program *(15)*. Because of the lack of randomized clinical trials assessing colorectal surveillance in UC, effectiveness only can be estimated through epidemiologic studies or decision analysis *(16)*.

The use of colonoscopy with multiple biopsies as a testing method is problematic. Because dysplasia can be present focally, as well as diffusely, biopsies must be taken throughout the colon. Sensitivity for detecting dysplasia is increased with a greater number of biopsies taken.

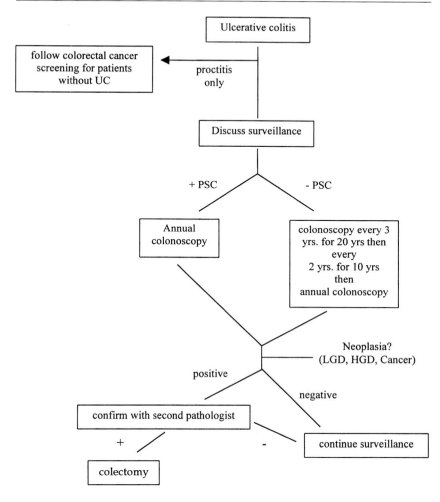

Fig. 1. Recommended method of surveillance for colorectal cancer surveillance in patients with UC.

However, the more biopsies taken, the worse the specificity, the higher the pathology costs, the longer the length of time of the procedure, and the greater the morbidity from the colonoscopy and sedation.

Rare cases of dysplasia and cancer in the ileoanal pouches of UC patients has led to the recommendation for annual sigmoidoscopic surveillance biopsies of the pouches that were created by stapling, which can leave a small amount of rectal mucosa behind in the newly formed pouch.

PATIENT UNDERSTANDING OF THE IMPLICATIONS OF SURVEILLANCE

There is little value in performing surveillance colonoscopy if a patient will refuse to have a proctocolectomy for a positive test (i.e., dysplasia). Rather than recommend prophylactic colectomy on all patients, surveillance is meant to identify the patients at very high risk of cancer mortality so colectomy can be selectively performed and allow patients with no dysplasia to continue in the cancer surveillance program. Failure to perform colectomy on patients with dysplasia will minimize the benefits of any surveillance program.

METHOD OF BIOPSY COLLECTION

The number of biopsies to be taken remains controversial. Dysplasia by its nature does not necessarily present with visible endoscopic findings. Any lesion that does not belong to the general contour of the surrounding mucosa should raise suspicion of a dysplasia-associated lesion or mass (DALM) and be biopsied. A complete set of surveillance biopsies for the large bowel only samples an estimated 0.05% of the total mucosal surface area—a huge sampling error. Fortunately, dysplasia, when present, can be detected in multiple regions of the colon and is not likely to be missed if a sufficient number of biopsies are taken. Sixty-four biopsies have a 95% probability of finding the highest grade of neoplasia in a colon containing dysplasia or cancer *(17)*. However, only 18 biopsies are needed to have a 95% certainty of finding either cancer or dysplasia in a patient who has a true malignancy present *(17)*. A reasonable approach is to take at least 32 biopsy specimens which amounts to two to four biopsies from each 10-cm segment of colon and raised lesions.

OPTIMAL INTERVAL BETWEEN EXAMINATIONS

The more tests that are performed in a lifetime of disease, the greater the chance that dysplasia will be uncovered and addressed prior to the development of cancer and, therefore, the lower the cancer-related mortality. However, a balance must be struck between benefits and cost/morbidity. Testing with uniform intervals is not the most efficient way of allocating tests over a lifetime of disease. Because the risk for developing dysplasia or cancer increases with longer disease duration, efficient surveillance calls for more frequent testing when the risk is highest *(18)*. One reasonable method calls for testing every 3 yr for the first 20 yr of disease, every 2 yr for the next 10 yr of disease, and yearly thereafter. Such an approach provides for at least 20 examinations over a 40-yr lifetime of disease. Most of the evaluations would be performed in the later yr when the risk is the highest.

The approximate time interval between the development of low-grade dysplasia and cancer, the lead-time, is 3 yr *(18,19)*. Testing at intervals longer than 3 yr should be discouraged because a majority of patients who develop cancer will not have the "opportunity" to have dysplasia detected prior to the cancer.

Implications of Dysplasia

Dysplasia is a neoplastic, premalignant lesion in UC. Dysplasia or cancer is found at initial endoscopy in 10% of patients *(20,21)*. If the initial endoscopy is negative for dysplasia, then only about 3% of patients will ultimately develop neoplasia when followed over time.

Experience has shown that if low-grade dysplasia is the indication for colectomy, a cancer already is present in 19% *(20)*. Patients with low-grade dysplasia undergoing further surveillance have a likelihood of progressing to a malignant lesion 16% of the time. If high-grade dysplasia is used as criteria for colectomy, a cancer is present in up to 45% *(20)*. These data suggest that the detection of high-grade dysplasia as a criterion for colectomy may be too "late" in the process of neoplastic progression to ensure colectomy prior to cancer development.

If the initial surveillance endoscopy is negative, the risk of progression to dysplasia or cancer when followed over time may be low. However, it has been reported that some patients were seen with cancer within 1 or 2 yr of their last negative surveillance colonoscopy *(21)*. In a historical cohort study comparing a group in a surveillance program to another group not having surveillance, neither cancer incidence nor cancer-related mortality was affected by surveillance *(22)*. There was a shift of cancer detected to an earlier Dukes' stage in the surveyed patients, but the effect was small and not associated with improved cancer-related survival.

Role of the Pathologist

Some pathologists do not accept what appears to be dysplasia as definite when biopsies are taken at a site of active inflammation. Therefore, the endoscopist should try to schedule surveillance examinations at times when there is little or no disease activity. As a result of high interobserver variability among pathologists interpreting dysplasia, two expert pathologists' agreement on a diagnosis of dysplasia is desirable. Interestingly, only 43% of physicians ask for a second morphologic opinion *(23)*.

Low-Grade, High-Grade Dysplasia, and DALMs

When evaluating biopsy specimens for dysplasia, the best criterion for a positive test is low-grade dysplasia because of its high sensitivity, rather than high-grade dysplasia with its high specificity. Approximately 20% of patients with low-grade dysplasia later develop high-grade dysplasia or carcinoma *(24,25)*. The current practice in most centers is that low-grade dysplasia with or without a mass should warrant a colectomy recommendation.

Physicians should have a high degree of concern for DALM lesions because the progression to cancer is very likely. A sessile adenoma in the area of colitis (even if the colitis is only found microscopically) is a DALM and not simply a benign adenoma *(23,26)*. Some, though, have disputed the ominous nature of the DALM *(27,28)*. What then should be the approach to DALMs or colon polyps in UC? If an older patient (greater than age 50) has a sessile adenoma in the colon clearly distinct from the area of colitis, it is more likely that this lesion is a sporadic adenoma and it is advisable to recommend polypectomy and not colectomy. For the sessile adenoma arising in an area of colitis, especially in patients younger than age 50 who usually do not have sporadic adenomas, it would be advisable to treat this lesion as a DALM and recommend a colectomy. However, peripolyp biopsies should be obtained, and if they reveal dysplasia, colectomy is indicated, regardless of the patient's age.

STRICTURES AND PSEUDOPOLYPS

Problematic issues involve pseudopolyps and strictures. It was found that dysplasia or cancer was a frequent occurrence in colonic strictures related to UC and dysplasia or cancer could not always be detected preoperatively *(29)*. If the strictured segment of bowel cannot be examined and biopsied endoscopically, strong consideration should be given to colectomy because this stricture is likely to harbor dysplasia or cancer. A patient with multiple pseudopolyps that cannot be adequately biopsied could easily have dysplastic tissue that eludes biopsy. These patients need to be informed of the inadequacy of surveillance and the benefits of prophylactic colectomy. There has been no study, though, to support this recommendation.

Crohn's Disease

Compared to the general population, patients with CD have a higher incidence of colonic carcinoma, although the exact magnitude is not well studied *(8)*. Most studies suggest that the risk increases with increasing disease duration *(3,7,30)*. The reported overall relative risk of developing cancer in CD compared with the general population is less than that seen with UC, ranging from 1.1 to 26.6 *(6–8)*. As in UC, population-based studies suggest that the overall risk associated with CD may be less than previously thought *(9)*. These studies were performed in patients with relatively short disease duration and highlight the need for studies with longer follow-up to better understand the true risk of cancer associated with CD. Compared to sporadic colorectal cancer, colorectal cancers in CD occur at an earlier age (48 vs 60 yr), are more often located in the right colon, and are more frequently multiple *(11)*. CD of the colon warrants attention to cancer risk and surveillance, particularly now that effective drug therapy is influencing a trend toward reduction or at least postponement of bowel resection *(15)*. Chronic, unresected disease is a risk factor for colorectal cancer development.

Compared to UC, programs of surveillance in CD are more difficult because of the prevalence of narrowed lumen, strictures, and fistulas preventing ready access to the colonoscope. Nevertheless, it is these sites of stricture and fistula formation that seem particularly prone to the development of carcinomas *(31)*. Surgery is indicated in patients with strictures that cannot be adequately traversed and biopsied, and the possibility of a chronic colonic stricture harboring a neoplasm despite negative biopsies must be seriously discussed with the patient. The same flat dysplasia found in biopsies of rectal and colonic mucosa of long-standing ulcerative colitis patients that serves as predictor of carcinoma also has been reported to occur in CD *(31–33)*. Unfortunately, unlike in UC patients, dysplasia is not widespread in the colon in CD and less likely to be detected.

SMALL INTESTINAL CANCER

Adenocarcinomas of the small intestine are rare and have an incidence <5% of that of colorectal carcinoma. The low incidence of carcinomas of the small intestine is intriguing because, in comparison to the rest of the gastrointestinal tract, the small intestine has a larger mucosal surface area and is exposed to a wider variety of potential carcinogens from ingested food *(34–40)*. Patients with CD are much more likely to develop small bowel carcinoma compared with the general population *(8)*. Most cancers of the small bowel in CD are adenocarcinomas, usually in the terminal ileum or jejunum, and they are difficult, if not impossible, to diagnose at a surgically curable stage. There is a lower average age at diagnosis of cancer in CD (45 vs 60 yr) than sporadic small bowel cancer. Compared to sporadic small bowel cancer, cancer in CD is located more often distally (76% vs 20% in the ileum) and the mean postoperative survival is shorter (8 mo vs 32 mo) *(11)*. As with UC, the incidence of cancer increases with duration of CD. At diagnosis of cancer, the mean duration of CD is 22 yr, 18 yr for cancers occurring in in-continuity bowel, and 28 yr for cancers occurring in excluded bowel *(11,41)*.

It has been postulated that prolonged untreated or unresected inflammation of the small bowel predisposes the patient to the development of cancer. In the past, patients with CD often were managed by bypassing diseased segments of the small bowel; the so-called Eisenhower operation named after the surgery done on President Eisenhower in 1956 for Crohn's disease. These segments then become exposed to prolonged periods of asymptomatic and untreated inflammation. When this surgery was more commonly practiced, up to 40% of small bowel cancers occurred within such bypassed segments. Such cancers tended to present at advanced stages because they went undetected by not producing classical symptoms of obstruction. Currently, bypassing segments of small bowel affected by CD is seldom recommended. Favorable prognostic variables in small bowel cancer include jejunal location, negative lymph nodes, and well-differentiated histopathology. Unfortunately, the majority of patients with CD who develop small bowel adenocarcinomas have either nodal or distant metastases at presentation and their 2-yr survival rate is 9%. In contrast, the 5-yr survival for patients with sporadic small bowel carcinoma ranges from 15% to 23%.

Thirty cases of intestinal adenocarcinoma arising in patients with CD have been described *(42)*. Most of the patients were male with the median age of diagnosis of CD and adenocarcinoma of 34 yr and 49 yr, respectively. In most cases, carcinoma was found incidentally at surgery. All carcinomas arose in areas involved by CD. The majority of cancers were found in the colon with only 27% found in the small bowel. Dysplasia was found adjacent to the carcinoma in the overwhelming majority of cases (87%). Most cases of CD-related intestinal adenocarcinoma have dysplasia in adjacent mucosa and 41% of those arising in the colorectum have distant dysplasia, supporting a dysplasia-carcinoma sequence in CD. Accumulation of *ras* oncogene and *p53* suppressor gene alterations occur during the adenoma-carcinoma sequence in small intestinal carcinogenesis, but a *ras*-independent pathway also may exist *(43)*. The infrequent loss of the adenomatous polyposis coli (*APC*) and deleted in colon cancer (*DCC*) suppressor gene function contrasts with sporadic colorectal carcinogenesis.

The usual clinical presentation of small bowel cancer is with signs and symptoms of obstruction. Diarrhea, weight loss, abdominal mass, and fistulas also are important features. Most of these symptoms are characteristic of the underlying CD, making diagnosis of cancer quite difficult. Small bowel cancer is rarely suspected, with the diagnosis being made preoperatively in less than 5% of patients. The occurrence of obstruction in a patient with long-standing CD should raise the question of possible malignant transformation.

Sporadic small bowel carcinoma is most common in the duodenum and other proximal segments. In the reported cases of carcinoma in CD, there has been a predominance of cancer in the ileum *(44)*. This finding supports the concept of chronically active CD predisposing to carcinoma. Numerous reports of carcinoma developing in chronic fistulas have been described *(35,36)*. Unfortunately, fistulas are common complications of CD and can be difficult to evaluate both radiographically and clinically. Fistulas that persist despite adequate therapy or that develop new symptoms of bleeding should be regarded with suspicion.

Role of Surveillance

The inaccessibility of small bowel to endoscopic examination, the difficulty of evaluating segments of bowel that are either bypassed or strictured, and the confusion of cancer symptoms associated with those of the underlying IBD make it difficult to propose a rational surveillance program for CD patients *(41)*. The smaller number of cases of colorectal cancer associated with CD vs UC may be related to a number of factors. It may be a reflection of the segmental nature of CD, small bowel disease without colonic involvement, or frequent surgical resections. Underreporting of cases prior to the late 1960s because the diagnosis of Crohn's colitis was not recognized, also has been implicated. Of note, there is an increasing number of patients at risk for developing cancer due to the rising incidence of CD in the general population *(45,46)*.

CANCER RISK IN IBD PATIENTS
WITH PRIMARY SCLEROSING CHOLANGITIS

Approximately 2–5% of UC patients develop primary sclerosing cholangitis (PSC) *(47)*. PSC patients with UC are at high risk for malignancies of the biliary tract *(48)*. Furthermore, PSC adds significantly to the already high risk of dysplasia and colorectal cancer in UC patients *(1,5,49)*. The high risk of cancer or dysplasia in PSC patients with UC should alter management. PSC patients should be tested more often, perhaps annually, than UC patients with the same duration of disease. Furthermore, since cancer surveillance is fraught with much uncertainty, prophylactic colectomy may offer the best alternative to UC patients with PSC in terms of life expectancy *(50,51)*.

An association between UC and various hepatobiliary lesions is well established. These lesions include fatty infiltration, cirrhosis, pericholangitis, and PSC. The association of cholangiocarcinoma and UC is uncommon but well recognized. The mean duration of colitis before the diagnosis of cholangiocarcinoma is 15.2 yr with a range of 1–30 yr. It also has been noted that cholangiocarcinoma is not influenced by colectomy, but there is an increased risk in patients with pancolitis, as opposed to disease restricted to a limited colonic segment, as well as those with a longer duration of disease. In all, the risk of cholangiocarcinoma in patients with UC is about 10 times greater than in the general population.

A similar association between CD and cholangiocarcinoma has not been well recognized, although cases have been documented in the literature. In general, cholangiocarcinoma in association with CD occurs at a young age after a long duration of disease. A female predominance has been noted in CD patients and concurrent colonic involvement has been less frequently reported. A lower rate of cholangiocarcinoma complicating CD may be explained by the lower rate of PSC in this patient population.

ESOPHAGEAL AND GASTRIC NEOPLASMS

The occurrence of esophageal cancer in patients with CD has been reported in the literature, but no evidence of CD involving the esophagus was identified in any of the patients before they developed carcinoma (52,53). The association between esophageal cancer and IBD is doubtful.

The coincidence of CD and gastric carcinoma has been described (54,55). Many of the patients documented in the literature presented with nonspecific symptoms referable to the upper gastrointestinal tract. Clinical evidence of active CD involving the stomach was absent in the majority of cases. Radiographic imaging with barium or CT can be important in establishing the diagnosis as endoscopy with biopsy may not always yield a clear result especially in areas of chronic inflammation. The reason for a lack of clinical information linking gastric neoplasm and CD is because of the rarity of gastric involvement with CD. This entity likely occurs in less than 3% of patients with CD. Although a relationship between CD and gastric or esophageal neoplasia is not well established, it is important to investigate symptoms referable to the upper gastrointestinal tract in patients with documented CD.

CANCER INVOLVING FISTULAS AND STOMAS

The occurrence of cancer in enterocutaneous, enteroenteric, and perineal fistulas is uncommon. Patients with carcinoma involving chronic fistulizing CD may have developed the malignancy as a result of chronic epithelial irritation (56,57). Alternatively, the carcinoma may actually be the cause of the fistula. The diagnoses of such carcinomas are often delayed because of the lack of specificity of symptoms and signs. The poor prognosis for both abdominal and perineal carcinomas associated with fistulas of CD reflects their advanced stage at diagnosis. An increase in pain, discharge, or bleeding associated with a perianal fistula warrants careful examination with biopsy of suspicious areas. Changes in symptoms and signs of abdominal disease also should prompt investigation. Biopsy or excision of fistulas should be considered in these settings.

Development of carcinoma involving an ileostomy stoma also has been described. Cancer in this area may not manifest for 30 yr or more after ileostomy construction. Persistent peristomal ulceration is worrisome and should be biopsied with wide local excision with relocation of the ileostomy stoma if carcinoma is identified.

CARCINOID TUMORS

Carcinoid tumors associated with IBD rarely have been reported with the most common site being the appendix. The average age at diagnosis was younger in the IBD patient compared with the general population (41 vs 53 yr). This is possibly because IBD patients come to surgery early for the underlying disease or its complications and a carcinoid tumor is discovered incidentally *(58)*. It is often difficult to differentiate between the symptoms of metastatic carcinoid and those of IBD because both conditions can produce diarrhea, bleeding, evidence of a mass, or intestinal obstruction *(59)*. Interestingly, a vast majority of carcinoid tumors in IBD patients are not metastatic and not recognized preoperatively. Carcinoid tumors in IBD patients are not increased in frequency or different in distribution, and, therefore, are not related to IBD.

IBD THERAPY AND MALIGNANCY

Immunosuppressive or immunomodulating agents including 6-mercaptopurine (6MP), azathioprine, methotrexate, cyclosporine, and infliximab have all raised concerns regarding malignancy, especially non-Hodgkins lymphoma, in the setting of treatment for patients with IBD. A large series of 755 patients followed for a median of 12.5 mo on immunosuppressive therapy found no cases of non-Hodgkins lymphoma *(60)*. Another series of 591 patients treated with 6MP for a at least 8 yr and followed for a mean of 17 yr found two cases of non-Hodgkins lymphoma, suggesting little, if any, increased risk *(61)*. The occurrence of lymphoma in transplant patients treated with cyclosporine appears to be dose-related and may regress with lower doses. The incidence of lymphoma in cyclosporine-treated renal transplant patients has been cited at 0.4%. Two cases of lymphoma were reported in patients who received infliximab *(62)*.

Although it remains true that these immunosuppressive agents all carry the potential for malignant lymphoproliferative disorders, the risk is small. Physicians considering the use of these agents should alert the patient to the small possibility of developing a malignancy even after therapy is discontinued. When discussing this issue, it is also equally important to stress the improved quality-of-life that may be achieved while on these medications. More information on the true incidence of malignancy with these agents will come as experience increases.

CONCLUSIONS

The association between IBD and gastrointestinal cancer is well established. What is yet to be elucidated is the optimal method of surveillance to accomplish the goal of maximally reducing cancer-related mortality. Further research in the area of molecular genetics to find complementary markers for dysplasia could assist the gastroenterologist in the early detection of premalignant lesions. For now, patients with UC should have surveillance colonoscopy every 1–3 yr with colectomy for dysplasia detected in any biopsy specimen. Surveillance in Crohn's colitis is only recommended if patients and physicians are aware of the limitations of surveillance and the relatively low effectiveness. Other malignancies have been associated with IBD, and the clinician should be aware that atypical presentations or a change in symptoms in patients with IBD warrants investigation for an etiology that may eventually uncover malignancy as a cause.

REFERENCES

1. Ekbom A, Helmick C. Zack M, et al. Ulcerative colitis and colorectal cancer. A population-based study. N Engl J Med 1990;323:1228–1233.
2. Greenstein A, Sachar D, Smith H, et al. A comparison of cancer risk in Crohn's disease and ulcerative colitis. Cancer 1981;48:2742–2745.
3. Choi PM, Zelig MP. Similarity of colorectal cancer in Crohn's disease and ulcerative colitis: Implications for carcinogenesis and prevention. Gut 1994;35:950–954.
4. Greenstein A, Sachar D, Pucillo A, et al. Cancer in universal and left sided ulcerative colitis: Clinical and pathologic features. Mt Sinai J Med 1981;46:25–32.
5. Gyde SN, Prior P, Allan RN, et al. Colorectal cancer in ulcerative colitis: A cohort study of primary referrals from three centers. Gut 1988;29:206–217.
6. Ekbom A, Helmick C, Zack M, et al. Increased risk of large bowel cancer in Crohn's disease with colonic involvement. Lancet 1990;336:357–359.
7. Gillen CD, Andrews HA, Prior P, et al. Crohn's disease and colorectal cancer. Gut 1994;35:651–655.
8. Greenstein A, Sachar D, Smith H, et al. A comparison of cancer risk in Crohn's disease and ulcerative colitis. Cancer 1981;48:2742–2745.

9. Weedon DD, Shorter RG, Ilstrup DM, et al. Crohn's disease and cancer. N Engl J Med 1973;289:1099–1102.
10. Mir-Madilessi SH, Farmer RG, Easley KA, et al. Colorectal and extracolonic malignancy in ulcerative colitis. Cancer 1986;58:1569–1574.
11. Greenstein AJ, Sugita A, Yamazaki Y. Cancer in inflammatory bowel disease. Jpn J Surg 1989;19:633–644.
12. Levin B. Lennard-Jones J, Riddell RH, et al. Surveillance of patients with chronic ulcerative colitis. WHO Collaborating Center for the Prevention of Colorectal Cancer. Bull WHO 1991;69:121–126.
13. Choi PM, Nugent FW, Schoetz DJ Jr, et al. Colonoscopic surveillance reduces mortality from colorectal cancer in ulcerative colitis. Gastroenterology 1993; 105:418–424.
14. Giardello FM, Gurbuz AK, Bayless TM, et al. Colorectal cancer in ulcerative colitis: Effect of a cancer prevention strategy on survival. Gastroenterology 1993;104:A705.
15. Korelitz B. Considerations of surveillance, dysplasia, and carcinoma of the colon in the management of ulcerative colitis and Crohn's disease. Med Clin N Am 1990;74:189–199.
16. Bernstein CN. Challenges in designing a randomized trial of surveillance colonoscopy in IBD. Inflam Bowel Dis 1998;4:132–141.
17. Rubin CE, Haggitt RC, Burmer GC, et al. DNA aneuploidy in colonic biopsies predicts future development of future dysplasia in ulcerative colitis. Gastroenterology 1992;103:1611–1620.
18. Lashner BA, Hanauer SB, Silverstein MD. Optimal timing of colonoscopy to screen for cancer in ulcerative colitis. Ann Intern Med 1988;108:274–278.
19. Lashner BA, Shapiro BD, Husain A, Goldblum JR. Evaluation of the usefulness of testing for p53 mutations in colorectal cancer for ulcerative colitis. Am J Gastroenterol 1999;94:456–462.
20. Bernstein CN, Shanahan F, Weinstein WM. Are we telling patients the truth about surveillance colonoscopy in ulcerative colitis? Lancet 1994;343:71–74.
21. Connell WR, Lennard-Jones JE, Williams CB. Factors affecting the outcome of endoscopic surveillance for cancer in ulcerative colitis. Gastroenterology 1994;107:934–944.
22. Lashner BA, Kane S, Hanauer SB, et al. Colon cancer surveillance in chronic ulcerative colitis: historical cohort study. Am J Gastroenterol 1990;85:1083–1087.
23. Bernstein CN, Weinstein WM, Levine DS, et al. Physicians perceptions of dysplasia and approaches to surveillance colonoscopy in ulcerative colitis. Am J Gastroenterol 1995;90:2106–2114.
24. Blackstone MO, Riddell RH, Rogers BH, et al. Dysplasia associated lesion or mass (DALM) detected by colonoscopy in longstanding ulcerative colitis: an indication for colectomy. Gastroenterology 1981;80:366–374.
25. Butt JH, Konishi F, Morson PC, et al. Macroscopic lesions in dysplasia and carcinoma complicating ulcerative colitis. Dig Dis Sci 1983;28:18–26.
26. Riddell RH, Goldman H, Ransohoff DF, et al. Dysplasia in inflammatory bowel disease: standard classification with provisional clinical applications. Hum Pathol 1983;14:931–968.
27. Engelsgjred M, Farraye FA, Odze RD. Polypectomy may be adequate treatment for adenoma-like dysplastic lesions in chronic ulcerative colitis. Gastroenterology 1999;117:1288–1294.
28. Rubin PH, Friedman S, Harpaz N, et al. Colonoscopic polypectomy in chronic colitis: conservative management after endoscopic resection of dysplastic polyps. Gastroenterology 1999;117:1295–1300.

29. Lashner BA, Turner BC, Bostwick DG, et al. Dysplasia and cancer complicating strictures in ulcerative colitis. Dig Dis Sci 1990;35:349–352.

30. Hamilton SR. Colorectal carcinoma in patients with Crohn's disease. Gastroenterology 1985;89:398–407.

31. Cooper DJ, Weinstein MA, Korelitz BI. Complications of Crohn's disease predisposing to dysplasia and cancer of the intestinal tract: Consideration of a surveillance program. J Clin Gastroenterol 1984;6:217–224.

32. Craft CF, Mendelsohn G, Cooper HS, et al. Colonic "precancer" in Crohn's disease. Gastroenterology 1981;80:578–584.

33. Warren R, Barwick KW. Crohn's colitis with carcinoma and dysplasia. Report of a case and review of 100 small and large bowel resections for Crohn's disease to detect the incidence of dysplasia. Am J Surg Pathol 1983;7:151–159.

34. Mittal VK, Bodzin JH. Primary malignant tumors of the small intestine. Am J Surg 1980;140:396–399.

35. Barclay THC, Shapira DV. Malignant tumors of the small intestine. Cancer 1983;511:878–881.

36. Johnson AM, Harman PK, Hanks JB. Primary small bowel malignancies. Am J Surg 1985;51:31–36.

37. DiSario JA, Burt RW, Vargas H, et al. Small bowel cancer; epidemiological and clinical characteristics from the population-based registry. Am J Gastroenterol 1994;89:699–701.

38. Seifert E, Schulte F, Stolte M. Adenoma and carcinoma of the duodenum and papilla of Vater: a clinicopathologic study. Am J Gastroenterol 1992;87:37–42.

39. Chow JS, Chen CC, Ahsan H, et al. A population-based study of the incidence of malignant small bowel tumors. SEER, 1973–1990. Int J Epidemiol 1996;25:722–728.

40. Parker SL, Tong T, Bolden S, et al. Cancer statistics, 1997. CA Cancer J Clin 1997;47:5–27.

41. Greenstein AJ, Sachar DB, Smith H, et al. Pattern's of neoplasia in Crohn's disease and ulcerative colitis. Cancer 1980;46:403–407.

42. Sigel JE, Petras RE, Lashner BA, et al. Intestinal adenocarcinoma in Crohn's disease. Am J Surg Path 1999;23:651–655.

43. Rashid A, Hamilton SR. Genetic alterations in sporadic and Crohn's-associated adenocarcinomas of the small intestine. Gastroenterology 1997;113:127–135.

44. Korelitz BI. Carcinoma of the intestinal tract in Crohn's disease: Results of a survey conducted by the National Foundation for Ileitis and Colitis. Am J Gastroenterol 1983; 8:44–46.

45. Binder V. Epidemiology, course and socio-economic influence of inflammatory bowel disease. Schweiz Med Wschr 1988;118:738–742.

46. Gollop JH, Phillips SF, Melton LJ, et al. Epidemiological aspects of Crohn's disease: A population based study in Olmsted County, Minnesota. Gut 1988;29:49–56.

47. Olsson R, Danilesson A, Jarnerot G, et al. Prevalence of primary sclerosing cholangitis in patients with ulcerative colitis. Gastroenterology 1991;100:1319–1323.

48. Mir-Madjlessi SH, Farmer RG, Sivak MV. Bile duct carcinoma in patients with ulcerative colitis. Dig Dis Sci 1987;32:145–154.

49. Marchesa P, Lashner BA, Lavery IC, et al. The risk of cancer and dysplasia among ulcerative colitis patients with primary sclerosing cholangitis. Am J Gastroenterol 1997;92:1285–1288.

50. Loftus EV, Sandborn WJ, Tremaine WJ, et al. Risk of colorectal neoplasia in patients with primary sclerosing cholangitis. Gastroenterology 1996;110:432–440.

51. Shetty K, Rybicki L, Brzezinski A, Carey WD, Lashner BA. The risk for cancer or dysplasia in ulcerative colitis patients with primary sclerosing cholangitis. Am J Gastroenterol 1999;94:1643–1649.

52. Kyle J. Carcinoma of the esophagus in patients with Crohn's disease. J R Coll Surg (Edinb) 1991;36:125–126.

53. Freedman PG, Dietrich ST, Balthazar EJ. Crohn's disease of the esophagus: a case report and review of the literature. Am J Gastroenterol 1984;79:835–858.

54. Gyde SN, Prior P, Macartney JC, et al. Malignancy in Crohn's disease. Gut 1980;21:1024–1029.

55. Glick SN. Gastric carcinoma in patients with Crohn's disease: report of four cases. AJR 1991;157:311–14.

56. Buchman P, Allan RN, Thompson H, et al. Carcinoma in a rectovaginal fistula in a patient with Crohn's disease. AM J Surg 1980;140:462–463.

57. Church JM, Weakley FL, Fazio VW, et al. The relationship between fistulas in Crohn's disease and associated carcinoma. Dis Colon Rectum 1985;28:361–366.

58. Greenstein AJ, Balasubramanian S, Harpaz N, Rizwan M, Sachar DB. Carcinoid turom and inflammatory bowel disease: a study of eleven cases and review of the literature. Am J Gastroenterol 1997;92:682–685.

59. Hsu EY, Feldman JM, Lichtenstein GR. Ileal carcinoid tumors stimulating Crohn's disease: incidence among 176 consecutive cases of ileal carcinoid. Am J Gastroenterol 1997;92:206205.

60. Connell WR, Kamm MA, Dickson M, Balkwill AM, Ritchie JK, Lennard-Jones JE. Long-term neoplasia risk after azathioprine treatment in inflammatory bowel disease. Lancet 1994;343:1249–1252.

61. Korelitz BI, Mirsky FJ, Fleisher MR, Warman JI, Wisch N, Gleim GW. Malignant neoplasms subsequent to treatment of inflammatory bowel disease with 6-mercaptopurine. Am J Gastroenterol 1999;94:3248–3253.

62. Bickston SJ, Lichtenstein GR, Arseneau KO, Cohen RB, Cominelli F. The relationship between infliximab treatment and lymphoma in Crohn's disease. Gastroenterology 1999;117:1433–1437.

15 Gender-Specific Issues in Inflammatory Bowel Disease

Sunanda V. Kane, MD

INTRODUCTION

The incidence of Crohn's disease (CD) in women has been increasing over the past few decades. It is not clear whether this is a result of improved diagnostic techniques, an increase in smoking habits by young women (patients with CD tend to be smokers compared to people without CD), or other factors not yet identified. However, the consequence of this trend is a growing population of patients with gender-specific needs and concerns related to their medical care. Every component of the reproductive cycle can potentially effect disease course or symptomatology. Because the diagnosis of CD or ulcerative colitis (UC) is

From: *Clinical Gastroenterology:*
Inflammatory Bowel Disease: Diagnosis and Therapeutics
Edited by: R. D. Cohen © Humana Press Inc., Totowa, NJ

often made in the childbearing years, fertility and pregnancy are important issues that previously have been handled exclusively by gynecologists. Gastroenterologists caring for women with inflammatory bowel disease (IBD) should be aware of these issues and their appropriate management.

SELF-IMAGE ISSUES

Maunder et al. reported consistently higher levels of symptom severity and rating of IBD patient concerns in women than men (1). Patient concerns that differed by gender included attractiveness, intimacy, and sexual performance. Women also had stronger concerns about self-image, feeling alone, and fearful of having children.

Active disease can lead to fatigue and loss of libido, in addition to the embarrassment of fecal incontinence. Corticosteroids to treat active disease leads to Cushingoid features along with weight gain and mood swings.

Perineal involvement in CD can be physically deforming, as well as resulting in dyspareunia and self-consciousness. The presence of an ostomy or other surgical scars can also lead to a lower self-esteem (2).

THE MENSTRUAL CYCLE

For girls diagnosed with IBD before or during puberty, the onset of menses (menarche) can be delayed. This can be secondary to chronic inflammation or a poor nutritional status that directly affects steroid hormone production. Menarche usually occurs once active disease is treated appropriately.

Disease activity can also affect the menstrual cycle after the onset of menarche. This can be manifested by irregular or skipped periods, or an increase in disease symptoms during the premenstrual or menstrual phase. A recent study corroborates this phenomenon (3). The premenstrual syndrome (PMS) includes gastrointestinal symptoms, but women with IBD complain of these symptoms above and beyond that found in the normal population. Some women consider these "mini-flares". In reality, this is a cyclic, predictable phenomenon, which is neither random or "all in the head". Rather than treating these symptoms as active IBD, conservative treatment to alleviate symptoms is more appropriate, as symptoms will tend to resolve in a few days' time. Table 1 lists those preparations that can be used as alternatives to standard medications to provide relief from menstrual-related symptoms.

Some women have such debilitating symptoms that the elimination of menses is the only way to provide relief. This can be achieved with the short-term injectable contraceptives (Depo-Provera®) or hormones

Table 1
Oral Preparations to Alleviate Menstrual Symptoms

Commercial Preparations	Supplements, Vitamins, and Herbs
Pamprin®	Calcium (1500 mg/d)
Doan's Pills®	Magnesium (up to 400 mg/d)
Pre-lief®	Vitamin E (400 mg/d)
Midol®*	Vitamin C (1000 mg/d)
	Vitamin B6 (100 mcg/d)
	Chamomile tea
	Black cohosh
	Evening primrose oil (1500 mcg/d)
	Dong quai
	Yam extract (480 mcg/d)

*Should be used with caution as this contains ibuprofen.

(Lupron®). At this time, a hysterectomy is not recommended for this indication, but those women who undergo this procedure for other gynecologic reasons find their IBD symptoms improve.

FERTILITY

Overall, the fertility rates for women with IBD are essentially the same as those of the normal population. Early studies showing lower fertility rates had not taken into account an increased voluntary childlessness rate in women with IBD.

Active CD, however, can reduce fertility in several ways, depending upon the location of inflammation. Active inflammation in the colon has been shown to decrease fertility, as well as any inflammation or scarring directly involving the fallopian tubes or ovaries. Women who have had any surgical resection are at risk for adhesions, which can also impair tubal function. Ileo-anal anastomosis has also been linked to decreased fertility in women.

None of the medications used to treat IBD has an effect on female fertility, but it is important to remember that sulfasalazine therapy reduces sperm motility and count in males. Although there is no minimum required time period with quiescent disease prior to a planned conception, the longer the better. Open discussions between patient and physician are the best way to ensure the best outcome of a pregnancy. If a woman is doing well and in remission, there is every reason to expect the pregnancy to proceed smoothly. If active disease is present, it is likely to continue through pregnancy and will place the pregnancy at greater risk for a complication (4). This risk appears to be higher in CD than in UC. The main priority is to establish and maintain remission before the patient conceives. One of the problems in CD is the accurate definition of remission. In CD, a patient may feel fine even though she has an elevated C-reactive protein (CRP), an abnormal colonoscopy, and/or X-ray.

Some women remain childless for fear of disease transmission to their offspring. Current data suggests that this risk is low; 7% if one parent has CD and less if one parent has UC. However, the risk of IBD increases as high as 37% if both parents have the disease. The risk of inheriting IBD is higher in Jewish (7.8%) than in non-Jewish (5.8%) families. It is important to remember that IBD is not a genetic disorder in a true Mendelian fashion. Even with genetic predisposition, other factors are necessary to produce expression of either disease.

CONTRACEPTION

The management of contraception in those women with IBD who do not wish to become pregnant differs from that for normal women. The most important goal still remains the selection of the most reliable method of birth control. Barrier methods of contraception are acceptable but are not as effective as alternatives. The use of intrauterine devices is not usually recommended, as any complaint of abdominal pain could potentially delay the correct diagnosis of active IBD vs pelvic inflammatory disease.

The data regarding the safety of oral contraceptives (OC) in IBD is conflicting. Early studies suggested an increased risk for the development of CD and UC, but did not account for tobacco use (5–8). Reports from Europe, where contraceptives contain a higher estrogen content, continue to show modest increases in risk for the development of CD after adjusting for cigarette use (odds ratios 1.2–2.0) (9).

Other data suggest that oral contraceptive use may exacerbate disease activity (10,11). Two small prospective studies have found an increased risk of disease recurrence after induction of remission in CD with OC use. No information is available for a possible similar risk in UC.

On the other hand, some physicians successfully use oral contraceptives to treat cyclic symptoms that appear to be related to the menstrual cycle, to tamper the effect of fluctuating hormone levels. At this time, no standard guidelines exist for oral contraception use, as there are many preparations available. The variable amounts of progesterone and estrogen are the factors that determine the side-effect profile. The choice of which oral contraceptive preparation to use has to be individualized, taking into consideration other factors including patient history, parity, and personal preferences. It does appear prudent to try to prescribe a formulation that contains the lowest amount of estrogen possible.

EFFECT OF IBD ON PREGNANCY

Women with IBD in remission are no more likely to experience spontaneous abortion, stillbirth, or children born with a congenital abnormality *(12)*. Figure 1 summarizes results of 24 published reports comparing outcomes in women with IBD vs the normal population. Some work has suggested that babies born to women with IBD are of smaller birth weight *(13)*. When a woman has active disease, premature birth is a greater concern.

The presence of IBD does not appear to have an impact on maternal complications related to pregnancy, including hypertension or proteinuria *(14)*. However, active perianal disease may worsen after a vaginal delivery. One retrospective of a study of women with CD found that 18% of those without previous perianal disease developed such disease after delivery, usually involving an extensive episiotomy *(15)*. Otherwise, the presence of IBD does not have a significant impact on the method of delivery, nor is it an indication for Cesarean section.

EFFECT OF PREGNANCY ON IBD

For women with quiescent UC, the rate of relapse is approx the same in pregnant vs nonpregnant patients. This is in contrast to the presence of active disease at the time of conception, which is associated with continued or worsening disease activity in approx 70% of women *(12)*. Comparable observations are seen in Crohn's disease. Figures 2 and 3 illustrate pregnancy-related disease activity as reported by Miller et al. *(4))*. The older literature suggested a trend for disease to flare in the first trimester, but this was documented prior to the accepted practice of maintenance therapy, continued even during pregnancy.

It is important to remember that hemoglobin and albumin levels decrease and ESR increase during pregnancy. Because of these normal physiologic changes, disease assessment during pregnancy should rely more on clinical symptoms than laboratory parameters. Ultrasound exams are clearly safe, and there is no evidence that if indicated, a sigmoidoscopy will induce premature labor *(16)*. Colonoscopy should only be performed when extent and severity of disease specifically need to be ascertained.

There is data that has suggested that a history of child bearing changes the natural history of CD *(17)*. Women who were pregnant had fewer resections or longer intervals between resections as compared to women

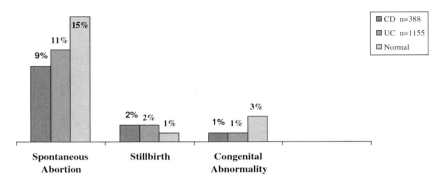

Fig. 1. Adverse outcomes in pregnancy in IBD vs normals.

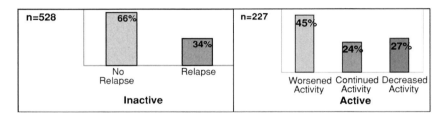

Fig. 2. Natural history of disease during pregnancy: UC.

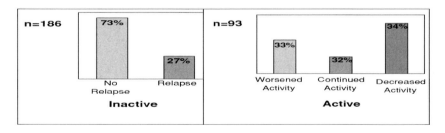

Fig. 3. Natural history of disease during pregnancy: CD.

who had not had children but otherwise similar disease. One possible explanation is the inhibition of macrophage function by relaxin. Relaxin is a hormone produced exclusively during pregnancy, which may result in less fibrosis and stricture formation by this inhibition of macrophages.

TREATMENT OF IBD DURING PREGNANCY

The key principle to management is to remember that the greatest risk to pregnancy is active disease, not active therapy. Because there are limited definitive data available on the safety of IBD medications in pregnancy, the focus, therefore, should be on establishing remission before conception and maintaining remission during pregnancy.

Sulfasalazine readily crosses the placenta, but has not been associated with any fetal abnormalities. However, patients taking sulfasalazine should also be supplemented with folic acid before conceiving to decrease the risk of neural tube defects. A dose of 1 mg bid would be appropriate.

The safety of mesalamine during pregnancy has been demonstrated in a number of trials (18,19). In two separate studies, women taking 2–3 g/d had no increased incidence of fetal abnormalities than that in normal healthy women. Topical 5-ASA agents are likewise safe during pregnancy.

The data regarding immunomodulator therapy (azathioprine, 6-MP) is more conflicting. There are no large studies on the use of these medications during pregnancy in women with IBD. To date, our information comes from the transplantation literature and from small retrospective series in IBD. It is generally believed by the most experienced IBD clinicians that immunosuppressives such as 6-MP, azathioprine, and cyclosporine can be used safely during pregnancy if the mother's health mandates therapy. Methotrexate, another immunomodulatory medication, is contraindicated in pregnancy. Infliximab was recently reclassified as a "Category B" drug in pregnancy, and open-label experience thus far has suggested that it may be safe to use.

Corticosteroids have not been associated with teratogenicity in humans and can be used as required to control disease activity. Prednisone crosses the placenta less efficiently than other steroid formulations such as betamethasone or dexamethasone. Only limited data is available regarding the safety of antibiotics as treatment for CD. Currently, ampicillin, cephalosporins, and erythromycin are believed safe, as well as ciprofloxacin. Metronidazole has been used to treat vaginitis in women during the first trimester of pregnancy but no controlled trials have definitively shown its safety. Table 2 details the safety of those medications used in IBD.

The medications known to be safe for breastfeeding include sulfasalazine, the mesalamine preparations (Asacol®, Pentasa®, Rowasa®, Colazal™, Canasa™) and corticosteroids. Negligible levels of infliximab (Remicade®) have been detected in breast milk. Mothers planning on nursing should discontinue the use of cyclosporine, metronidazole, ciprofloxacin, and methotrexate. No data is available regarding the thiopurines and should be discussed on a case-by-case basis. Table 3 summarizes the safety data regarding medications and their use during breastfeeding. Current studies are underway studying medication levels in breast milk, to assess for any increased risk of immunosuppression of the infant.

SURGERY AND PREGNANCY

The indications for surgery during pregnancy are identical to that of nonpregnant patients. These include obstruction, perforation, abscess, and hemorrhage. Pregnancy has not been shown to complicate stoma function. Women may experience some prolapse as a result of abdominal pressure, but no increased risk to the pregnancy is encountered.

For those women who have had ileoanal pull through procedures, an increase in the number of bowel movements during pregnancy has been reported, but no increased risk for pouchitis or delivery complications has been reported (20).

SURGICAL OUTCOMES

There has been a varying incidence of dyspareunia following pelvic surgery, ranging from 0 to 26%. This variation may be due to the heterogeneous nature of surgeries or underreporting of symptoms to physicians (21–23). After ileo-anal anastomosis, one report found 15% incidence of dyspareunia, and an increase in menstrual problems (2). Fertility may also be decreased following such surgery.

MENOPAUSE

Menopause, whether natural or surgical, leads to many physiologic changes in a woman's body. Just as oral contraceptives can help with controlling symptoms, there is data to suggest that some of the gastrointestinal symptoms associated with IBD have decreased in women who have achieved menopause.

Women with UC are at no greater risk for an early menopause than women without IBD. There is some data that suggest that women with CD may enter menopause earlier than normal women, but a mechanism has yet to be established (7).

What is certain however, is that the risk for osteoporosis is substantially higher because of steroid exposure, decreased dairy product consumption secondary to lactose intolerance, and malabsorption related to inflamed gastrointestinal mucosa. It is recommended, therefore, that

Table 2
Safety of IBD Medication During Pregnancy

Safe to Use When Indicated	Limited Data	Contraindicated
Oral Mesalamine	Olsalazine	Methotrexate
Topical Mesalamine	Azathioprine	Thalidomide
Sulfasalazine	6-mercaptopurine	
Ciprofloxacin*	Cyclosporine	
	Infliximab	
Corticosteroids	Metronidazole	

* Ciprofloxacin's use should be delayed until after the first trimester, if possible.

Table 3
Safety of IBD Medications During Breastfeeding

Safe to Use When Indicated	No Data	Contraindicated
Oral Mesalamine	Olsalazine	Methotrexate
Topical Mesalamine	Azathioprine	Thalidomide
Sulfasalazine	6-mercaptopurine	Cyclosporine
Corticosteroids		Ciprofloxacin
Infliximab		Metronidazole

every woman with IBD undergo a bone density scan to assess for bone loss. If present, then replacement calcium and vitamin D are essential, with the addition of bisphosphonates as indicated.

The issues regarding hormone replacement therapy (HRT) are identical to those in normal women for bone loss and cardioprotection. Family history for any breast or uterine cancer, or a personal history of either these or thromboembolic events need to be taken into consideration when deciding on HRT.

SUMMARY

- The menstrual cycle can affect IBD symptoms.
- Fertility is not affected in UC, but can be in active CD.
- There is no increase in bad outcome with quiescent IBD.
- Active disease at conception increases the risk for adverse outcomes.
- The majority of medications for IBD are safe in pregnancy and breastfeeding.
- Active disease is more deleterious than active therapy.

REFERENCES

1. Maunder R, Toner B, de Rooy E, Moskovitz D. Influence of sex and disease on illness-related concerns in inflammatory bowel disease. Can J Gastroenterol 1999; 13:728–732.
2. Counihan TC, Roberts PL, Schoetz DJ Jr, Coller JA, Murray JJ, Veidenheimer MC. Fertility and sexual and gynecologic function after ileal pouch-anal anastomosis. Dis Colon Rectum 1994;37:1126–1129.
3. Kane S, Sable, K, Hanauer, S. The menstrual cycle and its effect on inflammatory bowel disease and irritable bowel syndrome: a prevalence study. Am J Gastro 1998;93:1867–1872.
4. Miller JP. Inflammatory bowel disease in pregnancy: a review. J R Soc Med 1986; 79:221–225.
5. Boyko EJ, Theis MK, Vaughan TL, Nicol-Blades B. Increased risk of inflammatory bowel disease associated with oral contraceptive use. Am J Epidemiol 1994; 140:268–278.
6. Lesko SM, Kaufman DW, Rosenberg L, et al. Evidence for an increased risk of Crohn's disease in oral contraceptive users. Gastroenterology 1985;89:1046–1049.
7. Lichtarowicz A, Norman C, Calcraft B, Morris JS, Rhodes J, Mayberry J. A study of the menopause, smoking, and contraception in women with Crohn's disease. Q J Med 1989;72:623–631.
8. Sandler RS, Wurzelmann JI, Lyles CM. Oral contraceptive use and the risk of inflammatory bowel disease. Epidemiology 1992;3:374–378.
9. Godet PG, May GR, Sutherland LR. Meta-analysis of the role of oral contraceptive agents in inflammatory bowel disease. Gut 1995;37:668–673.
10. Timmer A, Sutherland LR, Martin F. Oral contraceptive use and smoking are risk factors for relapse in Crohn's disease. The Canadian Mesalamine for Remission of Crohn's Disease Study Group. Gastroenterology 1998;114:1143–1150.
11. Cottone M, Camma, C, Orlando, A, et al. Oral contraceptive and recurrence in Crohn's disease. Gastroenterology 1999;116:A693.
12. Yang H, McElree C, Roth MP, Shanahan F, Targan SR, Rotter JI. Familial empirical risks for inflammatory bowel disease: differences between Jews and non-Jews. Gut 1993;34:517–524.
13. Moser MA, Okun NB, Mayes DC, Bailey RJ. Crohn's disease, pregnancy, and birth weight. Am J Gastroenterol 2000;95:1021–1026.
14. Porter RJ, Stirrat GM. The effects of inflammatory bowel disease on pregnancy: a case-controlled retrospective analysis. Br J Obstet Gynecol 1986;93:1124–1131.
15. Ilnyckyj A, Blanchard JF, Rawsthorne P, and Bernstein CN. Perianal Crohn's disease and pregnancy: role of the mode of delivery. Am J Gastro 1999; 94:3274–3278.
16. Cappell MS, Colon VJ, Sidhom OA. A study at 10 medical centers of the safety and efficacy of 48 flexible sigmoidoscopies and 8 colonoscopies during pregnancy with follow-up of fetal outcome and with comparison to control groups. Dig Dis Sci 1996;41:2353–2361.
17. Nwokolo C, Tan WC, Andrews HA, Allan RN. Surgical resections in parous patients with distal ileal and colonic Crohn's disease. Gut 1994;35:220–223.
18. Diav-Citrin O, Park YH, Veerasuntharam G, et al. The safety of mesalamine in human pregnancy: a prospective controlled cohort study. Gastroenterology 1998; 114:23–28.
19. Marteau P, Tennenbaum R, Elefant E, Lemann M, Cosnes J. Foetal outcome in women with inflammatory bowel disease treated during pregnancy with oral mesalazine microgranules. Aliment Pharmacol Ther 1998;12:1101–1108.

20. Juhasz ES, Fozard B, Dozois RR, Ilstrup DM, Nelson H. Ileal pouch-anal anastomosis function following childbirth. An extended evaluation. Dis Colon Rectum 1995;38:159–165.
21. Tiainen J, Matikainen M, Hiltunen KM. Ileal J-pouch—anal anastomosis, sexual dysfunction, and fertility. Scand J Gastroenterol 1999;34:185–188.
22. Damgaard B, Wettergren A, Kirkegaard P. Social and sexual function following ileal pouch-anal anastomosis. Dis Colon Rectum 1995;38:286–289.
23. Bambrick M, Fazio VW, Hull TL, Pucel G. Sexual function following restorative proctocolectomy in women. Dis Colon Rectum 1996;39:610–614.

16 Economics of Inflammatory Bowel Disease

Russell D. Cohen, MD

Contents

INTRODUCTION

Advances in the medical and surgical care of patients with inflammatory bowel disease (IBD) have been geared toward improving the quality of care and quality of life of persons with this disease. Attention to cost-containment has traditionally taken a backseat to these objectives. However, in this ever-changing world of medical economics, it is reasonable to consider the economic impact of these diseases and their therapies. Economic outcomes are increasingly being requested by many parties: insurers, hospitals, the government, physicians, and, of course, the patients.

Medical therapies for IBD have flourished in the late 1980s and 1990s, with the introduction of multiple nonsulfa-containing aminosalicylates, advanced steroid-preparations, immunomodulators, and biological therapies, all of which have afforded more options, in some instances greater efficacy, but in all cases greater medication costs. The

From: *Clinical Gastroenterology:*
Inflammatory Bowel Disease: Diagnosis and Therapeutics
Edited by: R. D. Cohen © Humana Press Inc., Totowa, NJ

potential of these agents to decrease overall costs by decreasing utilization of medical services, and avoiding complications associated with the use of traditional steroids, has seldom been considered in response to their expensive price tags (1).

The cost-saving impact of surgical advances is perhaps more apparent, as bowel-sparing and minimally invasive approaches raise the potential for shorter hospitalizations, lower morbidity, and in some instances, a decrease in the number of surgeries a patient must endure over a lifetime of IBD. Attention to improving patient quality of life and decreasing the disability as a result of these diseases will likely impact indirect costs, which may contribute substantially to overall patient costs.

This chapter reviews the IBD economic studies to date and discusses the application of this information toward the modern day treatment of patients with IBD from the view of the patient, physician, financial planners, and payers.

IBD ECONOMICS

Joel and Alan Hay published the first landmark article on IBD economics in 1992. Appearing as two companion studies (2,3), their methodologies and results are often referenced by subsequent investigators. The Hays first studied IBD practice patterns and costs, and then applied them to a practice algorithm to estimate the diseases' overall impact. Two different approaches were utilized to calculate the estimated costs associated with the care of IBD patients: decision costing algorithms and medical claims database analysis.

The first approach was the creation of two separate medical decision costing algorithms, one for Crohn's disease and one for ulcerative colitis. Information on likely costs and outcomes of 100 hypothetical Crohn's and 100 hypothetical ulcerative colitis patients was derived from an extensive literature review of many characteristics of the disease. Included were disease incidence and prevalence rates, initial diagnostic work-up, annual outpatient care, cancer risks, colonoscopic surveillance, colectomy rates, surgery rates (including complications), hospitalization rates, medication utilization, ileostomy costs, and complications. As most topics were examined by multiple different studies, the authors selected rates that seemed to be either in the middle of the range of those studies, or most consistent with practice patterns in the United States at the time. Prices quoted were in 1990 dollars. Costs were determined by multiplying charges by 0.65 (locally consistent at the time).

The Hays then applied these costs to 100 hypothetical Crohn's and 100 hypothetical ulcerative colitis patients, resulting in estimated average annual costs of $6561 (Crohn's) and $1488 (ulcerative colitis) per patient. U.S. annual costs for each disease were calculated at $1.0–$1.2 billion (Crohn's) and $400,000–$600,000 (ulcerative colitis). Our group updated the Crohn's figures to 1996 dollars in a recent review to more than $9000 per patient, and $1.7 billion U.S. costs (4).

The majority (80%) of Crohn's costs were accounted for surgery and hospitalization (Fig. 1A). For ulcerative colitis (UC), 47% of costs were for surgery and hospitalizations, although the 29% listed for complications includes the high costs of patients with coexistent UC and primary sclerosing cholangitis who underwent liver transplantation (Fig. 1B). These findings suggest that substantial cost savings can only be realized by decreasing hospitalizations and surgeries. Attempts at limiting medication costs would have a minimal impact upon the overall cost of disease. This was further emphasized by a regression analysis that showed the impact of a new medication that doubled medication costs but, presumably because of its efficacy, decrease utilization of other healthcare services by 20%, was to decrease overall Crohn's costs by 12.9% and UC costs by 10.9%.

The second approach to determining IBD costs consisted of evaluation of the medical claims submitted to a large commercial insurer (CIGNA Corporation) for the 1-yr period extending from 1988 to 1989. More than 4000 patients submitted claims for Crohn's and 770 for UC, accounting for charges exceeding $25 million and $3 million, respectively. The top 2% of Crohn's patients accounted for 29% of charges and 34% of dollars paid! However, the most expensive cases also coded for liver cirrhosis; those patients presumably had liver transplantation to account for their inordinate costs. The top 2% of UC patients accounted for 36% of total charges and 39% of dollars paid, whereas the expenditures accrued for by more than one-half of the patients accounting for less than 7% of the total!

A more recent retrospective claims analysis was published in 2000 by Feagan et al. (5). These authors utilized a 1994 claims database from Hewitt Associates, a benefits firm that processes medical and pharmacy claims from employees of 50 of the largest U.S. employers. All Crohn's related claims (defined as ICD-9 code 555) from October 1994 through September 1995 were included. Patients were stratified into three groups defined by disease severity. Group I required an in-patient hospitalization with a primary or secondary diagnosis of Crohn's disease (CD). Group 2 were labeled as those requiring aggressive medical therapy, defined as chronic glucocorticoid use at a daily dose of at greater than 10 mg (presumably of prednisone) or immunosuppressive (a purine antimetabolite or methotrexate). Group 3 included all other patients. A separate analysis of patients with fistulizing CD was also conducted.

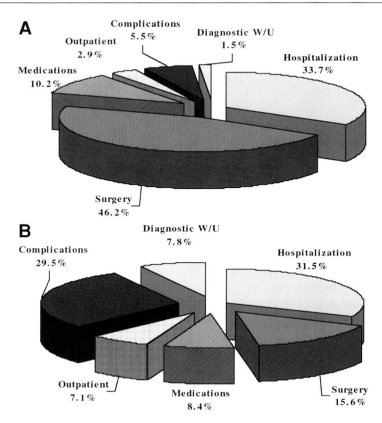

Fig. 1. **(A)** Estimated annual medical care costs for patients with CD. Data from Hay et al. *(2)*. **(B)** Estimated annual medical care costs for patients with UC. [Data from Hay et al. *(2)*.]

The results for the three main groups have been summarized in Table 1. Patients requiring a Crohn's hospitalization had more than triple the annual average charges than those in the aggressive therapy group, and nearly six times that of other patients in Group III. Annual median charge differences were even higher. The impact of hospitalization on charges was impressive: 57% of all charges were a result of hospitalization (nearly the same finding as the 56% of costs found in the Hays' study), and among those patients who did require hospitalization, those charges accounted for more than 75% of their overall charges! Similarly, in patients with fistulizing disease, inpatient care was responsible for 71% of their average charges.

Twenty-five percent of patients accounted for 80% of the overall charges. This imbalance mirrors the findings of the Hays study *(2,3)*.

Table 1
Characteristics of Each Group of Patients with CD.
Values Shown are per Patient, Annually. Data from Feagan et al. *(5)*

	Group I	*Group II*	*Group III*	*All Patients*
Group Characteristic	Hospitalized	Aggressive	All Others Therapy	—
% of patients	19%	5%	76%	—
Average Annual Charges	$ 37, 135	$ 10,033	$ 6277	$12,417
Median Annual Charges	$ 21,671	$ 5581	$ 2703	$3668

The disparity where a small percentage of sick patients consume a disproportionate share of resources also suggests that medical or surgical advances that substantially improve the condition of these patients may have a dramatic effect on lowering overall costs. In chronic, relapsing diseases such as CD and UC, questions often arise whether earlier diagnosis or more aggressive therapies administered earlier in the disease may alter its course. Determining which patients are at risk for aggressive disease, perhaps through genetic means or clues from studying the disease course in other patients with aggressive disease, may help guide a more aggressive therapeutic regimen to a high-risk patient.

This is of particular interest with the emergence of the first biological therapy for CD, infliximab. Extremely effective in patients with lumenal and fistulizing CD, much debate has centered over the high cost of the drug (currently approx $2300 for each infusion in a 70 kg person). This is the exact scenario hypothesized by the Hay's in the early 1990's, whereby an effective but expensive therapy might be cost saving, if it reduced utilization of health care resources.

With this in mind, we studied the impact of infliximab upon use of health care resources in the CD population at the University of Chicago *(6)*. All CD patients receiving infliximab within the first year of its release were analyzed to determine whether their rate of utilization of services changed after their first infusion of the drug. The incidence of hospitalizations, hospitalized days, surgeries, endoscopies, and radiographs were analyzed, as well as visits to the outpatient clinics and the emergency room.

Decreases were seen across the board in most areas. Surgeries declined by 38%, gastrointestinal surgeries by 18%, endoscopies by 43%, radiographs by 12%, visits to the emergency room by 66%, and to the outpatient clinics by 16% (20% for GI clinics). In addition, hospitalizations decreased by 59% among patients with CD fistulas, and there was a trend towards a decrease in hospitalized days for the combined groups of lumenal and fistulizing patients (declined 9%, $p = 0.06$). Changes were seen in both genders, and across all age spectrums.

It remains to be seen whether decreasing utilization of such resources proves to be cost-savings. One important area not included in the study, savings in indirect costs, has been a largely ignored, but likely important contributor to overall cost savings. To gain a better understanding of the different areas contributing to costs, each are more fully discussed later.

HOSPITALIZATIONS

The first analysis of actual cost and resource utilization of hospital resources in Crohn's disease was conducted by our group at the University of Chicago, a quaternary referral center for inflammatory bowel disease (7). The study looked at the cost, charges, revenues (reimbursements), and utilization of resources for all patients hospitalized at the University with a primary diagnosis of CD over a 1-yr period from July 1996 through June 1997.

There were 175 CD hospitalizations among 147 patients over that one-yr time period. Mean costs, charges, and reimbursements were $12,528, $35,378, and $21,968, respectively. Fifty-seven percent of the hospitalizations were surgical admissions, indicating that a primary CD—related surgical procedure was performed during the hospital stay. There was a great disparity in all three economic parameters between medical and surgical admissions, as shown in Fig. 2.

Surgery-related costs resulted in nearly 40% of all costs, with only minimal contribution of endoscopy, radiology, and laboratory tests to overall costs. Pharmacy costs accounted for nearly 19% of overall costs, with a disproportionate amount owing to total parenteral nutrition (TPN). Although TPN was administered in only 27% of hospitalizations, it accounted for 63% of the total pharmacy costs. Medical admissions requiring TPN were nearly three times longer than non-TPN admissions, at nearly four times the cost.

Physician charges were also disproportionately weighted toward surgical charges. Surgeons accounted for 18% of the number of charges, but 56% of the total dollar amount charged. General Medicine, in contrast, provided more physician services (20%) but only 9% of the dollars charged. Overall, surgery accounted for 57% of admissions, 40% of costs, and nearly three-quarters of overall charges and revenues.

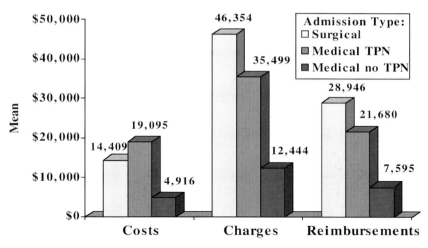

Fig. 2. Average costs, charges, and reimbursements per CD hospitalization. Data from Cohen et al. *(6)*.

These findings were echoed in a Canadian study of hospitalized patients with CD (197), UC (115), or indeterminate colitis (13). Utilizing a patient costing system at the Saint Boniface General Hospital in Manitoba, Bernstein et al. evaluated the cost of care among these 325 IBD patients (362 hospital admissions) hospitalized over the 2-yr period of 1994–1995 *(8)*. Surgery accounted for nearly 50% of admissions, 58% of hospital days, and 61% of costs.

Patients were also subcategorized by diagnosis-related group (DRG); those with a digestive system disease DRG had shorter mean lengths of stay (Fig. 3A) and lower mean costs (Fig. 3B) than those with nondigestive DRGs. At the time of their study, the average exchange rate between Canadian and U.S. dollars was $1 Canadian = $0.73 American. Patients who repeatedly required admission (at least twice over the 2-yr period) were not substantially more costly per admission than those only admitted once.

TPN was utilized in 9.5% of cases (7.1% in CD, 13.9% in UC) accounting for 27% of overall costs (21% CD, 36% UC) and 11% of the total costs for those patients that received TPN. As was the case in the University of Chicago study, the mean length of stay for medically treated IBD patients was over four times longer at approx five times the mean cost for TPN users. Comorbidity rates were also higher in the TPN patients, where over 58% had six other diagnoses listed in hospital discharge abstracts.

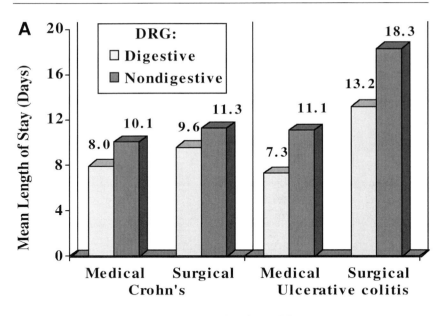

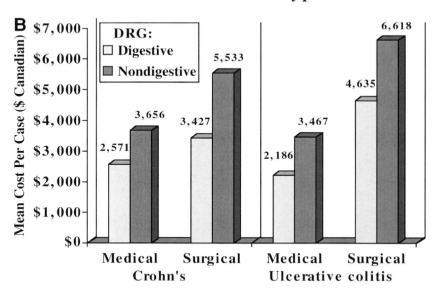

Fig. 3. (A) Mean length of stay for hospital admissions for CD and for UC. Data from Bernstein et al. (7). (B) Mean costs for hospital admissions for CD and for UC. $1 Canadian = $0.73 US. Data from Bernstein et al. (7).

CLINICAL COURSE AND COSTS

Costs for IBD medications, at doses generally used at the University of Chicago's Inflammatory Bowel Disease Center, and/or published in peer-reviewed literature (9–21) are shown in Table 2 (22). (Average Wholesale Prices [AWP] as of April, 2000.) Medication costs must be interpreted in the appropriate setting; for example, the very low cost of prednisone does not take into account the long-term costs of complications directly resulting from this medication.

One approach to determining the overall costs associated with CD has been to examined the projected clinical course of disease, and it's associated costs, based upon retrospective analysis of population-based data. Utilizing the principles of Markov Modeling (23–25), a consortium of American and Canadian investigators evaluated the clinical course of disease in Crohn's patients in Olmstead County, Minnesota (26).

The researchers defined seven possible disease severity states, depending upon the medical or surgical therapy, and the patients' response to therapy (Table 3). After reviewing the medical records from all 174 CD patients in Olmstead County over the 24-yr period extending from 1970–1993, they constructed a chronological course for each patient. They then applied their Markov model to this information to calculate the likelihood of transition between the different Markov states.

Medical charges were calculated as the difference in medical charges between the CD cohort and a control cohort (10 age- and sex-matched controls without Crohn's), and costs were derived from their charge data. Median monthly charges (1995 $US) were much higher in the surgery state ($7438) than in all other states combined; the next closest state was severe, drug responsive at $619. More revealing is the projected cost and clinical course data. Utilizing the median age at diagnosis (28.1 yr) of their population as the starting point, projected lifetime clinical course and costs are shown in Figs. 4A,B, respectively.

The projected future life expectance of 46 yr would be spent mostly in remission; either postsurgical remission (40%) or medical (25%), or on first-line therapies with mild disease (27%). Given the historically low use of immunosuppressive agents in IBD in the years of the study, one must wonder whether this evaluation is truly applicable to the state of medical affairs in IBD today.

Projected lifetime costs for the representative 28-yr-old was nearly $40,000 in charges, the largest proportion due to surgery (44%). Surgery resulted in the longest remission, raising the purely economic issue of the costeffectiveness of earlier surgery in CD However, the predisposition of CD patients to have disease recurrence postoperatively has

Table 2
Average Wholesale Price (AWP) of Drugs Commonly Used in CD *(22)*

Drug Name: generic (Brand)	Unit	AWP/dose	Doses/d	Cost/yr
Antibiotics				
ciprofloxacin (Cipro®)	500 mg	$4.40	2	$3212
clarithromycin (Biaxin®)	500 mg	$3.77	2	$2752
metronidazole	500 mg	$0.47	3	$515
metronidazole (Flagyl®)	500 mg	$2.97	3	$3252
Aminosalicylates				
mesalamine (Asacol®)	400 mg	$0.74	10	$2701
mesalamine (Pentasa®)	250 mg	$0.43	16	$2511
mesalamine enema (Rowasa®)	4 g		$12.32	1
$4497				
mesalamine suppository (Rowasa®)	500 mg	$3.90	2	$2847
olsalazine (Dipentum®)	250 mg	$0.98	12	$4292
sulfasalazine	500 mg	$0.20	8	$584
Sulfasalazine (Azulfidine-EN®)	500 mg	$0.34	8	$993
Steroids				
hydrocortisone enema (Cortenema®)	100 mg	$13.78	1	$5030
hydrocortisone foam (Cortifoam®)	900 mg	$5.11	2	$3730
prednisone	10 mg	$0.07	2	$51
Immunomodulators				
azathioprine	50 mg	$1.31	2	$956
azathioprine (Imuran®)	50 mg	$1.46	2	$1066
cyclosporine, intravenous[a]	100 mg	$10.56	—	$305
cyclosporine (Neoral®[b])	100 mg	$6.12	—	$857
cyclosporine (Neoral®[b])	25 mg	$1.53	—	$428
combined iv and oral cyclosporine[c]	—	—	—	$1590
combined cyclosporine + azathioprine[d]	—	—	—	$2546
6-mercaptopurine (Purinethol®)	50 mg	$3.15	2	$2300
methotrexate injectable[e]	25 mg	$3.43	1/wk	$179
infliximab (Remicade®)[f]	100 mg	$641.28	—	$8978

[a]Intravenous cyclosporine 4 mg/kg × 70 kg = 280 mg/d, mean duration 10.3 d.

[b]Oral cyclosporine 2 mg/kg for 70 kg person = 140 mg = 1–100 and 2–25 for a mean of 20 wk.

[c]Intravenous cyclosporine followed by oral cyclosporine, dosed as detailed above.

[d]Intravenous cyclosporine followed by oral cyclosporine and oral azathioprine (100 mg/d).

[e]Methotrexate 25 mg intramuscular or subcutaneous, dosed once weekly.

[f]Infliximab 5 mg/kg × 70 kg = 350 mg, given q 3mo.

Table 3
CD Severity States. Data from Islverstein et al. *(26)*

Disease Severity State	Characteristics
Remission/no medication	No medication, other than antidiarrheals.

Mild disease	Therapy with:
	    * 5-ASA compounds[a]
	    * Antibiotics[b]
	    * Topical therapy

Severe Disease, drug-responsive	Improvement with:
	    * Oral corticosteroids
	    * Immunosuppressives[c]

Severe disease, drug-dependent	Improvement with >6 mo of:
	    * Oral corticosteroids
	    * Immunosuppressives[c]

Severe disease, drug-refractory	No improvement after:
	    * 2 mo of corticosteroids
	    * 6 mo of immunosuppressives[c]

Surgery	Inpatient hospitalization for Crohn's surgery + 6 wk post-hospitalization convalescence.
Postsurgical Remission	No treatment for Crohn's after Crohn's surgery.
Death	Death from any cause.

[a]5-ASA includes mesalamine, sulfasalazine, olsalazine.
[b]Antibiotics include metronidazole or ciprofloxacin.
[c]Immunosuppressives includes 6-meracaptopurine, azathioprine, methotrexate, cyclosporin A.

since led to the adaptation of postoperative prophylaxis with various medications *(27–31)*, questioning the long-term cost savings that would be realized.

These authors also evaluated the impact upon overall lifetime costs by more costly (but more efficacious) medications. Sensitivity analysis suggested that a dollar increase in the price of minimally effective aminosalicylates increased projected lifetime costs by nearly 10-times the dollar amount than would result from a similar one-dollar increase in the more effective immunosuppressives. This analysis did not include the new biological agent infliximab. These findings are along the same reasoning as that first presented in the Hay study *(2)* and subsequently studied by our group *(6)*, whereby regression analysis

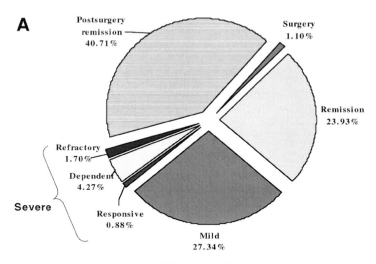

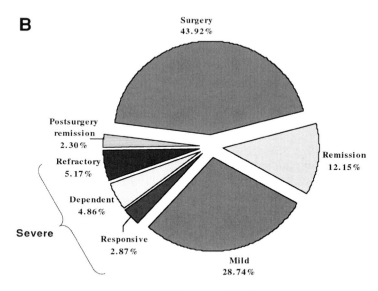

Fig. 4. **(A)** Projected lifetime clinical course for patients with CD. Data from Silverstein et al. *(25)*. **(B)** Projected direct medical costs for patients with CD. Data from Silverstein et al.*(25)*.

suggested that an expensive but highly effective medication could lead to overall cost savings.

SURGERY

The disproportionate contribution of surgery to overall costs in IBD raises the question as how to decrease surgical costs. This can be accomplished in three ways: decreasing the need for surgeries, decreasing the need for repeat surgeries, or decreasing the costs associated with surgery.

DECREASING THE NEED FOR SURGERY

Surgery has been considered inevitable for a large proportion of patients with CD. Approximately 70% of CD patients require at least one surgical operation *(32–34)*, and 45% ultimately require a second surgery *(35)*. CD typically recurs at the site of the surgical anastomosis at rates of 8–10% annually *(36,37)*.

In UC, the rate of surgery varies from 14–61%, depending upon the extent of disease *(38)*. Surgery typically consists of a total procto-colectomy followed by formation of either an ileal-anal anastomosis (IAA) or an ileostomy. The IAA is the procedure of choice in most patients, but often requires two or three surgeries, each accompanied by a 6-wk convalescence *(26)*.

How does one decrease the need for surgeries? Medication trials in IBD do not typically included "surgery" sparing as an outcome. Intra-venous cyclosporin has been shown to help severely ill UC patients avoid surgery in the short *(39)* and long term *(40)*. Initial results from our group have suggested that infliximab may lead to a decrease in surgeries in CD patients *(6)*, but clearly more studies are needed in this regard.

Decreasing the Need for Repeat Surgeries

The issue of repeat surgeries is quite different for patients with UC, where efforts have been to decrease the number of surgeries required for the typical proctocolectomy with ileoanal anastomosis, and CD, where the emphasis has been on preventing recurrence of disease symptoms necessitating surgery.

Patients with UC who require surgery almost always undergo complete removal of the colon and rectum, and in many instances formation of an ileal - anal pouch anastomosis. Traditionally a three-stage surgery, with a multiple month hiatus between stages and a 6-wk convalescence after each state, many procedures can be done in two or even one-stage in select patients. The benefit in decreased both the direct and indirect costs are apparent. Long-term follow-up of patients receiving one-stage proctocolectomy with ileoanal anastomoses will need to show that subsequent surgeries (i.e., adhesions, pouch failure) are not more common in this group of patients. Pouch failure leading to take-down are exceedingly rare events following the more traditional two- or three-stage procedures *(41)*.

CD patients who undergo partial resection of the small or large bowel face the near inevitability of eventual postoperative recurrence. There is now growing evidence that postoperative prophylaxis with mesalamine-based agents *(27–30)*, antibiotics *(31)*, or immunosuppressives *(27)* may lead to a delay in clinical relapse, but these studies have not all been convincing, and the outcome of delaying a repeat surgery has not been studied. To date, infliximab has not been formally studied in this regard, other than the results from our analysis suggesting a decrease in surgeries in patients with lumenal and fistulous CD, some of which were repeat surgeries *(6)*. Newer bowel-sparing surgical approaches in CD patients such as intestinal strictureplasty hold the promise of altering the inevitable cycle of serial bowel resection and ultimately short-bowel syndrome, in some individuals *(42,43)*. Long-term follow-up of more than 250 patients accounting for nearly 1000 strictureplasties has shown surprisingly little evidence of escalation of disease or need for reoperation *(44–48)*.

Decreasing the Costs Associated with Surgery

One of the keys to decreasing surgical costs is decreasing the length of hospitalization following surgery, through techniques decreasing morbidity, complication rates, and the need for inpatient acute convalescence. Laparoscopic surgeries are gaining wider acceptability in patients with IBD, although inherent difficulties from Crohn's-related abscesses, inflammatory masses, and enteric fistulae limit the opportunities to utilize a laparascopic approach *(42,49–53)*. Many cases are "laparoscopic-assisted" procedures, requiring small abdominal incisions. Initial studies of the impact upon hospitalization length and postoperative recovery times have had mixed results *(52,54)*, although it is anticipated that as these procedures achieve wider use and as surgeons gain more experience in performing laparoscopic IBD surgery that the times will shorten and cost-saving realized.

Changes in the techniques of administration of anesthesia from the use of traditional general anesthetics to epidural administration also may result in decreased postoperative recovery time and duration of hospitalization *(55,56)*, although one study showed a net 14% *increase* in charges when compared to narcotic injections *(57)*.

INDIRECT COSTS AND DISABILITY

Indirect costs, including the costs associated with disability, missed work or school, time spent with family, and so on, have been increasingly recognized as an important contributor to the overall costs of disease. In fact, in IBD, indirect costs may account for the lion's share of overall costs. A Swedish study of the impact of IBD upon indirect costs found that 68% of overall costs are indirect (approx equally caused by sick leave and early retirement) *(58)*. Among direct costs, 58% were due to hospitalizations, similar to the North American data *(7,8)*. Sick leave was more common in CD patients (0.39 per prevalent patient) than UC (0.09), with a mean duration of 45 d. The incidence of early retirement (1994 data) was 2.5 per 100,000, with an average duration of 14 yr, with 1% of CD and 0.03% of UC patients receiving early pensions.

The impact of disability was studied in West German patients, where high rates of disability were reported in young persons, disproportionately so in women (CD only) and in white-collar workers (both CD and UC) *(59)*. These findings were echoed in results from a Scottish study of the impact of juvenile onset of IBD upon education and future employment. Fifty percent of the UC and sixty percent of the CD patients reported an adverse impact of their disease upon their education. Significant work-time loss caused by their illness was claimed by 74% and 70%, respectively *(60)*.

The Hays' studies *(2,3)* estimated that 5–10% of IBD patients are disabled from working annually, although their results were an adaptation of the results reported in various other studies, mostly Scandinavian. The estimated annual cost to the U.S. system ranged from $400 to $800 million (1990 dollars). It is anticipated that infliximab's efficacy in clinical outcomes and quality of life evaluations will translate into decreased disability associated with CD, and perhaps substantial savings of indirect costs.

QUALITY OF LIFE

Quality of life is an important outcome in IBD. The unique characteristics of these diseases, which are often diagnosed at a relatively young age, follow a chronic, relapsing course, yet with a normal life expectancy, results in patients needing to balance their disease along with the other demands upon their life and lifestyle. Unlike other diseases, where patient quality of life scores generally parallel disability directly caused by their disease, these individuals have not shown such consistency with physical outcomes. In studies that compare these patients to HMO controls, IBD patients have significant functional impairment in work, sleep, recreation, social interaction, and emotional behavior, whereas physical dysfunction was not significantly different. This is in contrast to patients who underwent hip replacement surgery or patients with rheumatoid arthritis, where quality of life limitations are more weighted toward the physical function *(61)*.

Quality of life in CD patients has been shown to be worse than in healthy controls *(61–63)*, often worse than in patients with UC *(61,64)*, and directly related to disease activity *(62,65,66)*. UC patients also show greater impairment than HMO controls *(61)*, and a direct relationship between quality of life and disease activity *(65,67)*. Issues of greatest concern include the need for an ostomy bag, the effects of medications, fear of surgery, and the uncertain nature of their disease *(68)*. Emotional and social functioning components of quality of life scales are often lower than the physical components, owing to issues such as body image and adaptation to a stoma *(61,69)*.

Many pharmacological studies now include formalized quality of life analyses. Improvement in health-related quality of life has been shown in patients treated with agents such as mesalamine *(70,71)*, infliximab *(20,72)*, cyclosporin *(9)*, methotrexate *(73)*, and budesonide *(74)*. In fact, there is some debate that formalized quality of life scales may be more accurate than traditional disease activity scores in the overall assessment of patient response to therapy.

CONCLUSIONS

The economics of IBD must be well understood before one can determine what interventions have the potential to be truly cost-saving. The temptation to conclude that the high-cost medications will result in sky-rocketing costs must be tempered by the evidence that surgical and hospitalization costs account for the vast majority of overall direct costs, raising the possibility of cost-savings as a result of better disease control. Innovations in surgical and anesthetic techniques have the potential to substantially decrease costs associated with these same areas, resulting in further cost savings. The potential of medical and surgical care upon improving quality of life and decreasing disease morbidity and the associated indirect costs may have the greatest impact of all of these factors upon the economics of IBD.

REFERENCES

1. Cohen RD. The cost of Crohn's disease: drugs or surgery? BioDrugs 2000; 14:331–44.
2. Hay JW, Hay AR. Inflammatory bowel disease: costs-of-illness. J Clin Gastroenterol 1992;14:309–317.

3. Hay AR, Hay JW. Inflammatory bowel disease: medical cost algorithms. J Clin Gastroenterol 1992;14:318–327.
4. Hanauer SB, Cohen RD, Becker RV, 3rd, Larson LR, Vreeland MG. Advances in the management of Crohn's disease: economic and clinical potential of infliximab. Clin Ther 1998;20:1009–1028.
5. Feagan BG, Vreeland MG, Larson LR, Bala MV. Annual cost of care for Crohn's disease: a payor perspective. Am J Gastroenterol 2000;95:1955–1960.
6. Rubenstein JH, Chong RY, Cohen RD. Infliximab decreases resource use among patients with Crohn's disease. J Clin Gastroenterol 2002;35:151–156.
7. Cohen RD, Larson LR, Roth JR, Becker RV, Mummert MM. The cost of hospitalizations in Crohn's disease. Am J Gastroenterol 2000;95:524–530.
8. Bernstein CN, Papineau N, Zajaczkowski J, Rawsthorne P, Okrusko G, Blanchard JF. Direct hospital costs for patients with inflammatory bowel disease in a Canadian tertiary care university hospital. Am J Gastroenterol 2000;95:677–683.
9. Cohen RD, Brodsky AL, Hanauer SB. A comparison of the quality of life in patients with severe ulcerative colitis after total colectomy versus medical treatment with intravenous cyclosporin. Inflamm Bowel Dis 1999;5:1–10.
10. Feagan BG. Methotrexate treatment for Crohn's disease. Inflamm Bowel Dis 1998;4:120–121.
11. Singleton JW, Hanauer SB, Gitnick GL, Peppercorn MA, Robinson MG, Wruble LD, Krawitt EL. Mesalamine capsules for the treatment of active Crohn's disease: results of a 16-week trial. Pentasa Crohn's Disease Study Group. Gastroenterology 1993;104:1293–1301.
12. Candy S, Wright J, Gerber M, Adams G, Gerig M, Goodman R. A controlled double blind study of azathioprine in the management of Crohn's disease. Gut 1995;37:674–678.
13. Korelitz BI, Adler DJ, Mendelsohn RA, Sacknoff AL. Long-term experience with 6-mercaptopurine in the treatment of Crohn's disease. Am J Gastroenterol 1993;88:1198–1205.
14. Cohen RD, Hanauer SB. Immunomodulatory agents and other medical therapies in inflammatory bowel disease. Curr Op Gastroenterol 1995;11:321–330.
15. Kornbluth A, Lichtiger S, Present D, Hanauer S. Long-term results of oral cyclosporin in patients with severe ulcerative colitis: a double-blind, randomized, multi-center trial. Gastroenterology 1994;106:A714.
16. Tremaine WJ, Schroeder KW, Harrison JM, Zinsmeister AR. A randomized, double-blind, placebo-controlled trial of the oral mesalamine (5-ASA) preparation, Asacol, in the treatment of symptomatic Crohn's colitis and ileocolitis. J Clin Gastroenterol 1994;19:278–282.
17. Messori A, Brignola C, Trallori G, Rampazzo R, Bardazzi G, Belloli C, d'Albasio G, De Simone G, Martini N. Effectiveness of 5-aminosalicylic acid for maintaining remission in patients with Crohn's disease: a meta-analysis. Am J Gastroenterol 1994;89:692–698.
18. Sutherland L, Singleton J, Sessions J, Hanauer S, Krawitt E, Rankin G, Summers R, Mekhjian H, Greenberger N, Kelly M, et al. Double blind, placebo controlled trial of metronidazole in Crohn's disease. Gut 1991;32:1071–1075.
19. Peppercorn MA. Is there a role for antibiotics as primary therapy in Crohn's ileitis? J Clin Gastroenterol 1993;17:235–237.
20. Rutgeerts P, D'Haens G, Targan S, Vasiliauskas E, Hanauer SB, Present DH, Mayer L, Van Hogezand RA, Braakman T, DeWoody KL, Schaible TF, Van Deventer SJ. Efficacy and safety of retreatment with anti-tumor necrosis factor antibody (infliximab) to maintain remission in Crohn's disease. Gastroenterology 1999;117:761–769.

21. Cohen RD, Woseth DM, Thisted RA, Hanauer SB. A meta-analysis and overview of the literature on treatment options for left-sided ulcerative colitis and ulcerative proctitis. Am J Gastroenterol 2000;95:1263–1276.
22. Average Wholesale Prices (AWP). Vol. 2000: McKesson Wholesaler Computer Database.
23. Beck JR, Pauker SG. The Markov process in medical prognosis. Med Decis Making 1983;3:419–458.
24. Inadomi J, Sonnenberg A. Cost-analysis of prophylactic antibiotics in spontaneous bacterial peritonitis. Gastroenterology 1997;113:1289–1294.
25. Silverstein MD, Albert DA, Hadler NM, Ropes MW. Prognosis in SLE: comparison of Markov model to life table analysis. J Clin Epidemiol 1988;41:623–633.
26. Silverstein MD, Loftus EV, Sandborn WJ, Tremaine WJ, Feagan BG, Nietert PJ,et al. Clinical course and costs of care for Crohn's disease: Markov model analysis of a population-based cohort. Gastroenterology 1999;117:49–57.
27. Korelitz B, Hanauer S, Rutgeerts P, Present D, Peppercorn M. Post-operative prophylaxis with 6-MP, 5-ASA, or placebo in Crohn's disease: a 2 year multicenter trial. Gastroenterology 1998;114:A1011.
28. Lochs H, Mayer M, Fleig WE, Mortensen PB, Bauer P, Genser D, Petritsch W, Raithel M, Hoffmann R, Gross V, Plauth M, Staun M, Nesje LB. Prophylaxis of postoperative relapse in Crohn's disease with mesalamine: European Cooperative Crohn's Disease Study VI. Gastroenterology 2000;118:264–273.
29. Camma C, Giunta M, Rosselli M, Cottone M. Mesalamine in the maintenance treatment of Crohn's disease: a meta-analysis adjusted for confounding variables. Gastroenterology 1997;113:1465–1473.
30. Caprilli R, Andreoli A, Capurso L, Corrao G, D'Albasio G, Gioieni A, et al. Oral mesalazine (5-aminosalicylic acid;Asacol) for the prevention of post-operative recurrence of Crohn's disease. Gruppo Italiano per lo Studio del Colon e del Retto (GISC). Aliment Pharmacol Ther 1994;8:35–43.
31. Rutgeerts P, Hiele M, Geboes K, Peeters M, Penninckx F, Aerts R, Kerremans R. Controlled trial of metronidazole treatment for prevention of Crohn's recurrence after ileal resection. Gastroenterology 1995;108:1617–1621.
32. De Dombal FT, Burton I, Goligher JC. Recurrence of Crohn's disease after primary excisional surgery. Gut 1971;12:519–527.
33. Farmer RG, Whelan G, Fazio VW. Long-term follow-up of patients with Crohn's disease. Relationship between the clinical pattern and prognosis. Gastroenterology 1985;88:1818–1825.
34. Sachar DB. Patterns of postoperative recurrence in Crohn's disease. Scand J Gastroenterol-Supplement 1990;172:35–38.
35. Kornbluth A, Sachar DB, Salomon P. Crohn's Disease. In: Sleisenger, Fordtran, eds. Gastrointestinal and Liver Disease: Pathophysiology, Diagnosis, Management. Saunders, Philadelphia, PA,1993:1270 –1304.
36. Greenstein AJ, Sachar DB, Pasternack BS, Janowitz HD. Reoperation and recurrence in Crohn's colitis and ileocolitis: Crude and cumulative rates. N Engl J Med 1975;293:685–690.
37. Sachar DB, Wolfson DM, Greenstein AJ, Goldberg J, Styczynski R, Janowitz HD. Risk factors for postoperative recurrence of Crohn's disease. Gastroenterology 1983;85:917–21.
38. Farmer RG, Easley KA, Rankin GB. Clinical patterns, natural history, and progression of ulcerative colitis. a long-term follow-up of 1116 patients. Dig Dis Sci 1993;38:1137–1146.
39. Lichtiger S, Present DH, Kornbluth A, Gelernt I, Bauer J, Galler G, Michelassi F, Hanauer S. Cyclosporine in severe ulcerative colitis refractory to steroid therapy. N Engl J Med 1994;330:1841–5.

40. Cohen RD, Stein R, Hanauer SB. Intravenous cyclosporin in ulcerative colitis: a five-year experience. Am J Gastroenterol1999;94:1587–1592.

41. Hurst RD, Molinari M, Chung TP, Rubin M, Michelassi F. Prospective study of the incidence, timing and treatment of pouchitis in 104 consecutive patients after restorative proctocolectomy. Arch Surg 1996;131:497–500.

42. Hurst RD, Cohen RD. The role of laparoscopy and strictureplasty in the management of inflammatory bowel disease. In: Lichtenstein GR, ed. Seminars in Gastrointestinal Disease. Inflammatory Bowel Disease. Vol. 11. Philadelphia: W.B. Saunders Company, 2000:10–17.

43. Fazio VW, Galandiuk S, Jagelman DG, Lavery IC. Strictureplasty in Crohn's disease. Ann Surg 1989;210:621–625.

44. Hurst RD, Michelassi F. Strictureplasty for Crohn's disease: techniques and long-term results. World J Surg 1998;22:359–363.

45. Michelassi F. Side-to-side isoperistaltic strictureplasty for multiple Crohn's strictures. Dis Colon Rectum 1996;39:345–349.

46. Fazio VW, Tjandra JJ, Lavery IC, Church JM, Milsom JW, Oakley JR. Long-term follow-up of strictureplasty in Crohn's disease. Dis Colon Rectum 1993;36:355–361.

47. Ozuner G, Fazio VW, Lavery IC, Milsom JW, Strong SA. Reoperative rates for Crohn's disease following strictureplasty. Long-term analysis. Dis Colon Rectum 1996;39:1199–203.

48. Serra J, Cohen Z, McLeod RS. Natural history of strictureplasty in Crohn's disease: 9-year experience. Can J Surg 1995;38:481–485.

49. Reissman P, Salky BA, Edye M, Wexner SD. Laparoscopic surgery in Crohn's disease. Indications and results. Surg Endosc 1996;10:1201–1203.

50. Ludwig KA, Milsom JW, Church JM, Fazio VW. Preliminary experience with laparoscopic intestinal surgery for Crohn's disease. Am J Surg 1996;171:52–55;discussion 55–6.

51. Liu CD, Rolandelli R, Ashley SW, Evans B, Shin M, McFadden DW. Laparoscopic surgery for inflammatory bowel disease. Am Surg 1995;61:1054–1056.

52. Chen HH, Wexner SD, Weiss EG, Nogueras JJ, Alabaz O, Iroatulam AJ, et al. Laparoscopic colectomy for benign colorectal disease is associated with a significant reduction in disability as compared with laparotomy. Surg Endosc 1998;12:1397–1400.

53. Wu JS, Birnbaum EH, Kodner IJ, Fry RD, Read TE, Fleshman JW. Laparoscopic-assisted ileocolic resections in patients with Crohn's disease: are abscesses, phlegmons, or recurrent disease contraindications? Surgery 1997;122:682–688.

54. Fleshman JW. Invited Editorial. Disease of the Colon and Rectum 1997;40:238–239.

55. Scott AM, Starling JR, Ruscher AE, DeLessio ST, Harms BA. Thoracic versus lumbar epidural anesthesia's effect on pain control and ileus resolution after restorative proctocolectomy. Surgery 1996;120:688–695.

56. Grass JA. The role of epidural anesthesia and analgesia in postoperative outcome. Anesthesiol Clin North America 2000;18:407–428, viii.

57. Welch JP, Cohen JL, Vignati PV, Allen LW, Morrow JS, Carter JJ. Pain control following elective gastrointestinal surgery: is epidural anesthesia warranted? Conn Med 1998;62:461–464.

58. Blomqvist P, Ekbom A. Inflammatory bowel diseases: health care and costs in Sweden in 1994. Scand J Gastroenterol 1997;32:1134–1139.

59. Sonnenberg A. Disability from inflammatory bowel disease among employees in West Germany. Gut 1989;30:367–370.

60. Ferguson A, Sedgwick DM. Juvenile-onset inflammatory bowel disease: predictors of morbidity and health status in early adult life. J R Coll Physicians Lond 1994;28:220–227.

61. Drossman DA, Patrick DL, Mitchell CM, Zagami EA, Appelbaum MI. Health-related quality of life in inflammatory bowel disease. Functional status and patient worries and concerns. Dig Dis Sci 1989;34:1379–1386.
62. Casellas F, Lopez-Vivancos J, Badia X, Vilaseca J, Malagelada JR. Impact of surgery for Crohn's disease on health-related quality of life. Am J Gastroenterol 2000;95:177–182.
63. Love JR, Irvine EJ, Fedorak RN. Quality of life in inflammatory bowel disease. J Clin Gastroenterol 1992;14:15–19.
64. Farmer RG, Easley KA, Farmer JM. Quality of life assessment by patients with inflammatory bowel disease. Cleve Clin J Med 1992;59:35–42.
65. Irvine EJ, Feagan B, Rochon J, Archambault A, Fedorak RN, Groll A, Kinnear D, Saibil F, McDonald JW. Quality of life: a valid and reliable measure of therapeutic efficacy in the treatment of inflammatory bowel disease. Canadian Crohn's Relapse Prevention Trial Study Group. Gastroenterology 1994;106:287–296.
66. Drossman DA, Li Z, Leserman J, Patrick DL. Ulcerative colitis and Crohn's disease health status scales for research and clinical practice. J Clin Gastroenterol 1992;15:104–112.
67. Hjortswang H, Strom M, Almer S. Health-related quality of life in Swedish patients with ulcerative colitis. Am J Gastroenterol 1998;93:2203–2211.
68. Moser G, Tillinger W, Sachs G, Genser D, Maier-Dobersberger T, Spiess K, Wyatt J, Vogelsang H, Lochs H, Gangl A. Disease-related worries and concerns: a study on out-patients with inflammatory bowel disease. Eur J Gastroenterol Hepatol 1995;7:853–858.
69. Meyers S, Walfish JS, Sachar DB, Greenstein AJ, Hill AG, Janowitz HD. Quality of life after surgery for Crohn's disease: a psychosocial survey. Gastroenterology 1980;78:1–6.
70. Robinson M, Hanauer S, Hoop R, Zbrozek A, Wilkinson C. Mesalamine capsules enhance the quality of life for patients with ulcerative colitis. Aliment Pharmacol Ther 1994;8:27–34.
71. Singleton JW, Hanauer S, Robinson M. Quality-of-life results of double-blind, placebo-controlled trial of mesalamine in patients with Crohn's disease. Dig Dis Sci 1995;40:931–935.
72. Hanauer SB, Feagan BG, Lichtenstein GR, Mayer LF, Schreiber S, Colombel JF, Rachmilewitz D, Wolf DC, Olson A, Bao W, Rutgeerts P, Group atAIS. Maintenance infliximab for Crohn's disease: the ACCENT I randomised trial. Lancet 2002;359:1541–1549.
73. Feagan BG, Rochon J, Fedorak RN, Irvine EJ, Wild G, Sutherland L, et al. Methotrexate for the treatment of Crohn's disease. The North American Crohn's Study Group Investigators. N Engl J Med 1995;332:292–297.
74. Irvine EJ, Greenberg GR, Feagan BG, Martin F, Sutherland LR, Thomson AB,. Quality of life rapidly improves with budesonide therapy for active Crohn's disease. Canadian Inflammatory Bowel Disease Study Group. Inflamm Bowel Dis 2000;6:181–187.

17 Pathologic Features of Inflammatory Bowel Disease

John Hart, MD

Contents

INTRODUCTION

The diagnosis of an idiopathic inflammatory bowel disease (IBD), ulcerative colitis or Crohn's disease, cannot be made reliably without pathologic examination of biopsy and/or surgical specimens. On the other hand, there are no histologic features that are by themselves diagnostically specific for either of these diseases. It is therefore obvious that optimal patient management requires close interaction between the treating clinician and the surgical pathologist. Nevertheless, in day-to-day practice, communication between these parties is often minimal, often only a few terse words jotted on a requisition form accompanying the specimen to be interpreted. This commonly produces frustration and dissatisfaction on both sides, and can hinder the diagnostic process. This chapter summarizes the key pathologic features of Crohn's colitis and ulcerative colitis and highlights areas in which optimal clinical practice can aid in the pathologic assessment of biopsy material. Several excellent chapters discuss these issues in a more comprehensive fashion *(1–3)*.

From: *Clinical Gastroenterology:*
Inflammatory Bowel Disease: Diagnosis and Therapeutics
Edited by: R. D. Cohen © Humana Press Inc., Totowa, NJ

BIOPSY DIAGNOSIS OF IBD

General Considerations

The histologic hallmarks of IBD are distortion of the normal crypt architecture and the presence of mixed inflammatory cell infiltrates in the lamina propria. The presence of both of these features, in the proper clinical context, is almost always a result of either ulcerative colitis or Crohn's disease. Differentiating between these two diseases requires the evaluation of a number of additional histologic features, as discussed in the following.

In normal colonic mucosa, the crypts are arranged in straight and evenly spaced rows, akin to test tubes in a rack. Even in the initial attack of IBD, with symptoms of short duration, biopsies of involved segments will usually exhibit distortion of this normal crypt architecture *(4–6)*. This is typically manifested by scattered branched and irregularly shaped crypts, as well as crypts that no longer extend all of the way down to the muscularis mucosae. It is much easier for the surgical pathologist to evaluate crypt architecture in well-oriented biopsies. In histologic sections of poorly oriented biopsies, the crypts are usually seen in cross section as doughnut-shaped profiles, making it difficult to evaluate branching and foreshortening. Biopsies that include strands of the muscularis mucosae are much easier to orient by the endoscopist's assistant or histology technician.

A feature often associated with crypt architectural distortion is the presence of Paneth cell metaplasia. Paneth cells are normally present in the mucosa throughout the small intestine but in the colon are limited to the mucosa of the cecum and ascending colon. In IBD, Paneth cells may appear in the more distal colon, and their presence is a good marker of chronic colitis. In patients with inactive disease of very long duration, crypt architectural distortion may become very subtle, to the point where the histologic (and endoscopic) appearance may be indistinguishable from normal. In this situation, review of biopsies obtained during previous colonoscopic procedures may be necessary to confirm a diagnosis of IBD.

Normal colonic mucosa consists of surface and crypt epithelium between which lies a mixture of inflammatory cells, including lymphocytes, plasma cells, eosinophils, and macrophages. Neutrophils, on the other hand, are not normally present, and if seen in significant numbers, indicate that active colitis is present. Rare, scattered neutrophils, particularly when limited to the surface epithelium and superficial lamina propria, can occur simply as a result of oral bowel preparation agents or enemas. To prevent the over-diagnosis of colitis, the use of such agents should be made known to the surgical pathologist. The degree of neutrophilic inflammation is an indication of disease activity. The infiltration of neutrophils between crypt epithelial cells is known as "cryptitis". When neutrophils completely transverse the crypt epithelium and accumulate within crypt lumens, the term "crypt abscess" is applied (Fig. 1). When effective medical therapy is instituted, the neutrophilic inflammation resolves first, followed by the lymphoplasmacytic infiltrates. During periods of disease quiescence, there may be no discernible increase in the number of lamina propria inflammatory cells, and the only residual histologic evidence of disease would be the distorted crypt architecture and Paneth cell metaplasia (Fig. 2).

Biopsy Diagnosis of Ulcerative Colitis vs Crohn's Colitis

As mentioned in the introductory comments, histologic distinction between ulcerative colitis and Crohn's disease can be quite difficult in some patients. The best discriminating feature is the presence of epithelioid granulomas (Fig. 3), which are highly characteristic of Crohn's disease *(7)*. Unfortunately, granulomas can be identified in biopsy specimens in less than 50% of Crohn's patients, limiting the utility of this feature. Granulomas can occur in association with ruptured crypt abscesses in ulcerative colitis, presumably in response to extravasated mucin (Figs. 4A and B).

The presence of skip areas of normal mucosa is also considered to be a specific feature of Crohn's disease. This may take the form of a segment of normal colon between two affected portions, or the presence of normal epithelium adjacent to epithelium exhibiting colitis in a single biopsy. Aphthous erosion or ulceration occurring in a background of normal mucosa represents the prototypic example of a skip lesion (Figs. 5A and B). (It should be noted that the resolution of the latest generation of colonoscopies is such that normal lymphoid aggregates may be confused with small aphthous erosions, leading to an apparent discrepancy between endoscopic and histologic findings.)

In the relatively recent era of routine colonoscopy and effective medical therapy for IBD, it has become clear that healing ulcerative colitis can appear quite patchy endoscopically, simulating the appearance of Crohn's colitis. Fortunately, microscopic examination of these apparent "skip areas" of endoscopically normal mucosa in patients with treated ulcerative colitis usually reveals evidence of quiescent disease, as indicated by the presence of (sometimes subtle) crypt architectural distortion. However, patchy areas of completely normal mucosa have been documented in longstanding ulcerative colitis *(7)*.

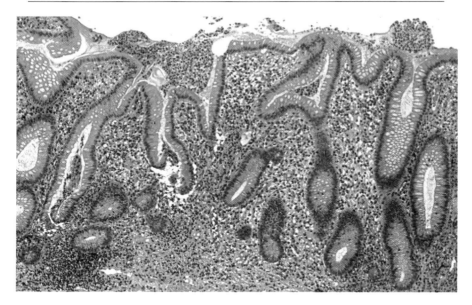

Fig. 1. Active ulcerative colitis. Note the distortion of normal crypt architecture, with branched crypts, and diffuse neutrophilic infiltrates, including a crypt abscess.

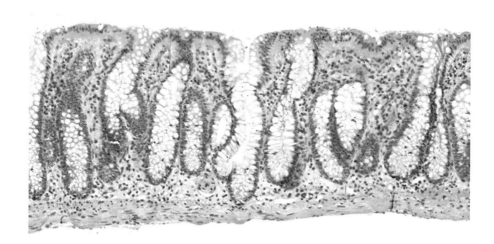

Fig. 2. Quiescent ulcerative colitis. There is marked crypt architectural distortion but no neutrophilic infiltrates. The lymphoplasmacytic infiltrates have also resolved.

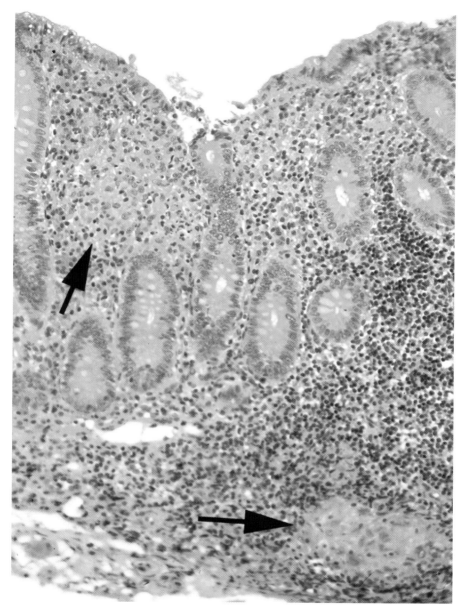

Fig. 3. Crohn's colitis. Two granulomas are evident within the lamina propria.

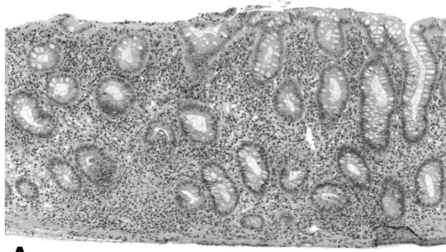

A

Fig. 4. Ulcerative colitis. (**A**) Low-power view demonstrating mild crypt architectural distortion, basal lymphoplasmacytic infiltrates, and diffuse neutrophilic infiltrates. (**B**) (*Opposite page*) High-power of the same biopsy revealing a granuloma adjacent to a ruptured crypt.

Transmural disease is another characteristic feature of Crohn's disease, but of course this feature cannot be assessed in endoscopic biopsy specimens. Inflammation can extend into the submucosa (or even deeper) in active ulcerative colitis, so the presence of inflammatory cells in the superficial portion of submucosa sometimes included in a biopsy specimen cannot automatically be assumed to be diagnostic of Crohn's disease. However, in ulcerative colitis, the inflammation of the overlying mucosa is always more severe than that of the submucosa. Therefore, a biopsy that exhibits marked inflammation of the superficial submucosa, with relatively little active inflammation in the overlying mucosa, would suggest a diagnosis of Crohn's colitis.

There are additional histologic features which, while not diagnostic, can be helpful in favoring a diagnosis of either ulcerative colitis or Crohn's colitis. For instance, the degree of crypt architectural distortion tends to be greater in ulcerative colitis. Thus, biopsies from ulcerative colitis patients often reveal significant mucosal atrophy with numerous branched crypts and marked alteration of the normal parallel arrangement of the crypts. Biopsies from patients with Crohn's colitis, in contrast, may exhibit only mild crypt architectural distortion with relatively

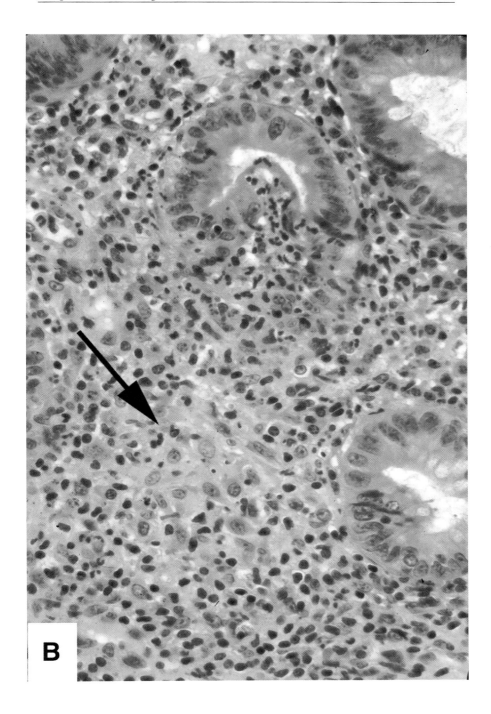

B

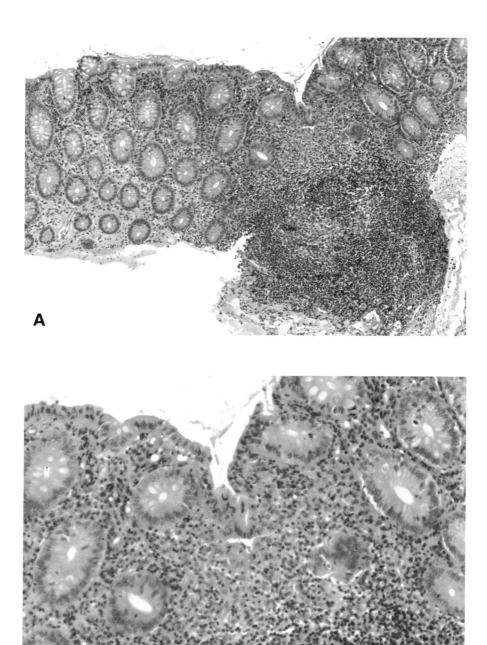

Fig. 5. Early Crohn's colitis. (A) Low-power view showing a lymphoid follicle. (B) High-power of the same biopsy reveals an early aphthous erosion, with focal neutrophilic infiltrate directly over the lymphoid follicle.

little atrophy. Moreover, biopsies from patents with active ulcerative colitis usually exhibit significant depletion of the normal mucin content of the crypt epithelial cells, while the mucin is often relatively preserved in active Crohn's disease *(7)*. Unfortunately there is considerable overlap in these features in biopsies from ulcerative colitis and Crohn's colitis patients, and their assessment is also subjective.

One can also take advantage of the fact that Crohn's disease can affect any portion of the gastrointestinal tract, while ulcerative colitis is essentially limited to the colon. Biopsies of the terminal ileum may reveal significant ileitis in some patients with Crohn's disease. The histologic features of Crohn's ileitis are essentially identical to those evident in colonic biopsies (Fig. 6). Although some ulcerative colitis patients with pancolitis may exhibit so-called "backwash ileitis," histologic assessment usually can allow distinction from Crohn's ileitis. Backwash ileitis generally consists only of scattered neutrophils in the lamina propria and surface epithelium, with relative preservation of the mucosal architecture. In Crohn's ileitis there is usually marked distortion of normal villous architecture at least focally, and the degree of active inflammation is often greater as well. Of course biopsies of the upper gastrointestinal tract may also be quite helpful in making a diagnosis of Crohn's disease if involvement can be documented. Even biopsies of endoscopically normal mucosa can reveal evidence of Crohn's disease (e.g., granulomas and focal inflammatory cell infiltrates).

Histologic Distinction Between IBD and Other Forms of Colitis

The histologic features of a number of other forms of colitis can overlap with those described previously for IBD. Definitive distinction usually requires correlation with the clinical history, laboratory test results and colonoscopic features. Depending on the amount of this clinical data made available to the pathologist, a firm histologic diagnosis of IBD may be possible in some cases, while in others only a differential diagnosis can be given. The histologic appearance of each form of colitis is discussed in the following, emphasizing features most useful in differentiating from IBD.

INFECTIOUS COLITIS

Most enteric bacteria (e.g., *Escherichia coli*, *Salmonella*, *Shigella*, *Yersinia*, and *Campylobacter*) produce a nonspecific form of colitis, which in the past has been termed "acute self-limited colitis." Histologically there are neutrophilic infiltrates in the lamina propria, and in more severe cases, there may be foci of cryptitis and crypt abscesses. These

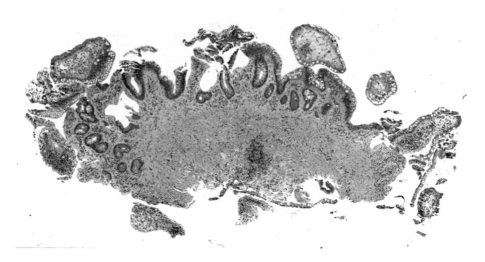

Fig. 6. Crohn's ileitis. There is prominent distortion of normal villous architecture.

features are quite similar to those of IBD, although in infectious colitis the neutrophilic infiltrates tend to be more superficial (Fig. 7). The key features in terms of distinction from IBD are the maintenance of normal crypt architecture and the lack of a basal lymphoplasmacytic infiltrate *(6,8,9)*. However, these two histologic findings are difficult to assess in poorly oriented biopsies. The inflammatory changes in infectious colitis may be patchy or diffuse, so this diagnosis must be considered in the differential with both ulcerative colitis and Crohn's colitis. Gram stains performed on biopsy specimens are not useful since luminal bacteria are abundant in health. Instead, confirmation of the diagnosis requires a positive stool culture, which is obtained in only a minority of cases. Without a positive stool culture, presumptive diagnosis rests on the self-limited clinical course or the resolution of symptoms with antibiotic therapy.

Colitis owing to *E. coli O:157H7* infection is histologically more distinctive, most often being right-sided and prominently hemorrhagic. Severe cases may be transmural and can be clinically confused with Crohn's disease. Stool cultures must be specifically sent for *E. coli O:157H7* and may be negative unless obtained soon after the onset of symptoms *(10,11)*. Colitis owing to *Entamoeba histolytica* infection is often segmental and may be transmural, closely simulating Crohn's disease clinically *(12)*. Stool ova and pararsites (O & P) examination

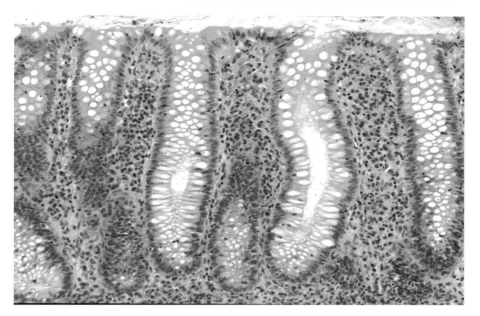

Fig. 7. Infectious colitis. Normal crypt architecture is well maintained. Scattered neutrophils are evident within the superficial lamina propria. A stool culture grew *Campylobacter jejuni.*

is usually diagnostic, although multiple specimens may need to be examined. If colon biopsies are obtained from the edge of an ulcer, the trophozoites can be seen within acute inflammatory cell exudate or necrotic debris, and highlighted with a PAS stain. Clinical suspicion of *E. histolytica* infection should be reported to the surgical pathologist so that a special effort is made to find the organism, which may be sparse.

Ischemic Colitis

While histologically distinctive, acute ischemic colitis may clinically and colonoscopically be confused with IBD. When patchy, particularly if focal ulceration develops, ischemic colitis can resemble Crohn's colitis. Segmental left-sided ischemic colitis has been described in young women and has been associated with the use of oral contraceptives *(13)*. Ischemia may not be considered clinically in these patients because of their young age and atypical disease distribution. Fortunately the histologic features of acute ischemic colitis are quite characteristic. There are only very minimal neutrophilic infiltrates, limited to areas of erosion or ulceration, and lymphoplasmacytic infiltrates are

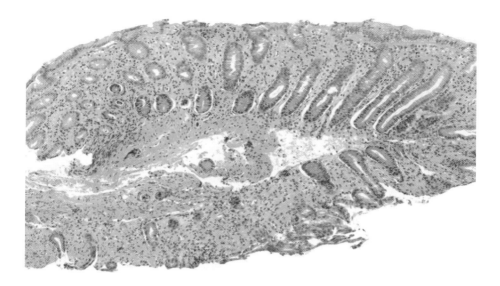

Fig. 8. Acute ischemic colitis. Normal crypt architecture is maintained, although detachment of the surface epithelium and withering of the superficial portions of the crypts is evident. Also note the lack of significant inflammatory cell infiltrates and the deposition of pinkish proteinaceous material in the lamina propria.

never present. Ischemia preferentially produces damage to the superficial portion of the mucosa, a pattern not seen in IBD. Hemorrhage and deposits of proteinaceous material within the lamina propria are also characteristic of acute ischemia and are not seen in IBD (Fig. 8).

Chronic ischemic colitis can result in focal ulceration or stricture formation, which can clinically and endoscopically resemble Crohn's disease. Again, ischemia may not be considered clinically because a watershed zone may not be affected. Ischemia owing to thrombosis, emboli, or vasculitis can involve any colonic segment, including so-called protected zones like the cecum and rectum. Biopsies will reveal significant crypt architectural distortion, similar to that seen in IBD, but will also demonstrate prominent lamina propria fibrosis. In addition, the neutrophilic and lymphoplasmacytic infiltrates typical of untreated IBD are never present in chronic ischemic colitis. Nonetheless, focal ulceration owing to chronic ischemia is sometimes misdiagnosed as Crohn's disease by the unwary pathologist and clinician. This is particularly true in cases with cecal involvement (solitary cecal ulceration), where ischemia may be one of several contributing factors (along with uremia, CMV infection, and/or drug toxicity).

NSAID COLITIS

The diagnosis of NSAID colitis is often not considered by either the clinician or pathologist. Patients may not be forthcoming regarding their usage of NSAIDs, and the endoscopist may not directly ask about these agents. The histologic features of NSAID colitis have not been completely documented, and some pathologists may not consider the possibility, particularly if a history of NSAID use is not mentioned in the pathology requisition form. Chronic NSAID use can result in the formation of a focal ulcer or stricture, and therefore a diagnosis of Crohn's colitis might be entertained *(14)*. NSAIDs can also produce diffuse mild colitis, which can be confused with ulcerative colitis colonoscopically *(15,16)*. Histologic examination reveals mild neutrophilic infiltrates, but maintenance of normal crypt architecture and an absence of a lymphoplasmacytic infiltrate in the lamina propria, ruling out IBD. In addition, there may be a patchy thickening of the subepithelial collagen layer, similar to that seen in collagenous colitis. However, the absence of a significant increase in intra-epithelial lymphocytes, the presence of colitis colonoscopically, and the absence of a history of chronic watery diarrhea eliminates collagenous colitis as diagnostic consideration.

OTHER FORMS OF COLITIS

Chronic radiation colitis and chronic graft vs host disease both produce crypt architectural distortion and therefore could be theoretical in histologic differential diagnosis of treated IBD. The clinical history would obviously be important in these cases, and there are other histologic features of these conditions that are helpful in arriving at the correct diagnosis. Drugs other than NSAIDs can rarely cause colitis and must be considered in problematic cases. Distal colitis can also be produced factitciously by the instillation of toxic agents via enema.

FULMINANT IBD AND INDETERMINANT IBD

Although a more common complication of ulcerative colitis, fulminant colitis and toxic megacolon can also occur in Crohn's disease or as a complication of various infections (*Shigella*, *Salmonella*, *Campylobacter*, and *Clostridium*) *(3)*. Unfortunately, many of the histologic features characteristic of either ulcerative colitis or Crohn's disease cannot be evaluated because of the presence of very severe inflammation and necrosis. Typically a colon affected by fulminant colitis exhibits confluent areas of deep ulceration. The remaining mucosa is severely congested, friable, and hemorrhagic. Ulceration often extends into the muscularis propria and sections from these areas may show inflammatory cells extending into the serosa. This transmural inflammation is merely a reflection of the severity of the acute disease and should not by itself prompt a diagnosis of Crohn's colitis. On the other hand, lymphoid aggregates in the muscularis propria or serosal tissues away from areas of deep ulceration are consistent with Crohn's colitis. Often in cases of fulminant ulcerative colitis, the mucosa of the rectum is grossly less affected in comparison with the sigmoid area, leading to a false impression of Crohn's colitis. However, histologic sections will show crypt architectural distortion, consistent with involvement by ulcerative colitis. In some cases, a diagnosis of indeterminate colitis must be rendered if no specific features of ulcerative colitis or Crohn's disease can be recognized. Of course, if the patient has a firm history of either ulcerative colitis or Crohn's colitis before the onset of the fulminant episode, then there is no reason to change the diagnosis to indeterminate colitis for the colectomy specimen. The problematic situation arises only in patients in whom an established diagnosis has not already been made.

Considerable confusion regarding the term indeterminate colitis has developed because it has been used in several different clinical and pathologic contexts. Endoscopists sometimes use the term when the findings observed are not specific for either ulcerative colitis or Crohn's colitis. Likewise, some pathologists use the term when the histologic features present in biopsy specimens do not allow clear distinction between the two diseases. It is probably best to restrict the term to those cases in which it is impossible to distinguish between ulcerative colitis and Crohn's disease, despite examination of a colectomy specimen (in a patient without a firm pre-operative diagnosis).

ATYPICAL HISTOLOGIC FEATURES IN ULCERATIVE COLITIS

Some patients with typical left-sided ulcerative colitis exhibit endoscopic and histologic evidence of an additional isolated focus of disease in the cecum, usually taking the form of a patch of inflamed mucosa near the appendiceal orifice and/or ileocecal valve. This so-called "cecal red patch" may be regarded as a skip lesion and therefore a feature favoring Crohn's disease by those not aware of its occurrence in ulcerative colitis (17). Histologic sections from these endoscopically abnormal patches reveal changes typical of mildly active ulcerative colitis, with crypt architectural distortion and mild mixed inflammatory cell infiltrates. It should be remembered, however, that cecal biopsies normally contain more intense lamina propria inflammatory cell infiltrates than are present in biopsies from other parts of the colon. In fact, rare neutrophils may even be present normally in cecal mucosa.

The possibility of patchy disease involvement in ulcerative colitis has already been mentioned. It is now well-documented that intensive medical therapy for symptomatic ulcerative colitis can lead to patchy healing, resulting in an endoscopic impression of skip areas. Biopsies from these endoscopically normal regions, which can include the rectum, may reveal no disease activity, but in most cases crypt architectural distortion is still evident, indicating prior disease involvement. In rare cases, the distortion of crypt architecture may be very subtle or simply not apparent *(18)*. There are also cases in which skip areas of normal mucosa are definitely present from the onset (typically a segment in the transverse or descending colon), and yet all other clinical and histologic features are consistent with the diagnosis of ulcerative colitis. The clinical course in such a patient is almost always that of typical ulcerative colitis.

DYSPLASIA IN IBD

The identification of dysplasia is one of the most important tasks of the pathologist in evaluating colonic biopsies from patients with IBD. Dysplasia is defined as an unequivocal neoplastic change in the colonic epithelium, without invasion past the basement membrane. This premalignant change has been shown to be a useful marker of a high risk for the presence or development of invasive adenocarcinoma, and is the basis of surveillance colonoscopy programs. The diagnostic criteria for the diagnosis of dysplasia were established by an international group of expert pathologists who blindly reviewed a collection of slides showing a range of reactive and dysplastic changes *(19)*. The panel recognized that significant interobserver and intraobserver variation was unavoidable, particularly in the distinction of low grade dysplasia from reactive changes that closely resemble dysplasia. The problem of interobserver variability in the diagnosis of dysplasia has in fact been confirmed in other studies *(20–22)*.

A variety of technical problems can hinder the ability of pathologists to make a reproducible diagnosis of dysplasia. Small, crushed, and poorly oriented biopsies are obviously difficult to interpret. Poor fixation, sectioning, and staining of the biopsies compounds the difficulty. In addition, the presence of marked active inflammation and/or ulceration produces cytologic alterations that closely simulate those seen in dysplasia. Even if large, well-oriented, and properly handled biopsies are obtained and prepared, there are still a variety of interpretational obstacles that prevent a high degree of precision and accuracy in the diagnosis of dysplasia. Dysplasia represents a biologic continuum which has been arbitrarily divided into low-grade and high-grade categories, and there will always be biopsies with features that fall at the dividing points between them. Some pathologists have little experience in diagnosing IBD-associated dysplasia, and therefore may be relatively unfamiliar with the fine points of the grading scheme. Also, in some biopsies there may be discordance between the cytologic and architectural features of dysplasia, or the focus of dysplasia may be extremely small. Clear-cut criteria for proper grading in these circumstances have not been agreed upon. For these reasons, consultation from an expert gastrointestinal pathologist is recommended in difficult cases and in cases where a management decision will be made based on the histologic diagnosis.

Although a variety of more objective markers for the diagnosis of dysplasia have been studied (e.g., flow cytometry for DNA ploidy and immunohistochemistry for Ki-67 and p53 protein), these techniques are not widely available and have not been well validated. There are also a variety of technical and interpretative problems with these techniques (23,24).

The light microscopic diagnosis of dysplasia rests on a combination of cytologic and architectural criteria, and the grade of dysplasia is judged based on the severity of the cytologic and architectural abnormality (19). Cytologic features of dysplasia include: increased nuclear cytoplasmic ratio, nuclear hyperchromasia, and nuclear pleomorphism. Unfortunately these changes are similar in many respects to those of reactive atypia caused by the presence of active inflammation. Architectural features, which are less affected by the presence of neutrophilic infiltrates, include loss of normal cell and nuclear polarity, crowding of glandular profiles, and the presence of cribiforming (back-to-back glands without intervening lamina propria). One key feature of dysplasia is the extension of abnormal cytologic changes from the deep aspects of the crypts all the way to the surface epithelium (Figs. 9 and 10). Optimal evaluation for the presence of this feature naturally requires proper biopsy orientation. One common situation leading to a diagnosis of "indefinite for dysplasia" is the presence of mild cytologic atypia in the deep aspects of the crypts, but without visible extension of these changes to the surface epithelium.

In many cases dysplasia is diagnosed in a random biopsy of mucosa with no distinctive endoscopic appearance. Dysplasia in a biopsy from an endoscopically recognizable lesion or mass (DALM) is of particular concern because the incidence of invasive tumor is much higher (25). Foci of IBD-associated dysplasia that are recognizable grossly are usually described as plaque-like areas of velvety mucosa. Recently there

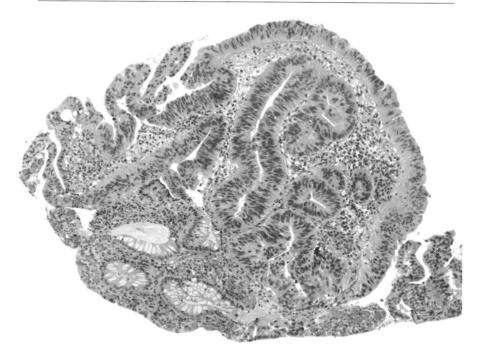

Fig. 9. Ulcerative colitis with low grade dysplasia. Compare the cytologic features of the non-dysplastic epithelium in the lower portion of the biopsy with the dysplastic epithelium above it. Note that the dysplastic changes extend to the surface epithelium at the top of the biopsy.

has been great interest in molecular markers that might allow better distinction between DALMs and sporadic adenomas (unrelated to the underlying history of IBD). Traditionally these two types of lesions have been separated based on clinical criteria, since there are no reliable light microscopic features that distinguish the adenomatous (dysplastic) epithelium of a sporadic adenoma from the adenomatous (dysplastic) epithelium of a DALM. Clinical findings considered to favor a diagnosis of DALM over sporadic adenoma include: age under 40–45 yr, location in a colonic segment affected by IBD, an atypical endoscopic appearance, and the presence of dysplasia in surrounding flat mucosa. Molecular techniques have been used by various investigators to analyze expression of p53, β-catenin, bcl-2, and loss of heterozygosity for p16 and at chromosomes 3p in sporadic adenomas and DALMs *(26–29)*. Significant differences in the expression of these markers have been documented, supporting the contention that both types of lesions may exist in the colons of IBD patients. Unfortunately, there is considerable

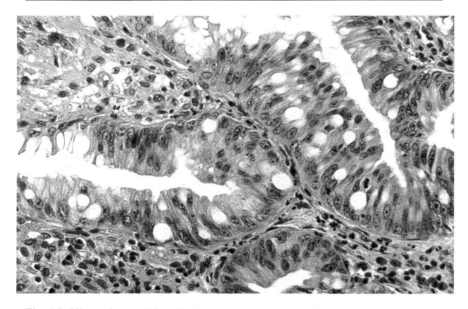

Fig. 10. Ulcerative colitis with high grade dysplasia. There is a greater degree of cytologic atypia in this biopsy that is evident in Fig. 9. The nuclei are greatly enlarged and have very irregular contours. There is also a loss of normal nuclear polarity.

overlap in the incidence of abnormal expression of these markers, making them unsuitable for use in routine clinical practice.

PRACTICAL ENDOSCOPY GUIDELINES

As mentioned in the introductory comments for this chapter, optimal evaluation of endoscopic biopsies from IBD patients is greatly aided by close interaction between the endoscopist and surgical pathologist. A concise and focused summary of the patient's clinical history and a copy of the endoscopic report (or summary of the pertinent findings) can allow the pathologist to move from a purely descriptive report to one that includes an interpretation and often a definitive diagnosis. Orientation of endoscopic biopsies can be very helpful if done properly. Orientation is best performed by the endoscopist or nurse since biopsies are difficult to orient once they have been placed in fixative. Oriented biopsies can be placed on any number of substrates, including millipore filter paper or plain paper towel. The larger the biopsy, the easier it is to orient properly. A dissecting microscopy might be helpful at the outset for training purposes, but its use is time-consuming and unnecessary once experience is gained. Training and feedback from the pathologist on proper orientation technique is very helpful. Proper fixation is also critical to optimal histologic evaluation, but any standard fixative can be used. (Formalin is most commonly used.) It is important that the biopsy is immediately placed in the fixative and not allowed to dry out. The biopsy container should be nearly filled with fixative to ensure that if it is tipped on its side during transport the biopsy remains submerged.

There are a number of indications for colonoscopy in IBD patients, including:

- Initial diagnosis of IBD (ulcerative colitis or Crohn's disease).
- Confirmation of the diagnosis of ulcerative colitis or Crohn's disease.
- Evaluation of the extent and severity of IBD.
- Re-evaluation of the histologic diagnosis of ulcerative colitis or Crohn's disease after new or conflicting clinical data is obtained.
- Surveillance for IBD-associated dysplasia.

The specific steps the endoscopist can take to aid the surgical pathologist depend on which of the above indications pertains to the patient being evaluated. These are outlined separately in the following discussion. The endoscopist should clearly state which of these indications the colonoscopy is performed for, and can ask that specific issues be addressed by the pathologist in the report.

Initial Diagnosis of IBD

The initial endoscopy in a patient with suspected IBD is critical to determine the correct diagnosis, since the patient is unlikely to have received medical therapy that might influence the histologic appearance. The differential diagnosis usually includes infectious (bacterial) colitis, and the histologic distinction depends mainly on the crypt architecture and presence of a basal lymphoplasmacytic infiltrate. Evaluation of these two features depends to a large extent on the orientation of the biopsies, so multiple biopsies should be obtained to ensure that at least some of them are properly oriented. Multiple biopsies also increase the likelihood that a granuloma will be identified, leading to a specific diagnosis of Crohn's colitis. If the colitis is patchy, then biopsies from affected and normal mucosa should be placed in separate containers that are labeled with the anatomic site. Biopsies from normal mucosa above the proximal extent of endoscopically evident colitis are also helpful for histologic verification of the extent of disease involvement. These biopsies should also be placed in a separate container labeled with the anatomic site. If a colonoscopy is being performed, biopsies of the terminal ileum should be obtained if possible.

Confirmation of the Diagnosis
of Ulcerative Colitis or Crohn's Disease

In this circumstance, the patient is likely to have received medical therapy for IBD, which can alter the histologic appearance of the biopsies (e.g., producing patchy healing). Submission of slides from any previous endoscopy performed at an outside institution can be very valuable to the pathologist in interpretation of the current material. Biopsies should be submitted in a manner similar to that discussed previously for the initial diagnosis of IBD.

Evaluation of the Extent and Severity of IBD

In this situation, the diagnosis of either ulcerative colitis or Crohn's disease has already been established. Biopsies from the involved segment(s) of colon can be submitted together in a single container. Biopsies from normal segments should be submitted separately so that the histologic extent of disease can be accurately determined. Biopsies from the cecum and ascending colon should be placed in a separate container labeled as such because mucosa from these sites normally contain scattered Paneth cells, while their presence in more distal colonic biopsies is indicative of IBD. Ileal biopsies can also be placed in this container unless there is active disease in both the cecum/ascending colon and ileum. In that case, the ileal biopsies may exhibit ulceration and/or severe villous blunting to the point where they can be confused with biopsies of colonic origin. Likewise, colonic biopsies may exhibit a villiform metaplasia that creates a resemblance with ileal mucosa.

Re-evaluation of the Diagnosis
of Ulcerative Colitis or Crohn's Disease

In some patients, new clinical findings may lead to a reconsideration of an established diagnosis of either ulcerative colitis or Crohn's colitis. For instance, a patient carrying a diagnosis of ulcerative colitis may develop perianal skin tags or a fistula. It is also possible that during a routine colonoscopy to document the extent or severity of disease atypical endoscopic features are unexpectedly discovered (e.g., aphthous-type ulcers in an ulcerative colitis patient). In these types of circumstances, the patient may very well be receiving medical therapy, which can alter the histologic appearance. The list of current medications should be made available to the surgical pathologist, as well as slides from any previous endoscopy performed at outside institutions. The new clinical or endoscopic data that has put the established diagnosis in doubt should also be concisely communicated. It is critical that biopsies from normal and affected areas in placed in separately designated containers. Ileal biopsies should be performed if possible.

Surveillance for Dysplasia in IBD Patients

Various proposals have been made regarding the minimum number of biopsies obtained during surveillance colonoscopy, but no standard has been accepted nationally. If significant active colitis is evident at the time of colonoscopy, biopsies should be postponed until after a trial of medical therapy. Some pathologists may not be comfortable diagnosing dysplasia in the face of active inflammation (because of possible confusion with reactive atypia), and a diagnosis of "indefinite for dysplasia" is made much more often in this situation than in patients with quiescent disease.

Biopsies of polyps and possible DALMs should be placed in separate containers labeled to anatomic site. Biopsies of the mucosa surrounding the lesion should be placed in another labeled container. These biopsies are helpful in documenting whether the lesion, if adenomatous, is arising in a background of normal mucosa (which supports a diagnosis of sporadic adenoma) or of IBD (which favors a diagnosis of IBD-associated dysplasia).

Random biopsies can be placed in separate containers by level (e.g., 90 cm, 80 cm, 70 cm, etc.) or grouped into regions (e.g., right colon, left colon, rectosigmoid), depending on institutional preference. In Crohn's disease patients, it may be possible to perform a right hemicolectomy if the random biopsy with dysplasia is known to be from the proximal colon. Also, knowledge of the site of origin of a random biopsy diagnosed as "indefinite for dysplasia" would allow numerous follow-up biopsies to be obtained from that same segment of the colon.

ACKNOWLEDGMENT

Color photographs provided through an unrestricted educational grant from Procter & Gamble Pharmaceuticals, as well as grants from Shire US Inc., Prometheus Laboratories Inc., and Salix Pharmaceuticals Inc.

REFERENCES

1. Riddell RH. Pathology of Idiopathic Inflammatory Bowel Disease. In: Inflammatory Bowel Disease (4th ed). (Kirsner JB and Sorter RG, eds), 1995. Williams & Wilkins, Baltimore, pp. 517–552.
2. Lewin KJ, Riddell RH, Weinstein WM. Inflammatory bowel Diseases. In: Gastrointestinal Pathology and Its Clinical Implications. 1992. Igaku-Shoin, New York, pp. 812–989.
3. Whitehead R (ed). Gastrointestinal and Oesphageal Pathology (2nd ed). Churchill Livingstone: New York, 1995, pp. 589–632.

4. Surawicz CM, Belic L. Rectal biopsy helps distinguish acute self limited colitis from idiopathic inflammatory bowel disease. Gastroenterology 1984;86:104–113.

5. Nostrant TT, Kumar NB, Appelman HD. Histopathology differentiates acute self-limited colitis from ulcerative colitis. Gastroenterology 1987;92:318–328.

6. Schumacher G, Sandstedt B, Kollberg B. A prospective study of first attacks of inflammatory bowel disease and infectious colitis. Scand J Gastroenterol 1994;29:265–274.

7. Tanaka M. Riddell RH, Saito H, Soma Y, Hidaka H, Kudo H. Morphologic criteria applicable to biopsy specimens for effective distinction of inflammatory bowel disease from other forms of colitis and of Crohn's disease from ulcerative colitis. Scand J Gastroenterol 1999;34:55–67.

8. Kleer CG, Appelman HD. Ulcerative colitis: pattern of involvement in colorectal biopsies and changes with time. Am J Surg Pathol 1998;22:983–989.

9. Schumacher G, Kolberg B, Sandstedt B. A prospective study of first attacks of inflammatory bowel disease and infectious colitis. Histologic course during the 1st year after presentation. Scand J Gastroenterol 1994;29:318–332.

10. Griffin PM, Olmstead LC, Petras RE. Escherichia coli O157:H7-associated colitis: a clinical and histological study of 11 cases. Gastroenterology 1990;99:142–149.

11. Ilnyckyj A, Greenberg H, Berstein CN. Escherichia coli O157:H7 infection mimicking Crohn's disease. Gastroenterology 1997;112:995–999.

12. Ellyson JH, Bezmalinovic Z, Parks SN, Lewis Jr FR. Necrotizing amebic colitis: a frequently fatal complication. Amer J Surg 1986;152:21–26.

13. Deana DG, Dean PJ. Reversible ischemic colitis in young women: association with oral contraceptive use. Am J Surg Pathol 1995;19:454–462.

14. Gargot D, Chaussade S, d'Alteroche L, et al. Non-steroidal anti-inflammatory drug-induced colonic strictures: two cases and literature review. Am J Gastroenterol 1995;90:2035–2038.

15. Bjarnason I, Hayllar J, Macpherson AJ, Russell AS. Side effects of nonsteroidal anti-inflammatory drugs on the small and large intestine in humans. Gastroenterology 1993;104:1832–1847.

16. Davies NM. Toxicity of nonsteroidal anti-inflammatory drugs in the large intestine. Dis Colon Rectum 1995;38:1311–1321.

17. D'Haens G, Geboes K, Peeters M, Baert F, Ectors N, Rutgeerts P. Patchy cecal inflammation associated with distal ulcerative colitis: a prospective endoscopic study. Am J Gastroenterol 1997;8:1275–1279.

18. Kim B, Barnett JL, Kleer CG. Appelman HD. Endoscopic and histological patchiness in treated ulcerative colitis. Amer J Gastroenterol 1999;94:3258–3262.

19. Riddell RH, Goldman H, Ransohoff DF, et al. Dysplasia in inflammatory bowel disease: standardized classification with provisional clinical applications. Hum Pathol 1983;14:931–968.

20. Dixon MF, Brown LJ, Gilmour HM, et al. Observer variation in the assessment of dysplasia in ulcerative colitis. Histopathology 1988;13:385–397.

21. Melville DM, Jass JR, Morson BC, et al. Observer study of the grading of dysplasia in ulcerative colitis: comparison with clinical outcome. Human Pathol 1989;20:1008–1014.

22. Eaden J, Abrams K, McKay H, et al. Inter-observer variation between general and specialist gastrointestinal pathologists when grading dysplasia in ulcerative colitis. J Pathol 2001;194:152–157.

23. Löfberg R, Broström O, Karlen P, et al. DNA aneuploidy in ulcerative colitis: reproducibility, topographic distribution, and relation to dysplasia. Gastroenterology 1992;102:1149–1154.

24. Wong NA, Mayer NJ, MacKell S, et al. Immunohistochemical assessment of Ki67 and p53 expression assists the diagnosis and grading of ulcerative colitis-related dysplasia. Histopathology 2000;37:108–114.

25. Blackstone MO, Riddell RH, Rogers BH, Levin B. Dysplasia-associated lesion or mass (DALM) detected by colonoscopy in long-standing ulcerative colitis: an indication for colectomy. Gastroenteology 1981;80:366–374.

26. Walsh SV, Loda M, Torres CM, et al. P53 and beta catenin expression in chronic ulcerative colitis-associated polypoid dysplasia and sporadic adenomas: an immunohistochemical study. Am J Surg Pathol 1999;23:963–969.

27. Mueller E, Vieth M, Stolte M, Mueller J. The differentiation of true adenomas from colitis-associated dysplasia in ulcerative colitis: a comparative immunohistochemical study. Human Pathol 1999;30:898–905.

28. Odze RD, Brown CA, Hartmann CJ, et al. Genetic alterations in chronic ulcerative colitis-associated adenoma-like DALMs are similar to non-colitic sporadic adenomas. Am J Surg Pathol 2000;24:1209–16.

29. Fogt F, Urbanski SJ, Sanders ME, et al. Distinction between dysplasia-associated lesion or mass (DALM) and adenoma in patients with ulcerative colitis. Human Pathol 2000;31:288–291.

Index